WOMEN IN THE HEALTH SYSTEM

Patients, providers, and programs

Issues and problems in health care

Paul R. Torrens, M.D., M.P.H., Series editor

School of Public Health,
University of California,
Los Angeles, California

Other available titles

Health Program Evaluation, Stephen M. Shortell, Ph.D., and
  William C. Richardson, Ph.D.
The American Health Care System: Issues and Problems,
  Paul R. Torrens, M.D., M.P.H.
Rural Health Care, Milton I. Roemer, M.D.
Elements of Planning for Area-Wide Personal Health Services,
  William Shonick, Ph.D.
National Health Policy and the Underserved: Ethnic Minorities, Women,
  and the Elderly, Jerry L. Weaver, Ph.D.
The Law and the Public's Health, Kenneth R. Wing, J.D., M.P.H.

ed for care cannot be measured yet. This
e monitoring and research.
  expanded and enhanced role for women
nts out, women have been far more likely
s extramarket providers of care than as
s mothers, wives, and daughters, in home
unacknowledged and uncounted compo-
iscrimination in opportunity for profes-
More subtle issues — attitudes and differ-
e less easily resolved. The greater num-
p. So will the better informed, question-
ne.
  of women and health. It fills a conspicu-
involvement of American women in the
idely and thoughtfully read.

Dorothy P. Rice
Director, National Center for Health Statistics

WOMEN IN
THE HEALTH SYSTEM

Patients, providers, and programs

HELEN I. MARIESKIND, Dr. P.H.

Executive Director, End-Stage Renal Disease Network Coordinating Council
2, Seattle, Washington, and Editor of *Women & Health*

With 62 illustrations

The C. V. Mosby Company

ST. LOUIS • TORONTO • LONDON   1980

will affect women's health status and ne
is only one of many areas that will requir

There are ample opportunities for ar
in health careers. As Dr. Marieskind poi
to be involved with the health system a
health professionals. Women's service, a
care of the sick and elderly is often an
nent of the economics of health care. D
sional training is being reduced by law.
ences in modes of medical treatment—ar
bers of women in the professions will he
ing consumers created by books like this

This book is the first full-length study
ous gap in the academic literature on the
health care system. I hope that it will be w

Copyright © 1980 by The C. V. Mosby Company

All rights reserved. No part of this book may be reproduced
in any manner without written permission of the publisher.

Printed in the United States of America

The C. V. Mosby Company
11830 Westline Industrial Drive, St. Louis, Missouri 63141

Library of Congress Cataloging in Publication Data

Marieskind, Helen I
    Women in the health system.

    (Issues and problems in health care)
    Bibliography: p.
    Includes index.
    1. Women—Health and hygiene—United States.
2. Women's health services—United States.   3. Women—
Diseases—United States.   4. Women in medicine—United
States.   I. Title.
RA564.85.M37   362.1'9'088042   80-19961
ISBN 0-8016-3106-8

C/CB/CB   9 8 7 6 5 4 3 2 1   . 02/D/282

Preface

This book presents facts and figures on women's health. It has developed from my years of teaching courses in women's health when I was frustrated by the scarcity of readily available data on the topic. Although many books dealt with important issues and relevant experiences, no one source, readily accessible to teachers and students, had a comprehensive perspective on the basic facts of women's involvement, both as providers and consumers, within the health care system. The need for such a book was further demonstrated to me through conversations with others working in the health field who were either unaware of the issues of women's health or who tended to think the concerns were only those related to reproductive health.

Women in the Health System: Patients, Providers, and Programs is an attempt to meet this need. The book presents data, services, and programs on many aspects of women's health without assuming an ideological position. Such a focus was chosen deliberately to allow the facts to speak for themselves, to enable teachers and students to analyze the material and develop policy perspectives, and to enable women and men reading the book to reach their own conclusions.

The book is intended for both men and women undergraduate and graduate students in the health professions and those in general women's studies programs. I also hope that the book will be read by other persons who are interested in women's health, and that comprehension and appreciation of women's needs will be strengthened, particularly among those responsible for training providers, administrators, and policy makers. Most important, I hope the book will be a useful tool to help women analyze their involvement with the health care system.

Many people have contributed to helping me write this book. I would like to thank the following people from the Department of Health, Education and Welfare, National Center for Health Statistics for helping with data: Donald Smith and Gloria Gardocki, Hospital Discharge Survey; Thomas Drury, Health Interview Survey; Robert Heuser, Audrey Jones, and Paul Placek, Natality; Mary Grace Kovar, Chief, Analytical Branch; Trena Ezzati, National Ambulatory Medical Care Survey; and Donald Greenberg, Mortality. Stephen Rawlings, Census Bureau; Mandy Curnutt, Census Bureau, Region X; Lois Moore, Office of the Secretary; Ralph Pardee, Maternal and Child Health Bureau; Mariley Ferenes, Region X Library; and Kathy Dry, Center for Disease Control, have also contributed. Numerous other people within the department sent material, and Marcy Maurer, Seattle, and William Parsons, Association of Schools of Public Health, have also helped with data; their time and efforts are most appreciated.

I have also received tremendous help from the reference librarians at the University of Washington Health Sciences Library, particularly Carole Stock and Diane McKenzie, and from Carol Schneider, Swedish Hospital Library, Seattle.

Several people helped with photographs for the book, particularly Randi Kobernick, University of Washington Health Sciences Information Service.

Dorothy Bradwin, whose constant good-humored editing and encouragement kept me going, Jacqueline Moscou, and Vicki Wery have all assisted with manuscript preparation. Patricia Reagan, University of Utah, and Deborah Oakley and Eugenia Carpenter, University of Michigan–Ann Arbor, have provided helpful comments and recommendations.

Clara Schiffer, Office of the Assistant Secretary, Planning and Evaluation/Health, Department of Health, Education and Welfare, has been a good friend and a loyal editor throughout. Andrew K. Dolan, Francesca and Melinda Gates, and Andrew P. Marieskind Dolan have enabled the cooperative family effort needed to write a book.

Thank you very much.

Helen I. Marieskind

Contents

5 Women and occupational health, 157

6 Health care for young women, 196

Chapter 1

Women's health status

OVERVIEW
General remarks

The United States health care industry is dependent on women. Women are the majority of the patients, and at all but the top levels, the majority of the providers. Women's consumption of products and services and their work, both paid and unpaid, sustain the viability of the health care system.

The significance of women's role as health care consumers in the United States is demonstrated by data from the National Center for Health Statistics. Women report higher morbidity than do men and have lower mortality rates. After age 14 they make about 25% more office visits to physicians than do men (see Chapter 2). Women as a group are hospitalized more often than men, although this does not hold true for all age categories. They receive about 63% of all surgical operations, and women 15 to 44 years of age experience surgery at about 2.5 times the rate of men of the same age. Women consume more drugs than men, particularly the psychotropics. They are also institutionalized more often than men, although most of this difference is accounted for by women over the age of 65 (discussed later).

As providers, women comprise about 80% of all health care workers and nearly 100% of extramarket caretakers—unpaid workers in the home caring for sick family members. For many women, particularly the unskilled, health care is one available avenue of employment.

The health care industry's dependence on women is today, by and large, mutual. Although opinion varies as to the causes of this mutual relationship and desirability of respective control, women continue to use the health care system as the principal caretaker for their physiological and emotional needs. Their use is governed by legislative mandate as well as social values. Because it presents data on women's health status, their consumption and provision of services, and their relationship to the United States health care system, this book can be used as a foundation from which an analysis and evaluation may be made as to the causes, costs, and benefits of this interdependence. Many books have dealt with the issues of women's health—this book presents the data behind the issues, leaving the facts to speak for themselves.

Historical development of women's health care as a specialty

Regardless of whether men or women were the practitioners, since earliest times health care specifically for women has been concerned with their obstetrical

1

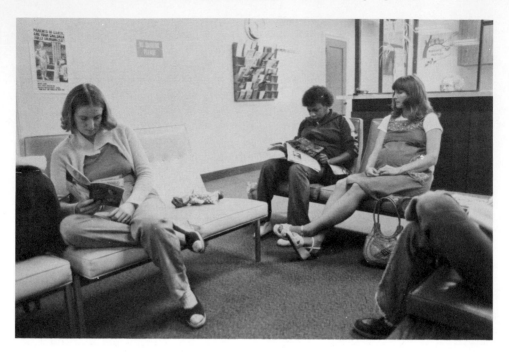

Fig. 1-1. Waiting for health care. (Courtesy Paul Temple.)

and gynecological needs. Ricci reasonably speculates that early midwives, seeing the relationship of menstruation, "its cyclical occurrence, its cessation during pregnancy and its profuse flow with miscarriages . . . included the administration of a rudimentary gynecological therapy" in their tasks.[105] Evidence of the antiquity of the specialty is contained in gynecological writings found in the Kahun Papyrus dating from 2500 BC, the Ebers Papyrus of 1500 BC, a book by Soranus of Ephesus (28 to 138 AD), and the work of Aspasia who lived in the early second century AD.[61]

Although obstetrics and gynecology were distinctly defined, they were viewed as one aspect of women's overall health needs. In this regard, Soranus summarizes the views of these early writers that, except for their reproductive tracts, women were essentially the same as men. He concluded that the

female has her illness in common with the male, she suffers from constriction or from flux, either acutely or chronically, and she is subject to the same seasonal differences, to gradations of disease, to lack of strength, and to the different foreign bodies, sores, and injuries. Only as far as particulars and specific variations are concerned does the female show conditions peculiarly her own, i.e., a different character of symptoms. Therefore she is subject to treatment generically the same.[124]

But the writings of Galen (ca. 130 to 200 AD), which in contrast deemed woman to be an "inside-out man" because she had insufficient body heat to force the genitals outside, were adopted by medieval anatomists. Greatly simplified, this idea of insufficiency combined with views on female sexuality rapidly was translated into female inferiority; the obviously different organs were viewed as the source of the inferiority and, subsequently, of all women's health problems.[17,54] There was scientific justification therefore, supported by laws and religious theory, for curative attempts on women's reproductive tracts. Although obstetrical procedures continued to be seen as generally normal and continued to be essentially managed by women until the seventeenth and eighteenth centuries, the vagaries of the "wandering uterus,"[17,123] vaginal "emissions," intercourse, and menstruation assumed a significance over the centuries that justified much medical study and ultimately the establishment of a separate specialty, gynecology. Male predominance in medicine could be well justified within this specialty as filling the need for superior beings to help the inferior. The assumption by men beginning in the seventeenth century of the work of the midwives, also placed them in a unique position for developing as gynecologists.

Particularly in the United States from 1845 on, the bulk of women's health concerns, whether physical or emotional, became firmly defined as caused by diseases of their reproductive organs, for which surgical intervention was the dominant therapy.[73,120] By the late nineteenth century, American gynecologists were internationally respected largely because of their adventurous use of sexual surgery. The diseases amenable to surgery were all-encompassing and included hysteria, insanity, dysmenorrhea, masturbation, atrophy of the genitals, vesicovaginal fistula, and ovarian and uterine disorders, as well as general slovenliness and disorderliness, which was demonstrated especially by agitation for education and the vote. Particular surgical techniques included hysterectomy, ovariectomy, and clitoridectomy.

The development of gynecology advanced the general respectability of medicine in the United States. Barker-Benfield notes that the gynecological operations "provided the material for the inauguration of specialized publications and institutions." J. Marion Sims, who was regarded as the father of this new medical specialty, published extensively and in 1855 established in New York the nation's first hospital for women. In 1869 *the American Journal of Obstetrics and Diseases of Women and Children* was founded; in 1920 it became the *American Journal of Obstetrics and Gynecology*. The American Medical Association constituted a "section" on obstetrics and diseases of women and children in 1873, and while Sims was president of the American Medical Association, the American Gynecological Society was founded in 1876.[12]

By the early 1900s the popularity of sexual surgery (except hysterectomy — see later) had begun to wane, and attention turned to the continuing prevalence of midwives. As a result of studies of varying quality, an emerging middle-class preference for physicians to attend birth, and a prevailing belief in the dirtiness and incompetence of midwives, childbirth in the United States by the 1920's became firmly the domain of the physician (see Chapter 4).[34,65] Now in charge of obstetrical and gynecological needs of women, the combined specialty assumed the format by which it is known today.

By the 1930s, residencies in obstetrics and gynecology were organized to concentrate on "the mechanism of labor, obstetric manipulations, management of obstetric complications, prevention of maternal mortality, and cancer detection."[158] Gradually research developments (still minor in comparison with other specialties), a stronger emphasis on nonsurgical gynecology, and advances in contraception have expanded the training in the specialty of obstetrics-gynecology. The current organization of obstetrical and gynecological services is discussed in Chapter 2.

Problems in measuring the health status of women

There are several factors impeding an accurate and comprehensive assessment of women's health status. Surveys and analyses have frequently ignored the variable of sex entirely so that distinctions in morbidity between men and women are not apparent. When women are presented as a separate group, data frequently do not distinguish among women of different ethnicities, age, education, economic status, sexual preference, marital status, or between those who work outside the home and those who do not. These are all factors known to affect morbidity and mortality. The socioeconomic variables particularly are increasingly significant in assessing health needs of specific populations, for example, minority women and women exposed to occupational hazards (see Chapter 5).

Furthermore, the traditional classification of health status and health care practices by the educational status of the head of household and by family income may greatly distort the data with their relevance to the women in the household. Failure to recognize the multiple roles of many women may inhibit accurate history taking and diagnoses and similarly distort the data.[87]

Surveys that have used self-administered questionnaires or interviews on health also may not accurately reflect health status. Women are believed to be more cooperative than men in completing such surveys, and their comparative cooperation may inflate their reported illnesses. Because it is socially acceptable for women to report illness, when they serve as proxy respondents for other family members, particularly husbands, they may underreport in comparison to reporting their own illnesses. Unwillingness to portray the provider as ill may also account for sexual differences shown by data.[67,151]

Data collected through employment-related insurance plans may also be sex-biased, since most women still work in jobs where this benefit, and therefore their access to health care, is less available than in men's.

Societal expectations and assumptions may also prevent accurate health status assessment. Assumptions that morbidity is psychological rather than physiological[7,69] may not only mean failure to treat but also that such conditions go unrecorded. Alternatively, morbidity such as attempted suicide, alcoholism, venereal disease, and abortion may also be underreported because of its incompatibility with societal expectations of women. This is particularly true when privacy concerning such morbidity cannot be guaranteed and, as Muller notes, not only affects health statistic reporting but also may deter health-seeking behavior. In addition, the role of providers' judgments in assessing emotional/behavioral phenomena and possible distortion of data has not been evaluated.[87]

Attempts are being made to provide a more accurate assessment of women's health status, as evidenced by the presentation of data by sex in *Health United States, 1978*,[143] and by a planned "elimination of sex-based stereotypes in census related statistics"[139] of the United Nations. At present, however, the paucity of accurate data and the limited validity of what do exist demand a cautious interpretation before generalizations on women's health status can be made.

Selected demographic characteristics of women

Various demographic variables such as age, race, income, education, marital status, and residence affect health needs and health status. Similarly, personal health characteristics—for example, weight, diet, whether an individual smokes, drinks, works, exercises, or is vaccinated—are correlated with outcome. These variables all affect measurements of women's health status, and the diversity of these characteristics in the female population affects the data on women's health status.

In 1978 there were over 112 million females in the United States (including armed forces overseas), comprising 51.3% of the population. Of these, 44.7% were aged 15 to 44 years, 20.4% were 45 to 64, and 12.7% were 65 and over. For the same age-groups, the percentages of men were 46.7%, 19.7%, and 9.2%, respectively (Fig 1-2).[140] Age differences alone affect which health services are needed, particularly in the 15 to 44 age bracket, in which most childbearing is done, and in the over-65 bracket, which is heavily dominated by women.

Among the total female population in 1978, 11.9% were black and 1.9% were of other races. By age category, 46.6% of black women were aged 15 to 44 years, 16.5% were 45 to 64, and 8.7% were 65 years and older. Of women of other nonwhite races, 50.8% were 15 to 44 years, 15.8% were 45 to 64, and 6.1% were 65 years and older.[140]

Most women live in metropolitan areas. A higher percentage of black women (55%) and women of Spanish origin (49%) live in central city areas than do whites (24%), but more white women (34%) live in nonmetropolitan (rural) areas than do blacks (25%) or women of Spanish origin (15.5%).[141]

Educational status is believed to affect health status either because people are better informed of appropriate health behavior (although possession of information is not necessarily reflected in healthier habits), or because education provides access to better jobs with higher incomes and that in turn provides the funds to seek needed medical care. By March, 1978, of all women 25 years and over, 34.8% had not finished high school, 39.6% had completed high school, 13.4% had completed 1 to 3 years of college, and 12.2% had completed 4 years or more of college. By comparison, 33.2% of men had less than 4 years of high school, 32.1% had completed high school, 14.9% had from 1 to 3 years of college, and 19.7% had 4 or more years of college.[141]

Of all children who are living with their mothers (either as a family head or spouse of family head), 10% live with mothers who are college graduates, 32% live with mothers who have not finished high school and 12% live with mothers who have not completed the eighth grade.[66]

Work may affect health status through exposure to occupational hazards and by providing increased access to health care. Most women of working age work— 50.1% as of January, 1979 (see Chapter 5). In 1978, of never-married women, 60.5% worked; of married women with their husbands present, 47.6% worked.

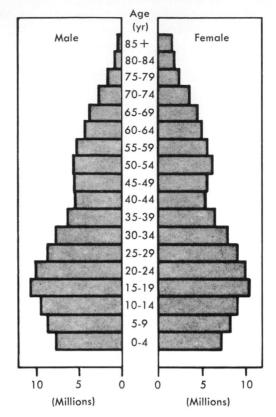

Fig. 1-2. Population profile of the United States: 1978. (From U.S. Department of Commerce, Bureau of the Census: Current population reports, series P-20, no. 336, April, 1979.)

Of the latter category, a lower percentage of women who had no children under 18 years worked (44.7%) than did women who had children 6 to 17 years of age only (57.2%). Of women who had children under 6 years and husbands present, 41.6% worked.

In 1978, 42.8% of widowed, divorced, and married but separated women worked; 71.2% of women in this category with children 6 to 17 years only worked. This percentage is comparable with the 69.9% of never-married women who worked and had children 6 to 17 years only.[141,162]

Marital status appears to affect health, although the causes and effects are not clear. According to the Health Interview Survey, divorced and separated people have the worst health status, followed by widowed people and never-married people. Married persons report the lowest rates of chronic limitation and disability and are assessed the healthiest.[150] In 1978, with 87.4 million women of marriageable age (defined as 14 years and over) in the civilian population, 23.9% were single, 6% were divorced, 11.6% were widowed, 3.6% were married with their husbands absent, and 54.8% were married with their husbands present.[104]

As with education, marital status, and employment, income may also affect health status because of the health services that can be purchased. In 1977, 74.8% of women had some income; among white women, 74.5% did so, 78.1% did so among black women, as did 66% of women of Spanish origin. For women of all races, the largest percentage (27.6%) had incomes of from $1 to $1999 in 1977, ranging from 26.7% of black women to 29.2% of women of Spanish origin. Only 0.6% of women had incomes over $25,000. By contrast, 8.6% of men had incomes of $25,000 and over, and only 11.6% were in the lowest income category.[141]

Personal health characteristics. Personal health characteristics, particularly those which reflect dietary intake and health behavior, are probably those which most profoundly affect health status but are the most difficult to measure accurately. People, including women, do not always tell the truth, particularly concerning sensitive areas such as food consumption, drug and alcohol consumption (see later), sexual behavior, and the degrees of stress under which they live. The effects of stress are increasingly important as more and more women enter the job market and must balance child care and work. The amount of stress, particularly on lower income women who do not have the resources to buy outside help, and its affects on health, are yet to be adequately researched.[64,134]

In 1976, 45.3% of the female population (51.3% of men) assessed themselves as being in excellent health, 40.7% thought their health was good, 10.6% fair, and 2.9% poor. Assessments of excellent and good health varied by family income, with 59.6% of families earning $15,000 or more believing their health was good, as contrasted with only 31.9% of families with incomes of less than $5,000.[143]

Exercise patterns among males and females aged 12 to 74 varied during the years 1971 to 1975. Of females, 50.9% reported they were "very active or had much exercise" (63.6% of males), 42.3% reported they were "somewhat active or had some exercise" (31.1% of males), and 6.8% stated they were "inactive or had little to no exercise" (5.3% of males).[143, Table 45, p. 217]

Correspondingly, more women reported they were obese and were found to be obese on examination than men. In 1974 women aged 45 to 64 years were self-assessed and confirmed as the most overweight group. White women generally assessed themselves as more obese than black women, but the latter were found to be more obese (31% as compared with 22%) on examination.[143, p. 202] Obesity in the United States appears more as a problem of the overconsumption of fats, sugar, salt, and alcohol than of simple overeating. Among men, obesity is more common above the poverty level and in women, below the poverty level. This holds constant by race (see Table 1-1). Obesity aggravates almost all other health conditions, and its gravity has tended to be downplayed by women's groups in a commendable effort to counteract social stereotypes of the thin, elegant woman being the only acceptable and/or beautiful woman. Obesity is harmful to women's health, and the obese place a greater drain on health resources (including their own) than do people of reasonable weights.

Correct dietary intake may also be affected by an individual's ability to chew,

Table 1-1. Obesity among persons 20 to 74 years of age, according to sex, race, age, and poverty level; United States, 1971-1974*†

| | Percent of persons | | | | | |
| | Male | | | Female | | |
Age and poverty level	All races	White	Black	All races	White	Black
All ages 20 to 74 years	13.0	13.3	11.6	22.7	21.8	31.2
Below poverty level	8.0	8.2	7.6	26.5	23.1	33.3
Above poverty level	13.8	13.9	13.4	22.6	22.1	30.0
20 to 44 years	14.2	14.2	13.3	19.7	18.4	25.6
Below poverty level	9.7	9.4	11.1	22.8	20.6	27.6
Above poverty level	14.7	14.9	14.6	18.8	18.3	24.0
45 to 64 years	12.1	12.2	10.2	29.0	27.6	43.0
Below poverty level	4.8	5.3	3.7	35.1	26.4	49.4
Above poverty level	13.2	13.2	12.4	29.2	28.5	40.0
65 to 74 years	11.0	11.5	5.8	20.5	19.8	27.7
Below poverty level	9.1	10.3	4.6	24.7	25.2	23.2
Above poverty level	10.8	11.1	7.0	20.1	19.2	36.3

*Based on data from Division of Health Examination Statistics, National Center for Health Statistics: Data from the Health and Nutrition Examination Survey.
†Data are based on physical examinations of a sample of the civilian noninstitutionalized population.
Note: Obesity measure is based on triceps skinfold measurements and is defined as falling above the sex-specific 85th percentile measurements for persons 20 to 29 years of age.

Table 1-2. Women 17 years and over who had had breast examination and/or Pap smear, United States, 1973*

Age	Number (000)	Breast examination only (%)	Pap smear only (%)	Both (%)	Neither (%)
All ages 17 years and over	75,161	5.2	3.8	70.7	15.5
17 to 24 years	15,062	7.3	3.1	57.5	27.0
25 to 44 years	25,862	2.2	2.9	86.4	5.2
45 to 64 years	22,370	4.8	4.6	73.4	12.1
≥ 65 years	11,867	10.0	4.9	48.0	29.7

*Based on data from use of selected medical procedures associated with preventive care, United States, 1973, Vital and Health Statistics, series 10, no. 110, March, 1977.

and this is particularly evident among the elderly. Among persons aged 12 to 74 years in the United States from 1971 to 1975, 14.6% were reported as having trouble with chewing steaks, chops, or other firm meats, biting apples or corn on the cob, or biting or chewing any other food. This 14.6% represents 16% of the female population and 13.1% of the male.[143, Table 41, p. 213]

Health-seeking behavior and disease prevention are believed to affect health status. Data from 1973 show that only 56.8% of women over age 40 had had an electrocardiogram compared with 64.6% of men. Of women 17 years and over, 21% never had had a Pap smear, with the largest group being women aged 65 and over (see Table 1-2). Although the value of the Pap smear is controversial (see Chapter 7), at this time it is still generally believed to be an important diagnostic tool in cancer prevention and is widely advocated as essential for all women.

Drinking, drug consumption, and smoking all affect health status and are discussed later. In 1976, 7% of women aged 20 or over used sleeping medications once a week or more, 26.9% took aspirins once a week or more, 15.9% consumed five or more cups of coffee per day, 32% were current smokers, and 20% smoked 15 or more cigarettes per day.[143, Table 51, p. 225] From 1971 to 1975, 3.9% of women reported they had at least one drink every day and 2% reported they did so "just about every day."[143, Table 50, p. 224]

The diversity of these characteristics combined with the problems discussed earlier in gathering data on women, suggest that the following data on women, generally defined in this chapter as females 20 years of age and over (see Chapter 6 for those under 20), should be evaluated with caution. While providing a useful overview, they also indicate data areas in which correlations, if any, need to be established, and highlight topics for additional detailed research.

HEALTH STATUS: SELECTED CHARACTERISTICS

In comparison with women in many other countries most women in the United States enjoy relatively good health. Although their health status may not be as good as that of women in some other industrialized nations, women in the United States, unlike millions of the world's women, do not confront on a daily basis threats to survival, whether from disease, starvation, or childbirth. For most United States women, health care issues are those of control, quality, and more equitable access.

Life expectancy

Females born in 1976 may expect to live an average of 76.7 years (7.7 years longer than males; see Table 1-3). Women alive at age 65 in 1976 have an expectancy of 18 years more of life, as compared with 13.7 years for men. Women other than white had a life expectancy in 1976 of 72.6 years (64.1 for men) and at age 65 in 1976, they may expect to live 17.6 years more (13.8 for men). After age 80, black females as a group have the lowest death rates. In comparison, white women born in 1900 had a life expectancy of 48.7 years (46.6 for males), whereas women of all colors could be expected to live 33.5 years (32.5 for males).[143, pp. 167-170]

Life expectancy has been increasing throughout the world (see Table 1-3). In 1975 the United States ranked ninth worldwide in female longevity. The most long-lived women were in Norway (77.6), Sweden (77.5), the Netherlands (77.2), France (76.4), Canada (76.36), Japan (76.31), Denmark (76.3), Switzerland (76.2), and the United States (75.9). Paraguay was forty-fourth with 63.6 years.[137]

Table 1-3. Life expectancy at birth and at 65 years of age, selected countries, selected years, 1969 to 1976*†

Country	Remaining number of years			
	At birth		At 65 years	
	Male	Female	Male	Female
Canada: 1970	69.3	76.2	13.7	17.4
1974	69.6	77.1	13.8	18.0
United States: 1969-1971§	67.0	74.6	13.0	16.8
1976	69.0	76.7	13.7	18.0
Sweden: 1970	72.3	77.4	14.4	17.2
1976	72.2	78.1	14.0	17.5
England and Wales: 1970	68.8	75.2	12.0	16.0
1976	69.7	75.8	12.3	16.3
Netherlands: 1970	70.9	76.6	13.6	16.6
1976	71.6	78.1	13.6	17.6
German Democratic Republic: 1970	68.9	74.2	12.9	15.4
1976	68.9	74.5	12.1	14.8
German Federal Republic: 1970	67.3	73.6	11.9	15.0
1975	68.1	74.7	12.2	15.7
France: 1970	69.1	76.7	13.4	17.4
1974	69.5	77.6	13.6	17.8
Switzerland: 1968-1973§	70.3	76.2	13.3	16.3
1976	71.7	78.3	14.0	17.7
Italy: 1970	68.5	74.6	13.0	16.1
1974	69.9	76.1	13.6	16.7
Israel‡: 1970	69.9	73.4	13.5	14.5
1975	71.0	74.7	14.0	15.5
Japan: 1970	69.5	74.9	12.7	15.6
1976	72.3	77.6	14.1	17.0
Australia: 1970	67.4	74.2	11.9	15.7
1975	69.3	76.4	13.1	17.1

*Based on data from World Health Organization: World health statistics, 1970, vol. 1, Geneva 1973, World Health Organization and vol. 1, 1978, United Nations: *Demographic yearbook 1976*, Pub. No. ST ESA STAT SER R4, New York, 1977, United Nations; National Center for Health Statistics: U.S. Decennial Life Tables for 1969-1971, vol. 1, no. 1, DHEW Pub. No. (HRA) 75-1150, Health Resources Administration, Washington, D.C., May, 1975, U.S. Government Printing Office; Final mortality statistics, 1976, Monthly vital statistics report, vol. 26. no. 12. supp. 2, DHEW Pub. No. (PHS) 78-1120, Public Health Service, Washington D.C., March 30, 1978, U.S. Government Printing Office.
†Data are based on reporting by countries. Countries are grouped by continent.
‡Jewish population only.
§Average for the period.

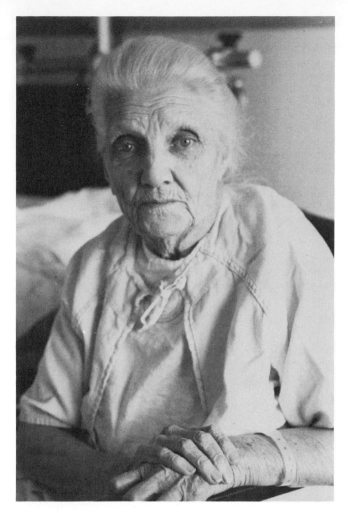

Fig. 1-3. Longevity. (Courtesy Health Sciences Information Service, University of Washington, Seattle.)

By 1977, females in Iceland enjoyed the longest life expectancy in the world: 79.2 years.

Lack of a clearly defined role for the elderly in the United States may reduce the benefits of longevity, especially for women, who generally outlive their mates and comprise the majority of nursing home residents (discussed later).

Mortality

Mortality rates for both males and females are affected by a number of factors, including race, age, education, occupational status, economic status, health-seeking behavior, personal health characteristics (e.g., weight), geography, and environmental factors.

Since the 1950s, mortality rates in the United States have remained relatively stable. In the 1970s they have dropped rapidly, with most of the gains in survival occurring among infants and the elderly, and with evidence that some of women's long-held mortality advantages are eroding.[149]

It is still true, however, that at every stage of life and for almost all causes women experience lower mortality than do men. Several reasons have been advanced for this, some or all of which may be contributory: females' genetic advantage, less exposure to occupational hazards, less aggressive socialization, less exposure to stress, and more frequent health-seeking behavior.[94,148,152]

In the 1900s the leading causes of mortality for women aged 15 to 44 years were tuberculosis, complications of childbirth, and heart disease (see Table 1-4). By 1977 most of the mortality of women aged 20 years and over was still from largely preventable causes: accidents, heart disease, malignant neoplasms, cerebral vascular disease, diabetes, and influenza (see Table 1-5). Among accidental deaths of women, motor vehicles accounted for 46.7% in 1976 and 48% in 1977.

Maternal mortality. Maternal mortality is defined as that resulting from complications of pregnancy, childbirth, and the puerperium up to 42 days postpartum, and also includes abortion-related mortality.[163] Until the last few decades maternal mortality was a leading cause of death among women. In the United States from 1915 to 1919 for every 100,000 live births, about 728 women died. By race, the rates were 700.3 for whites and 1253.5 for minorities. Today, the average woman has a 94% chance of surviving from the birth of her first child to the marriage of her last.[77] Maternal mortality had dropped by 1977 to 11.2 per 100,000 live births; the rate for whites was 7.7 and for minorities, 26.0 (see Table 1-6).

The discrepancy between maternal mortality of white and minority women suggests that it could be reduced. Data from other industrialized countries, which, despite popular opinion, do not have totally homogeneous populations to which their low rates can be attributed, confirm this, as shown by the number of deaths per 100,000 live births: Sweden (1975), 2.0; Denmark (1976), 1.5; Belgium (1976), 5.0; Netherlands (1976), 5.1; Norway (1977), 9.8; Puerto Rico (1977), 2.9; Switzerland (1977), 4.4; Northern Ireland (1977), 3.9; New Zealand (1976), 4.1; Israel (1976), 8.1; and Canada (1977), 6.1.[138] (When maternal deaths are less than 30 per 100,000 live births, one or two deaths can substantially alter the annual rate.)

According to the Center for Disease Control (CDC), Abortion Surveillance Branch, abortion-related mortality rose in 1977 for the first time since 1972. (CDC reports more abortion-related deaths than does the National Center for Health Statistics; see Table 1-7.) In 1972 there were 24 deaths from legal abortions; this dropped to 11 in 1976 and rose to 15 in 1977. In 1972 there were 39 deaths from illegally induced abortion; this figure dropped to 2 in 1976 and rose to 4 in 1977. Of women who had spontaneous abortions, 25 died in 1972, 13 in 1976, and 14 in 1977.[25] With the continued lack of governmental support for abortion (see Chapter 3), maternal mortality for this cause may rise as women resort to illegal or self-induced abortion.

Table 1-4. Number of deaths of women from 15 to 44 years of age, 1913*

Abridged international list no.	Cause of death	Number of deaths
13,14,15	Tuberculosis of lungs, tuberculous meningitis, other forms of tuberculosis	26,265
31,32	Puerperal septicemia (puerperal fever, peritonitis) and other puerperal accidents of pregnancy and labor	9,876
19	Organic diseases of heart	6,386
29	Acute nephritis and Bright's disease	5,741
16	Cancer and other malignant tumors	5,065
22	Pneumonia	4,167
35	Violent deaths (suicide excepted)	3,262
1	Typhoid fever	2,706
30	Noncancerous tumors and other diseases of female genital organs	2,669
26	Appendicitis and typhlitis	1,620
36	Suicide	1,562
23	Other diseases of respiratory system (tuberculosis excepted)	1,458
18	Cerebral hemorrhage and softening	1,398
24	Diseases of stomach (cancer excepted)	940
27	Hernia, intestinal obstruction	854
28	Cirrhosis of liver	598
9	Influenza	489
17	Simple meningitis	484
8	Diphtheria and croup	330
12	Other epidemic diseases	312
6	Scarlet fever	307
5	Measles	304
3	Malaria	250
21	Chronic bronchitis	184
20	Acute bronchitis	90
33	Congenital debility and malformations	24
11	Cholera nostras	18
4	Smallpox	16
7	Whooping cough	9
2	Typhus fever	2
10	Asiatic cholera	0
37	Other diseases	11,688
38	Unknown or ill-defined diseases	458

*Computed from figures in Mortality Statistics, 1913, pp. 338-349, in which causes of death are given by registration area according to the detailed International List of Causes of Death. Reproduced from Meigs, G. L.: Maternal mortality from all conditions connected with childbirth in the United States and certain other countries, Miscellaneous series no. 6, Bureau Pub. no. 19, U.S. Department of Labor, Washington, D.C., 1917, U.S. Government Printing Office.

Table 1-5. Leading causes of mortality, United States, 1977*

Cause	Total	White		Other	
		Female	Male	Female	Male
20 to 24 years					
All causes	23,543	5018	16,255	1478	3792
Accidents	12,939	2140	9180	346	1273
Suicide	3694	637	2638	86	333
Homicide	3299	399	1273	328	1299
Malignant neoplasms	1422	434	804	82	102
Heart disease	622	154	260	89	119
Influenzas and pneumonias	272	75	126	29	42
Cerebral vascular disease and stroke	304	98	129	50	27
Congenital anomalies	301	101	152	23	25
Diabetes	103	36	43	15	9
Anemias	83	14	14	23	32
Benign neoplasms	64	28	29	4	3
25 to 44 years					
All causes	101,898	25,646	50,527	8930	16,795
Accidents	22,399	3805	14,536	864	3194
Malignant neoplasms	16,485	7592	6277	1473	1143
Heart disease	14,393	2380	8725	1148	2140
Suicide	8823	2331	5625	219	648
Homicide	8554	829	3317	795	3613
Cirrhosis of liver	5058	1015	2203	681	1153
Cerebral vascular disease and stroke	3737	1315	1236	596	590
Influenzas and pneumonias	2027	561	771	275	420
Diabetes	1477	463	619	188	207
Congenital anomalies	740	293	342	†	†
45 to 64 years					
All causes	446,096	133,666	242,808	27,411	42,211
Heart disease	158,069	33,791	102,703	8216	13,359
Malignant neoplasms	130,993	52,841	60,593	7305	10,254
Cerebral vascular disease and stroke	24,630	8634	10,200	2800	2996
Accidents	19,000	4647	11,264	758	2331
Cirrhosis of liver	17,821	4938	10,036	983	1864
Suicide	8546	2640	5541	†	†
Influenzas and pneumonias	8010	2311	3974	540	1185
Diabetes	8006	2958	3042	1224	782
Homicide	3837	†	1603	305	1419
65 years and over					
All causes	1,242,342	563,929	565,194	55,137	58,084
Heart disease	548,352	253,601	249,968	23,008	21,775
Malignant neoplasms	232,226	95,373	114,851	8795	13,207
Cerebral vascular disease and stroke	154,623	83,117	55,916	8777	6813
Influenzas and pneumonias	39,871	18,045	18,507	1345	1974
Arteriosclerosis	27,371	15,590	9936	1019	826
Accidents	24,092	10,640	11,189	899	1364
Diabetes	23,599	12,564	7835	2119	1081
Bronchitis, emphysema, and asthma	16,288	4010	11,549	†	550
Cirrhosis of liver	8622	3022	4950	†	406
Nephritis and nephrosis	5834	†	†	589	601
Suicide	4763	†	3567	†	†
Hypertension	4511	†	†	347	†
Hernia and intestinal obstruction	4186	2390	†	†	†
Septicemia	4144	†	†	365	†

*Based on data provided by Donald Greenberg, Statistician, Mortality Statistics Branch, Division of Vital Statistics, Washington, D.C., National Center for Health Statistics.
†Not a leading cause in this age, color, or sex category.

Table 1-6. Maternal mortality rates by color: birth-registration states, United States, 1915-1977*†

Year	Total	White	All other	Year	Total	White	All other
1915 to 1919	727.9	700.3	1253.5	1957	41.0	27.5	118.3
1920 to 1924	689.5	649.2	1134.5	1958	37.6	26.3	101.8
1925 to 1929	660.6	515.0	1165.7	1959	37.4	25.8	102.1
1930 to 1934‡	636.0	575.4	1080.7	1960	37.1	26.0	97.9
1935 to 1939	493.9	439.9	875.5	1961	36.9	24.9	101.3
1940	376.0	319.8	773.5	1962§	35.2	23.8	95.9
1941	316.5	266.0	678.1	1963§	35.8	24.0	96.9
1942	258.7	221.8	544.0	1964	33.3	22.3	89.9
1943	245.2	210.5	509.9	1965	31.6	21.0	83.7
1944	227.9	189.4	506.0	1966	29.1	20.2	72.4
1945	207.2	172.1	454.8	1967	28.0	19.5	69.5
1946	156.7	130.7	358.9	1968	24.5	16.6	63.6
1947	134.5	108.6	334.6	1969	22.2	15.5	55.7
1948	116.6	89.4	301.0	1970‖	21.5	14.4	55.9
1949	90.3	68.1	234.8	1971‖	18.8	13.0	45.3
1950	83.3	61.1	221.6	1972‖¶	18.8	14.3	38.5
1951	75.0	54.9	201.3	1973‖	15.2	10.7	34.6
1952	67.8	48.9	188.1	1974‖	14.6	10.0	35.1
1953	61.1	44.1	166.1	1975‖	12.8	9.1	29.0
1954	52.4	37.2	143.8	1976‖	12.3	9.0	26.5
1955	47.0	32.8	130.3	1977‖	11.2	7.7	26.0
1956	40.9	28.7	110.7				

*Based on data from Final mortality statistics and vital statistics of the U.S., II, 1915-1977, Division of Vital Statistics, Washington, D.C., National Center for Health Statistics.
†Prior to 1933, data are for birth-registration states only. Rates are per 100,000 live births in specified group. Deaths are classified according to the International Classification of Diseases in use at the time.
‡For 1932 to 1934, Mexicans are included with "All other."
§Figures by color exclude data from residents of New Jersey.
‖Excludes deaths of nonresidents of the United States.
¶Deaths based on a 50% sample.

The data in Table 1-6 show two periods when a rapid drop in maternal mortality occurred. One suggested explanation for the drop between 1930 and 1935 (636.0 to 493.9) is the growing use of hospitals and physicians for childbirth; for example, in 1900 less than 5% of women had delivered in hospitals, but by 1935 over 30% did so.[95] (See Chapter 2 for location of births and attendants.)

Another large drop in maternal mortality occurred from 1940 to 1949, when the rate dropped from 376.0 in 1940 to 90.3 in 1949. This decline coincided with the official establishment in March, 1943, of the Emergency Maternity and Infant Care Program (EMIC) which provided obstetrical (including payments for deliveries) and pediatric care to the wives and children of World War II servicemen. The federally funded program was administered through the maternal and child health divisions of the health departments, and when it ended in 1947, the program had done much to influence maternal and child health services provided by the states through Title V of the Social Security Act (see Chapter 3).[121]

The various causes of maternal mortality in 1977 are displayed in Table 1-7. In the United States, data on maternal mortality are not collected by mode of delivery, but the recent rise in cesarean section incidence, with its increased risks to the mother, indicate that these data are needed (see Chapter 7). Preliminary data suggest a maternal mortality rate of 1 per 1000 live births by cesarean section.[26, 144] This is to be contrasted with the 11.2 per 100,000 live births in 1977. The relatively long-standing very low rates of some other countries indicate that maternal mortality may never be totally eradicated but that it can be diminished.

Hospitalization

In 1977 women as a group were hospitalized more often than men — 196 per 1000 women and 141 per 1000 men. When deliveries were excluded, rates for

Table 1-7. Maternal deaths and maternal mortality rates for selected causes, United States, 1977*

Cause of death	ICDA code	Number of deaths			Mortality rate		
		Total	White	All other	Total	White	All other
Complications of pregnancy, childbirth, and the puerperium	630 to 678	373	208	165	11.2	7.7	26.0
Ectopic pregnancy	631	44	15	29	1.3	0.6	4.6
Toxemias of pregnancy and the puerperium, except abortion with toxemia	636 to 639	55	33	22	1.7	1.2	3.5
Hemorrhage of pregnancy and childbirth	632, 651 to 653	56	35	21	1.7	1.3	3.3
Abortions	640 to 645	20	8	12	0.6	0.3	1.9
Induced for legal indications	640, 641	6	3	3	0.2	0.1	0.5
Induced for other reasons	642	3	-	3	0.1	-	0.5
Spontaneous	643	4	1	3	0.1	0.0	0.5
Other and unspecified	644, 645	7	4	3	0.2	0.1	0.5
Sepsis of childbirth and the puerperium	670, 671, 673	70	44	26	2.1	1.6	4.1
All other complications of pregnancy, childbirth, and puerperium	630, 633 to 635, 654 to 662, 672, 674 to 678	128	73	55	3.8	2.7	8.7
Delivery without mention of complications	650	-	-	-	-	-	-

*From National Center for Health Statistics: Monthly Vital Statistics Report, **28**, May 11, 1977.

women were still higher, although they dropped to 166 per 1000, compared with 141 for men. When age-specific data are examined, in the under-15 and over-65 age-groups, hospital discharge rates for men were higher.

Once hospitalized however, if delivery and pregnancy-related disorders are included, men had longer average lengths of stay than did women (7.8 and 7.0 days, respectively). When deliveries (usual length of stay 2 to 3 days) are excluded, women's average length of stay rises to 7.6 days.[53]

A woman's socioeconomic status affects the likelihood of her being hospitalized. Data from 1975 to 1976 demonstrated that the wealthier a woman was, the less often was she likely to be hospitalized and the shorter was her length of stay. For example, among families with less than $5000 annual income there were 230 hospital discharges per 1000 population and the average length of stay per discharge was 9.5 days; the rate of discharges among families with $15,000 or more was 129 with a 6.6-day average length of stay. Among white families with incomes less than $5000 the rate was 237 per 1000 and 210 for "all others"

Table 1-8. Leading diagnoses for women discharged from nonfederal short-stay hospitals, United States, 1977*

Diagnosis	Total annual discharges (to the nearest thousand)
15 to 44 years	
All diagnoses	10,627
Delivery without complications	2377
Delivery with complications	935
Abortion	475
Complications of pregnancy	342
Special conditions and examinations without sickness, or tests with negative findings	337
Intermenstrual bleeding	253
Neuroses and personality disorders, excluding anxiety neuroses	154
45 to 64 years	
All diagnoses	4562
Chronic ischemic heart disease	158
Diabetes mellitus	124
Cholelithiasis (gallstones)	122
Malignant neoplasm of breast	102
Uterine fibromyoma and other benign neoplasm of uterus	96
65 years and over	
All diagnoses	4690
Chronic ischemic heart disease	408
Cerebral vascular disease	265
Cataracts	159
Diabetes mellitus	136
Congestive heart failure	123

*Based on data provided by Gloria Gardocki, Survey Statistician, Hospital Care Statistics Branch, Washington, D.C., National Center for Health Statistics.

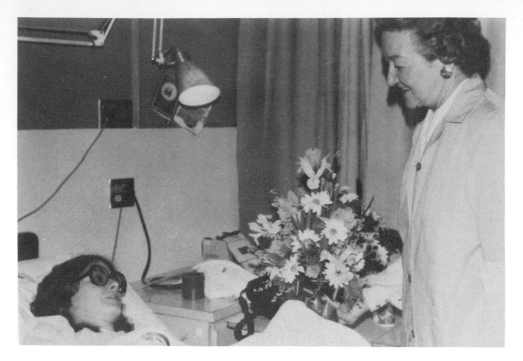

Fig. 1-4. Volunteer and hospitalized patient. (Courtesy Health Sciences Information Service, University of Washington, Seattle.)

(includes blacks), who, averaging 10.3 days, had the longest length of stay in that income group. In the high-income group, "all others" also had the longest length of stay, 10.5 days, and the lowest rate (94 per 1000) of discharges. This is compared with a rate of 130 per 1000 population and 6.5 days for high-income whites.[143, Table 106, p. 316]

In 1977 the leading discharge diagnoses for women aged 15 to 44 years were associated with delivery or abortion; for women 45 to 64 years the leading diagnosis was chronic ischemic heart disease. Women aged 65 and over were most frequently admitted for heart disease and cerebral vascular disease, although the incidence of the latter appears to be declining[48] (see Table 1-8).

Infection rates for nosocomial infections (ones that occur during hospitalization but were not present or incubating on patient's admission) are not available by sex. However, from the National Nosocomial Infection Study conducted by the CDC, it is estimated that one third of all infections in hospitalized patients are nosocomial. About 1.5 million patients annually develop nosocomial infections, and the direct cost of medical care services for this problem exceeds 1 billion dollars. By service, infection rates for 1975 to 1976 were 1% in pediatrics, 1.5% in newborn nurseries, 1.9% in obstetrical, 3.1% in gynecological, 3.7% in medical, and 5% in surgical services. Although the infection rate has remained fairly constant for the past several years, the study noted that for gynecological services, the rates had decreased from about 5.1% in 1972 to 3% in 1976.[24]

Surgery

As noted earlier, women in 1975 and 1976 experienced 63% of all surgical operations, and in the 15 to 44 age-group, women had surgery at 2.5 times the rate of men in the same age-group.[143, Table 108, p. 318] Much of this difference was due to sex-specific procedures such as dilation and curettage (D&C) of the uterus, hysterectomy (discussed later) and cesarean section (see Chapter 7). However, when gynecological procedures as a surgical category are included in the rates for both sexes of all ages, they still are the leading surgical category (see Table 1-9).

The proportions of surgery performed were the same for whites as for "all others" or larger in 1977, except in the categories of gynecological surgery and obstetrical surgery and for the procedures within those categories.[53] Other data have also shown that blacks are 2.2 to 4.3 times more likely to be placed under the care of surgeons in training than are whites; at the time of the study, this pattern had remained unchanged for the past two decades.[38]

In 1975 and 1976 for women aged 15 to 44, the leading operations per 1000 population were D&C of the uterus, hysterectomy, ligation and division of fallopian tubes (bilateral), cesarean section, biopsy, D&C after delivery or abortion, and oophorectomy/salpingo-oophorectomy. For women in 1975 and 1976, aged 45 to 64 years, the leading operations per 1000 population were D&C of the uterus, biopsy, hysterectomy, oophorectomy/salpingo-oophorectomy, cholecystectomy, plastic repair of cystocele and/or rectocele, excision of lesion of skin and subcutaneous tissue, and partial mastectomy. For women 65 years and over for the same time period, the leading operations were biopsy, extraction of lens (cataract surgery), reduction of fracture with fixation, cholecystectomy, excision of lesion of skin and subcutaneous tissue, D&C of the uterus, closed reduction of fracture without fixation, resection of small intestine or colon, hysterectomy, and insertion or replacement of electronic heart device.[143]

Surgery on women, and particularly the frequency of hysterectomy, has been strongly criticized and extensively evaluated. Despite numerous audits,[68,81] demonstrations of lower rates in other countries,[18,37] recommendations and plans for second opinions,[62] governmental hearings,[84] and popular press reports on unnecessary hysterectomies,[28,115] the procedure continues to be the second most frequent major surgical procedure. In 1976, 705,000 hysterectomies were performed;[53] estimates are that 62 of every 100 women living in 1978 have undergone or will undergo hysterectomy.

Greatest concern is about hysterectomies that are performed for birth-control measures when a safer tubal ligation would suffice,[19,57] as a means to relieve pregnancy anxiety, and as a general preventive measure against cancer. The costs, physiological in terms of mortality and morbidity, as well as economic and psychological,[11,42,82,101] are such that the Department of Health, Education

Table 1-9. Rate of leading operations for patients discharged from short-stay hospitals, United States, 1977*†

Surgical category/procedure	All ages			15 years and over (both sexes)
	Both sexes	Female	Male	
All operations	9972.1	12,021.3	775.1	11,854.4
All gynecological surgery	1884.4	3642.1	NA‡	2472.5
Abdominal surgery	1384.4	1396.0	1372.0	1640.7
Orthopedic surgery	1345.9	1244.9	1454.1	1616.4
Otorhinolaryngology	839.6	810.9	870.3	595.1
Urological surgery	782.2	429.9	1159.9	888.5
Obstetrical procedures§	665.1	1285.5	NA	869.0
Biopsy	552.8	699.1	396.1	709.4
Vascular and cardiac surgery	520.1	395.9	653.3	652.4
Plastic surgery	514.8	480.1	551.9	591.2
Dilation and curettage of uterus (diagnostic)	469.1	906.6	NA	617.5
Ophthalmology	394.8	425.7	361.7	460.7
Hysterectomy	332.2	642.0	NA	436.5
Tonsillectomy with or without adenoidectomy	290.8	318.6	261.1	126.5
Ligation and division of fallopian tubes (bilateral)	275.9	533.2	NA	363.9
Proctological surgery	270.3	242.3	300.3	349.2
Repair of inguinal hernia	251.0	59.3	456.5	265.4
Oophorectomy; salpingo-oophorectomy	215.7	416.8	NA	283.3
Cesarean section	214.4	414.3	NA	281.3

*Based on data from Vital and Health Statistics, series 13, no. 41, Washington, D.C., March, 1979, National Center for Health Statistics.
†Numbers per 100,000 population.
‡*NA* = Not applicable.
§Excludes some obstetrical procedures (ICDA codes 75.0 to 75.6 and 75.9) for inducing or assisting delivery.

Table 1-10. Live births and birth and fertility rates, United States, 1966 to 1978*

Year	Number of live births	Birth rate	Fertility rate
1966	3,606,274	18.4	91.3
1967	3,520,959	17.8	87.6
1968	3,501,564	17.5	85.7
1969	3,600,206	17.8	86.5
1970	3,731,386	18.4	87.9
1971	3,555,970	17.2	81.8
1972	3,258,411	15.6	73.4
1973	3,136,965	14.9	69.2
1974	3,159,958	14.9	68.4
1975	3,144,198	14.8	66.7
1976	3,167,788	14.8	65.8
1977	3,326,632	15.4	67.8
1978	3,290,000	15.3	66.4 (estimate)

*Based on data from Final natality statistics, Washington, D. C., 1966-1978, National Center for Health Statistics.

and Welfare, in an effort to reduce unnecessary hysterectomies, has refused to fund them when they are performed for purposes of sterilization or for non-medical reasons.[146]

Fertility and related characteristics

Fertility. After many years of steady decline from 91.3 in 1966, the United States fertility rate rose in 1977 to 67.8, but it is expected to drop back to 66.4 in 1978 (see Table 1-10). Much of the increase could be accounted for by the phenomenon of delayed childbearing in older women 24 to 34 years of age, who, having postponed childbirth, are now having their first babies (see Table 1-11).

Most babies however, are still born to women 20 to 24 years of age, and almost half of the babies born are born to mothers who worked during their pregnancies.[56] In 1976 in almost all age-groups, the black fertility rate was higher than that of whites, but for ages 25 to 29 years it was lower. The rate for "all others" was consistently higher than that for whites and exceeded that of blacks after age 25. For example, in 1976 the rate among whites aged 25 to 29 was 108.4, for "all others" it was 111.6, and for blacks it was 105.5.[143, Table 10, p. 155] As with other years, more triplets and twins were born to blacks than to whites. Nearly one fifth of all infants were born to women younger than 20 (see Chapter 6).

Data from 1973 suggest that currently married women aged 40 to 44 expected to have an average of 3.3 children, but those aged 20 to 24 expected to have an average of only 2.3 children.[15] However, according to other data from 1973, one fifth of all births to women aged 15 to 44, both black and white, were reported as unwanted, or probably not wanted prior to conception. Women with the highest parities reported the highest percentage of unwanted births. By 1979, improved job opportunities, increased access to contraception,[88] and spiraling costs of children were contributing to smaller family size.[50,59]

Obstetrical care. In 1976, 5.7% of women had no prenatal care or little (obtained care only in the last trimester); most of these women were in the group at highest risk—under age 15. Among black women, 9.9% had little or no prenatal care, and those under 15 (19.7%) were again the largest group in this category. Similarly, the rate of little or no care for whites under age 15 was 23.6% (see Table 1-12), but for all white women, only 4.8%. Because these are national aggregate data, they may obscure specific ethnic groups, age-groups, or geographical areas where rates of little or no prenatal care are even higher.

Despite increased numbers of women receiving prenatal care[133] or perhaps because of it, the numbers of deliveries defined as with complications, are increasing (see Table 1-13). Reasons for this increase have not been explored and may include seemingly contradictory explanations: for example, that women are increasingly sicker; that a greater number of women with medical problems are becoming pregnant (true, but still a small minority); that physicians are more skilled at defining complications; that physicians are less skilled and not detecting

Table 1-11. Live first births by age of mother, United States, 1966 to 1977*

Year	Under 15 years	15 to 19 years	20 to 24 years	25 to 29 years	30 to 34 years	35 to 39 years	40 to 44 years	45 to 49 years	Percentage over 20 years and under 29 years
1966	7830	465,356	541,968	151,038	39,332	15,392	3692	178	43.4%
1967	8252	445,483	562,231	160,017	36,286	12,754	3082	169	41.1
1968	9216	455,006	597,052	191,254	41,130	14,260	3350	192	39.8
1969	9926	463,982	622,442	200,682	40,256	12,036	2786	168	39.1
1970	10,932	498,388	652,530	212,102	42,404	11,704	2442	178	39.5
1971	10,944	485,158	613,822	210,852	41,822	10,640	2286	144	40.0
1972	11,179	473,260	531,945	217,992	42,863	9954	1998	66	41.8
1973	11,412	454,684	492,607	226,685	46,434	9639	1798	99	42.1
1974	11,838	462,107	517,467	257,569	52,897	10,433	1782	101	41.0
1975	11,976	451,586	516,528	269,668	56,677	10,901	1671	99	40.3
1976	11,321	431,219	517,376	288,086	63,396	11,654	1666	93	39.2
1977	10,833	430,622	544,194	310,507	76,485	12,766	1674	62	38.4

*Based on data from Final natality statistics. Washington, D.C., 1966-1977, National Center for Health Statistics.

Table 1-12. Percent distribution of prenatal care according to month of pregnancy care began, United States reporting areas, 1976*†

| Race | Month of pregnancy prenatal care began | | | | No prenatal care |
	First or second	Third	Fourth to sixth	Seventh to ninth	
TOTAL‡	13.8	18.0	46.7	15.7	5.7
TOTAL UNDER 15 YEARS	46.7	26.7	20.8	4.3	1.4
Total white	49.6	27.2	18.4	3.7	1.1
Under 15 years	14.4	17.7	44.3	17.3	6.3
15 to 19 years	30.2	26.5	33.4	7.7	2.2
20 to 24 years	49.3	27.9	18.2	3.6	1.1
25 to 29 years	57.6	26.9	12.7	2.2	0.7
30 to 34 years	55.3	27.1	14.2	2.5	0.8
35 to 39 years	47.2	27.7	19.4	4.1	1.5
40 years and over	37.5	26.7	26.9	6.2	2.7
Total black	33.2	24.5	32.4	7.0	2.9
Under 15 years	13.5	18.2	48.6	14.4	5.3
15 to 19 years	23.4	23.1	40.7	9.3	3.5
20 to 24 years	34.5	25.1	31.0	6.6	2.8
25 to 29 years	42.7	25.4	24.8	4.9	2.2
30 to 34 years	41.3	25.5	25.8	5.2	2.2
35 to 39 years	34.7	25.0	30.5	6.5	3.3
40 years and over	28.3	25.4	34.6	7.8	3.9

*Based on data from Health United States, 1978, Washington, D.C., Dec., 1978, U.S. Department of Health, Education and Welfare.
†In 1976 the month of pregnancy during which prenatal care began was reported by 44 states and the District of Columbia.
‡Includes all other races not shown separately.

Table 1-13. Deliveries with and without complications, United States, 1968 to 1977*

Year	Number without complications (000)	Number with complications (000)	Percent of complications
1968	2697	738	21.5
1971†	2771	668	19.9
1972	2625	727	21.7
1973	2457	781	24.1
1974	2392	901	27.4
1975	2345	983	29.5
1976	2302	1027	30.9
1977	2390	1161	32.7

*Based on data provided by Donald Smith from Hospital discharge survey, Washington, D.C., National Center for Health Statistics.
†Data from 1969-1970 unavailable because collection system was altered.

complications until delivery and/or providing poor care so that complications occur; and that the declining birthrate produces a need to expand "business."

Contraceptive utilization. During the 1960s and 1970s there was an increase in use of highly effective contraception by married couples, particularly sterilization.[44,156] By 1976, 30.2% of couples in which the woman was aged 15 to 44 years were considered sterile; of the rest, 48.6% were using contraceptive methods, 13.4% were pregnant, at the postpartum stage, or trying to get pregnant, and 7.7% were classified as nonusers of contraception (in Chapter 7 see Table 7-1 and discussion of contraception risks). This group was only slightly smaller than in 1973 (8.7%), and was comprised mainly of older women.[44]

Among widowed, divorced, and separated 15 to 44-year-old women in the United States in 1976 (an estimated 3.6 million), about one third (1.2 million) reported they were sterile, while nearly one half (1.6 million) reported they were using a contraceptive method. By contrast, in 1973 about one fifth of women in this group reported they were sterile, and 30% reported using a contraceptive method.[45]

Sterilization (see Chapter 3 for discussion of abuse), either for women (tubal ligation) or for men (vasectomy) is more common among whites than blacks and other minorities. It is generally selected by couples in which the wife is in her thirties, reaching a peak at ages 35 to 39, and after 15 to 19 years of marriage. Among whites the prevalence of sterilization in 1975 was about equally divided among males and females, 17% and 19%, respectively.[156]

Abortion. In 1977 more than 1 million legal abortions were reported to the CDC.[25] Data from the Alan Guttmacher Institute, which reports 1.3 million abortions in 1977, show that 28% of all pregnancies in that year were terminated by abortion. Of these, about one third were in women under age 20, one third were in women 20 to 24 years of age, and the rest were in women 25 years and older; approximately 75% of these women were unmarried. About 30% of women who wanted abortions in 1977 were unable to obtain them, primarily because only about one fifth of all United States counties have abortion providers. Over 40% of women who obtained abortions traveled out of county or out of state to do so. Most abortions (61%) were performed in nonhospital clinics.[46]

Access to abortion is being increasingly curtailed by restrictive legislation and by cutbacks in federal and state funding for Medicaid payments for abortion (see Chapter 3).[14,98] Of the 4.6 million Medicaid-eligible women, 57% are at risk of unintended pregnancy.[1] Access may also be curtailed by physician attitude,[89] the organized opposition of antiabortion forces,[13] or the methods available in relation to the length of the pregnancy.

Women have always used abortions and generally for economic reasons.[2,33] They are likely to continue to do so, and restrictive funding and access may be expected to affect the safety of the procedure.[25,99]

Mental health

The National Center for Health Statistics estimates that mental disorders affect 15% of the United States population annually. Included in the definition

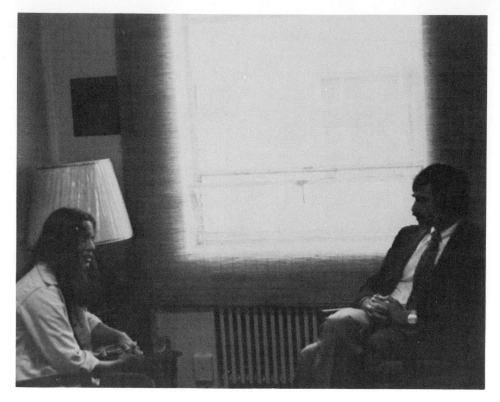

Fig. 1-5. Mental health setting.

of mental disorders are organic and functional psychoses, neuroses, personality disorders, alcoholism, drug dependence, behavioral disorders, and mental retardation. Excluded are "problems of living" and emotional symptoms,[135] although psychiatric care is frequently sought for these.

Among females, women aged 25 to 64 are most likely to be admitted for mental care. Minority women are more likely to be admitted than are white women, and their care setting is more likely to be a state or county mental hospital, community mental health center, or an outpatient psychiatric service.[135]

When Veterans Administration hospitals are included in overall data on admissions for psychiatric reasons, more men than women are shown to be admitted, but female admissions outnumber those for males in outpatient psychiatric services and in private inpatient facilities such as private mental hospitals and private general hospitals.[21,135] Once admitted to any type of facility, however, women stay longer than men.[41] This is particularly true in state and county mental hospitals, where the average length of stay for women in 1975 was 33 days, compared with 23 days for men. This difference may be explained in part by alcoholic disorders, which usually require shorter lengths of stay and which are more common among men. Another contributing factor may be, understandably, a woman's unwillingness, conscious or unconscious, to return to a situation that she asso-

Table 1-14. Distribution of admissions to private mental hospitals, United States, 1975*

Primary diagnosis	All races (%)			White (%)			Races other than white (%)		
	Total	Female	Male	Total	Female	Male	Total	Female	Male
Alcohol disorders	8.3	3.7	14.5	8.4	3.7	14.9	7.2	3.8	11.0
Drug disorders	2.4	1.7	3.3	2.3	1.6	3.2	3.4	2.1	4.9
Organic brain syndromes	4.0	4.1	3.9	3.9	4.0	3.8	5.0	5.3	4.7
Depressive disorders	42.5	49.0	33.7	43.6	50.1	34.6	29.7	35.8	23.0
Schizophrenia	21.8	21.7	21.9	20.8	20.9	20.8	33.0	32.3	33.5
Neuroses	5.6	5.0	6.4	5.7	5.1	6.4	4.9	3.8	6.1
Personality disorders	5.1	4.5	5.9	5.1	4.5	6.0	4.6	4.5	4.8
Childhood disorders	1.2	0.9	1.6	1.1	0.8	1.5	2.3	†	3.1
Transient situational disorders of adolescence, adult, and late life	6.0	6.1	5.8	6.0	6.1	5.8	6.4	6.9	5.8
Social maladjustment	0.1	†	0.2	0.1	†	0.2	†	†	†
No mental disorder	0.6	0.7	0.5	0.6	0.7	0.5	†	†	†
All other	2.4	2.5	2.3	2.4	2.4	2.3	2.7	3.0	2.4

*Based on unpublished data from Division of Biometry and Epidemiology, National Institute of Mental Health, Washington, D.C.

†Five or fewer sample cases—estimate not shown because it does not meet standards of realiability.

ciates with ill health, which therefore prolongs her hospitalization. White women generally have a shorter length of stay than minority women in all but private facilities, where the reverse is true.[135]

In all types of inpatient units, women are hospitalized most frequently for depressive disorders, schizophrenia, and alcoholism, although the relative rates for each diagnosis vary by type of institution[40,78] (see Table 1-14).

Women's mental health is particularly influenced by societal expectations and social roles,[27] and since these expectations are also frequently held by mental health professionals,[16,154] women's mental health problems are compounded.[10,118] Role conflicts, internally and externally imposed, may both cause and aggravate mental illness. Marriage, motherhood, and career goals in a society that provides inadequate support for the optimal pursuit of all three, may be constantly in conflict.[9,52,103] Traditional therapeutic measures that sought to "adjust" the woman to her situation, to help her lower her expectations and find contentment, or to medicate her to cope[136] are slowly giving way to radical and feminist approaches that seek to reduce conflict by recognizing the need for society and families to adjust to a woman's goals.[8,47,79,106]

Drug consumption

PRESCRIPTION. The National Institute on Drug Abuse (NIDA) reported that in 1977 tranquilizers were prescribed for 32 million women (42%), sedatives for 16 million (21%), and stimulants for 12 million (17%). For men the prescriptions were, respectively, 19 million (26%), 12 million (17%), and 5 million (8%).[92] Of first prescriptions of these drugs for women, 8.5 million were for tranquilizers, 3 million were for sedatives, and almost 1 million were for stimulants.[92]

The differences in prescribing patterns are believed to be caused by physicians' more frequent perceptions of women's reported morbidity as psychosomatic,[7,30,69,97] women's greater frequency of physician visits[86] (see Chapter 2), women's more frequent reporting of anxiety and stress,[75] the frustration caused by conflicts between women's goals and expected social roles for which drugs are prescribed to help women cope,[93,159] and the focus on women by drug industry advertising and promotion.[83,102,125]

Many women become addicted to these prescription drugs. Some estimates approach 20 million,[31] although the NIDA states that an estimated 1 to 2 million women have problems because of prescription drugs.[92] Statistics from the Client Oriented Data Acquisition Process (CODAP) operated by NIDA, to which all federally-funded drug abuse treatment and rehabilitation units report, show that in 1976, 62,981 (26%) of all admissions were for women. Of these women, 35% were 21 to 25 years old, 22% were 26 to 30 years old, and 16% were over 30 (14% were under 18 and 13% were aged 18 to 20). Most women admitted were whites (57%); blacks accounted for 33%, and Hispanics 9%.[90]

For the majority of the females (62%), the primary drug problem was opiates (heroin); marijuana accounted for 9% of admissions, barbiturates 6%, amphetamines 6%, and other sedatives 5%.[90]

The Drug Abuse Warning Network (DAWN) sponsored by the Drug Enforcement Administration and NIDA, which gathers data from emergency rooms on emergency drug-related episodes (as opposed to patients), reported a

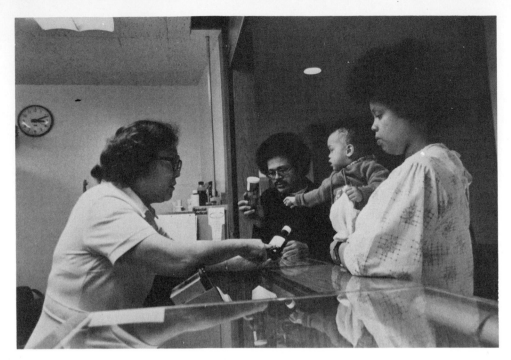

Fig. 1-6. At the pharmacy. (Courtesy Health Sciences Information Service, University of Washington, Seattle.)

total of 118,311 episodes from May, 1975, to April, 1976. Women accounted for 59% of these, and over 50% of the episodes were related to a suicide attempt or gesture (see Table 1-15 for 1976 to 1977 data).[91]

Although controversy exists over whether Valium (diazepam) (the most commonly prescribed drug in the United States and most frequently prescribed to women) and Librium (chlordiazepoxide) are dangerous or addictive,[60] Valium accounted for the largest number of emergency room reports (21%) in 1976 and 1977. Librium, also frequently prescribed for women, accounted for 3.6% of emergency room reports in the same years.[143, Table 96, p. 299] NIDA notes that "when either Valium or Librium appear in an emergency room crisis, they have been used in combination with alcohol or some other drug more than half of the time."[91] In 1976 and 1977, alcohol in combination with other drugs accounted for 18.3% of emergency room reports;[143, Table 96, p. 299] presumably the majority of these were for women.

Women accounted for 43% of drug-related deaths in 1977; most of these were from narcotics, sleeping pills, tranquilizers, and pain relievers. Of the Valium-related deaths, 94% also involved alcohol or another drug. Women accounted for 35% of drug-related deaths among blacks and 45% among whites. Among black males and females and white males, the median age at drug-related death was 28 years in 1977; for white females, it was 43 years.[92]

Efforts being made to prevent prescribing of fatal drug combinations or

Table 1-15. Emergency room reports of drug abuse patients, United States reporting areas, May, 1976, to April, 1977*

Age, sex, and race	Number of emergency room reports	Motivation for taking substance (%)				
		Psychic effects	Dependence	Suicide attempt or gesture	Other	Unknown or non-response
TOTAL	123,164	20.8	16.1	38.8	2.4	21.9
Age						
Under 10 years	121	9.9	—	15.7	28.1	46.3
10 to 19 years	25,418	28.1	5.8	38.8	2.1	25.2
20 to 29 years	53,789	21.7	21.2	34.7	2.1	20.3
30 to 39 years	23,291	17.3	18.3	41.8	2.4	20.3
40 to 49 years	11,190	14.2	14.2	47.0	2.9	21.6
50 years and over	7930	11.7	10.3	48.6	4.7	24.7
Unknown	1425	14.0	16.8	29.6	1.5	38.2
Sex						
Male	51,129	25.4	24.7	25.5	2.3	22.0
Female	71,832	17.5	9.9	48.3	2.5	21.8
Unknown	203	24.6	19.7	32.5	1.0	22.2
Race						
White	74,455	20.9	11.2	44.1	2.4	21.4
Black	28,698	23.2	31.0	25.5	2.7	17.6
Other races	4782	22.6	21.7	36.3	2.0	17.4
Unknown	15,229	15.3	9.8	38.7	2.2	34.0

*Based on data from Project DAWN V, Drug Enforcement Administration, U.S. Department of Justice, and National Institute on Drug Abuse, U.S. Department of Health, Education and Welfare. Data include only medical emergencies related directly or indirectly to drug ingestion. One emergency room episode can involve more than one drug. Each drug included in an episode constitutes a drug report. Data are for 24 standard metropolitan statistical areas and are based on reporting by a sample of hospital emergency rooms.

"doctor shopping" to satisfy legal addiction include computerizing prescriptions,[29] and Pills Anonymous,[43] run similarly to Alcoholics Anonymous. Drug advertising and promotion of drugs for women, drug company profits from sales to women, and questionable marketing practices, particularly in the Third World, appear to continue unabated, however[119] (see Chapter 7).

ILLEGAL DRUG USE. There are no data specifically on illegal drug use among adult women. (Data on women in federally funded drug treatment programs, and their drug usage, which includes illegal drugs was given earlier.) The most commonly used illegal drug is heroin; among female clients at federally funded drug abuse centers, heroin was the principal drug of 82% of black women, 76% of Hispanic women, and 41% of white women.[90] In contrast to the data on prescription drugs, data on emergency room episodes reported by DAWN for 1975 and 1976 show that more men (71%) than women (29%) have emergent episodes with heroin. By 1977, heroin- and morphine-related episodes were the third most common drug-related reason for emergency room visits, accounting for 12% of the total. Marijuana or hashish accounted for 3.4%, methadone 3.2%, PCP 1.7%, and cocaine 1.4%.[143]

Of the 62% of women admitted to treatment in federally funded centers who reported heroin as their primary drug problem, 75% reported daily use of opiates. In addition to the primary drug problem reported, 34% of women admitted reported a secondary drug problem; for 9% of women it was marijuana, and for 4%, cocaine.[90]

Almost one third (31%) of opiate abusers had first used opiates by age 17, and by age 20, 62% had. Among women who abused inhalants, 72% had first used them by age 15; this was also true for 65% of women who abused marijuana and 59% of hallucinogen abusers.[90]

Although health problems of women drug addicts are only beginning to be studied, initial data suggest that in addition to the complications of the drug use (e.g., for heroin, hepatitis, hepatic cirrhosis, infection), women have additional problems, some of which may be related to support of the drug habit (e.g., venereal disease). Major categories of problems reported among women drug addicts are dental (broken teeth), genitourinary (e.g., vaginitis), nervous system (especially diseases of the eye, ear, and nose), and circulatory system (e.g., disturbances of blood pressure, varicose veins).[5]

Drug use, whether prescription or illegal, is particularly harmful during pregnancy. Pregnant women addicts frequently place their offspring in increased jeopardy because, fearful they will be judged unfit mothers and lose their children, they do not seek prenatal care.[93] Babies born to drug abusers are generally also addicted.[22,51,63,131]

Alcoholism. There are an estimated 3 to 5 million women alcoholics in the United States, who come from all socioeconomic strata (see Chapter 6 for teenage alcoholism). Only about 5% of all alcoholics fit the "skid row" stereotypes, and 70% of alcoholics hold down steady jobs and have family lives and ties with the community,[111] but such data are not yet available specifically for women alcoholics. Women represent from 35% to 50% of the nation's total alcoholics, and now account for nearly one in every three new members of Alcoholics Anonymous. Alcoholism treatment centers report seeing one woman for every three men as opposed to one for every six men about 5 years ago.[4]

Men appear to drift into alcoholism, but women who become alcoholics frequently pinpoint a specific event in their lives that they believe precipitated their drinking. Generally, the event is related to societal stereotypes of women as perfect wives and mothers, feminine and sexy, and the event (e.g., divorce, widowhood, postpartum depression) is related to a sense of inadequacy in one of these roles.[4] Lesbian women report a particularly high rate of alcoholism.[35] Women alcoholics are often stereotyped as silent drinkers at home, and although many are housewives, many also work outside the home. If a woman has a propensity for alcoholism, being relatively isolated at home can provide an environment for easy access to liquor, and this may contribute to a higher rate of alcoholism in housewives.

Mortality from alcoholism is difficult to measure because of unwillingness to list it on death certificates. However, in data from 1973 and 1974, death rates per 100,000 women aged 20 years and over were 5.7 for white women and 16.2 for nonwhite women. This represented an increase of 36% and 71%, respectively, from 1963 and 1964.[76]

Alcoholism in women is particularly devastating because of the possible effects on the fetus. Babies born to alcoholic mothers may be born addicted and frequently suffer from fetal alcohol syndrome (an estimated 1 out of every 2000 new born babies, 1 out of every 100 infants of alcoholic women). Characteristics of this syndrome are small size (length and weight), including an abnormally small head, mental retardation, facial peculiarities (i.e., protruding forehead, narrow, slitlike eyes, narrow upper lip that gives the mouth a fishlike shape, receding chin, deformed ears, short, upturned nose). In addition, there may be other deformities of the joints, genitals, and heart.[108,130]

Smoking. In 1955 an estimated 24% (13.1 million) of women 20 years of age and older smoked; by 1965 this had risen to 32% (19.7 million) and had dropped to 29% (21 million) by 1975. By race, in 1976 33.5% of black women smoked, compared to 29.8% of white women. Overall, absolute numbers of women who smoke have risen steadily.[23] In 1976, of women over 17 years who smoked, 19.4% smoked 25 cigarettes or more per day; in 1975, of women 21 years and older, 22.8% smoked 25 or more cigarettes per day.[107]

In the past decade there has been a 2.6% reduction in the number of women who smoke but a 13.6% reduction in the number of men.[107] For reasons that are not clear, women appear to experience more difficulty giving up smoking than do men.[155]

Among women morbidity that is related to smoking is increasing. Lung cancer has increased 5 times among women since 1955 (discussed later). Women who smoke have 45% more days of absence from work than do nonsmokers. They have 21% more acute conditions and 9% more chronic conditions. Women who smoke and use oral contraceptives are particularly at risk of heart disease[107] (see Chapter 7).

As with drugs and alcohol, the fetus is also affected by cigarette smoke. On the average, babies born to smokers weigh 200 grams less than those born to nonsmokers, and their overall dimensions are smaller. The ratio of placenta weight to birth weight increases with increasing levels of maternal smoking, and this may be due to lower oxygen availability caused by carbon monoxide presence. Long-term studies indicate that smoking "may affect physical growth, mental development, and behavior characteristics of children at least up to the age of 11."[107]

Suicide. Women attempt suicide about three times as often as men, but they actually commit suicide about four times less often. With increasing age, the disparity widens; by age 85, 12 men commit suicide for every woman. This difference is believed to be partly because women use less lethal methods such as pills, gas, and poisons, whereas men tend to use guns. It may also be because women use a suicidal gesture as a plea for help, feeling more comfortable with seeking help than do men.

In 1977, suicide was among the 10 leading causes of death for both black and white women aged 20 to 44 and for white women aged 45 to 64. Although rates for all women have increased in the last 10 years, rates have dramatically risen for black women 20 to 24 years of age and for women with careers in medicine and psychology, who show a suicide rate three times higher than for women in the general population.[72,126] These increases are attributed to the new opportunities for women that have increased pressures and present more opportunities for failure, loss of self-esteem, or being fired.

Wife abuse. The number of wives who are physically assaulted is unknown; one legal aid center reported seeing 1000 victims of ongoing severe wife beating annually.[96] A national survey estimated that out of the nearly 50 million couples living together in the United States, 1.7 million spouses have experienced violence involving the use of a knife or gun, and more than 2 million have experienced one spouse physically assaulting the other.[129]

Differing explanations as to the cause of wife abuse include abuse being an expression of social and cultural norms, being imitative behavior by either a husband or a wife who witnessed wife abuse as a child, or being the result of frustration and inability to communicate verbally.[49,70,114,128,153] Although the cause is undefined, the traditional view of spousal violence has been to regard it as a domestic issue; police and social agencies have therefore been reluctant to intervene. As a result, refuges for battered women and children are lifesaving.[112]

Chronic diseases

A chronic disease is one that is marked by long duration or frequent recurrence; most chronic conditions are present in persons 45 years of age and older. In 1976, women of all ages comprised 51.7% of persons with some degree of activity limitation due to a chronic condition.

Arthritis and rheumatism accounted for most limitation; 31.6% in women aged 65 and over, 24.2% in women aged 45 to 64, 8.8% in those 17 to 44 years of age, and 1.9% in those under age 17. Heart conditions and hypertension were the next most frequent; in women 45 to 64 years of age they accounted for 22.2% of limitation; in women 65 years and over, 25.3%; but only 2.5% in those under 17; and 3.9% in those aged 17 to 44. Overall, hypertension was the third chronic cause of limitation for all women in 1976 (8.9%); most of this was in women aged 45 and over. Impairment of the back and spine accounted for 14.5% of the limitation for women aged 17 to 44, but only 7.9% and 3.8%, respectively, for women aged 45 to 64 and those 65 years and older.[143, Table 56, p. 236]

In comparison, males of all ages were most frequently limited by heart conditions (16.7%), arthritis and rheumatism (11.4%), and impairments of the back and spine (7.2%). As with women, back and spine impairments affected the 17 to 44 age-group (13.9%).[143] In general more chronic conditions are reported by low-income families and families in which the head has completed less than 12 years of education.[113,157]

Selected chronic conditions

HYPERTENSION. In 1975 it was estimated that 17% of white females and 28% of black females aged 20 and over suffered from hypertension; for white and black men the respective rates were 13% and 25%.[55] High blood pressure can result in stroke, congestive heart failure, or kidney failure, and is a major risk factor in coronary artery disease. In most cases (90%), although it is easily detectable and controllable, the causes of hypertension are unknown, but stress, salt intake, and diet may be related.

CANCER. Although some cancers are acute, most are chronic, requiring lengthy treatment and close observation. Among women, breast cancer occurs most frequently. It is estimated that there were about 90,000 new cases of breast cancer in 1978 and 33,800 deaths. All cancers of the digestive organs affected 83,200 women, with 50,000 deaths. Within this group there were an estimated 39,000 cases of cancer of the colon and rectum, with 22,300 deaths. The third most frequent cancer for women in 1978 was cancer of the genital organs, of which 69,200 new cases were estimated, with 22,500 deaths.[20] Lung cancer, discussed earlier as being on the rise,[74,127] affected 23,000 women and caused 21,900 deaths. Cancer incidence for 1978 by site and sex is estimated for women (in ascending order of frequency) as follows: skin, 1%; mouth, 2%; pancreas, 3%; urinary organs, 4%; ovary, 5%; lung, 7%; leukemia and lymphomas, 7%; uterus, 14%; colon and rectum, 15%; breast, 26%; and all others, 16%. For men the incidence estimates are as follows: skin, 1%; pancreas, 3%; mouth, 5%; leukemia and lymphomas, 9%; urinary organs, 9%; colon and rectum, 14%; prostate, 16%; lung, 22%; and all others, 21%. Cancer deaths in ascending frequency, by site are, for women: skin, 1%; mouth, 1%; urinary organs, 3%; pancreas, 5%; uterus, 6%; ovary, 6%; leukemia and lymphomas, 9%; lung, 12%; colon and rectum, 15%; breast, 19%; and all others, 23%. For men they are as follows: skin, 2%; mouth, 3%; pancreas, 5%; urinary organs, 5%; leukemia and lymphomas, 9%; prostate, 10%; colon and rectum, 12%; lung, 33%; and all others, 21%.[20]

HANDICAPPED WOMEN. Because data are "educated guesses" until more accurate statistics are derived from the 1980 census, it is believed that there are approximately 36 million handicapped persons (defined as functional inability to perform in some areas) in the United States. In general, the handicapped population is older, less educated, and holds lower status jobs than does the population overall; one fourth of the handicapped population are below the poverty level. In the 1970 census, 5.3 million women of working age were defined as handicapped, and only a small percentage of these women earned over $10,000 per year. Among handicapped women who are single, 15% have some earned income; among those married, 24% depend on spousal support.[32]

Both handicapped men and women seek independence provided by job training, rehabilitation services (less than 15% of severely handicapped women aged 18 to 54 receive these services in contrast with 25% of men in this category),[32] home health care workers, and recognition of their sexuality. Handicapped women's sexuality has been unresearched and their needs only recently addressed.[116,117]

Nursing homes. Prior to the Social Security Act of 1935 and the 1965 Medicare and Medicaid Amendments, there were few nursing homes. By 1976 there were 20,185 homes of all types nationwide.[143, Table 142, p. 373] In 1975 and 1976,

Table 1-16. Nursing home residents and discharges, United States, 1976 and 1977*

Age, sex, race, and marital status	1977 residents		1976 discharges	
	Number	Percent distribution	Number	Percent discharged alive
TOTAL	1,287,400	100.0	973,100	74.2
Age				
Under 65 years	189,500	14.7	135,400	89.9
65 to 74 years	202,000	15.7	161,200	73.4
75 to 84 years	470,600	36.6	381,800	75.9
85 years and over	425,300	33.0	294,700	65.3
Sex				
Male	369,400	28.7	349,700	74.8
Female	918,000	71.3	623,400	73.9
Race				
White†	1,180,300	91.7	‡	‡
All other	107,100	8.3	‡	‡
Marital status§				
Married	160,800	12.5	192,100	80.1
Widowed	743,700	57.8	552,300	71.8
Divorced or separated	87,600	6.8	84,700	86.2
Never married	265,900	20.7	106,300	69.4
Unknown	29,400	2.3‖	37,700	65.8‖

*Based on data from National Center for Health Statistics: Comparison of nursing home residents and discharges, 1977 National Nursing Home Survey, by E. Hing and A. Zappolo; and from Advance data from vital and health statistics, No. 29, Pub. no. (PHS) 78-1250, U.S. Department of Health, Education and Welfare, Hyattsville, Md., May 1978. Public Health Service. Data are based on resident records in a sample survey of nursing homes.
†Excludes Spanish-American (Hispanic).
‡Data not available.
§For resident data, marital status at time of data collection. For discharge data, marital status at time of discharge.
‖Data do not meet standards of reliability or precision.

71% of the 1.3 million residents of nursing homes were women (see Table 1-16); this accounts for the preponderance of women in data on total institutionalizations in the United States.[143, pp. 322-324, Table 114, p. 327]

Most women in nursing homes are over age 65, and data from 1973 and 1974 showed that 80% were over age 75 compared with 63% of male residents. Because women live longer than men and have lower incomes than men, they have fewer resources for companionship, housing, and food and possibly are in greater need of nursing homes. In 1973 and 1974, 73% of female nursing home residents were widowed.[132]

Most (70% to 75%) nursing home residents stay from 1 to less than 3 years, regardless of the sex or age category examined, and most enter for physical reasons. In 1973 and 1974, 81.8% of women entered for physical reasons, 6.4%

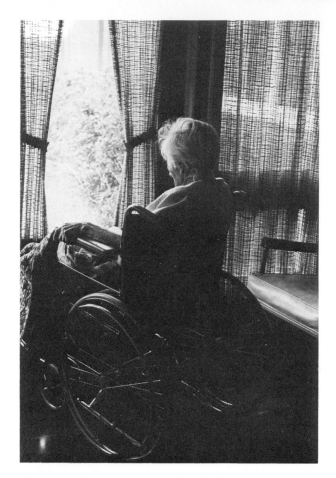

Fig. 1-7. Nursing home resident. (Courtesy Health Sciences Information Service, University of Washington, Seattle.)

for social reasons, 10.9% for behavioral reasons, and 0.9% for economic reasons.[132] In 1977, 73.9% of the female population of nursing homes were discharged alive[143] (see Table 1-16).

Although sex-specific data are not yet available, of all nursing home residents in 1977, the most frequent primary diagnoses per 1000 residents at last examination were as follows: diseases of the circulatory system, 370.8; and mental disorders and senility without psychosis, 223.4.[58]

MINORITY WOMEN

In general, minority women are poorer, less educated, and have a lower employment rate and less money than do white women. Thirty percent of black women are considered heads of households, as are 14% of Hispanic women; of these, about 66% of black households and nearly 60% of Hispanic households live in poverty, compared with 42% of whites.[85,142,160] As data in this chapter demonstrate, minority women also are in poorer health than white women (see particularly maternal mortality differentials in Table 1-6), and are subject to more sterilization abuse (see Chapter 3).[3,36,39,109,147]

Black women

Health status characteristics particularly evident among black women include hypertension, obesity, heart disease, atherosclerosis, kidney disease, diabetes, nutritional deficiencies, especially low hemoglobin levels, arthritis, gout, digestive problems such as ulcers, gastritis, and cirrhosis of the liver, and for lower income black women, higher mortality rates from cervical and breast cancer than are reported in the general population. In addition, black women experience higher levels of family violence than do white women.[80]

Black women, especially if they are poor, are likely to have less access to health care than whites. This is particularly true for rural black women whose health care needs are likely to be compounded by extreme poverty, poor sanitation, inadequate water supplies, and malnutrition.[110]

Hispanic women

Women of Spanish or Hispanic origin are those who indicate their ethnic background is, for example, Mexican, Puerto Rican, Cuban, or Central or South American.[160] For many of these, the English language is a formidable barrier to access to health care.

The problems of poverty as it relates to health are frequently compounded for the large numbers of women in this group who are migrant farm workers. Not only do these women (and their families) have few regular sources of care, but they are exposed to potentially harmful pesticides (see Chapter 5) when working in the fields. In addition, one study in Utah found the most frequent health problems among migrants were pharyngitis or tonsillitis, upper respiratory tract infections, minor trauma, and dermatitis.[6] Conditions that may affect them as adults, such as high cholesterol levels, overweight, anemia, and low height for age, have been found among Mexican-American children.[164]

Native American women

According to the 1970 census, there were 798,119 Native Americans; the American Indian population comprised 763,594 of this total, the remainder being composed of Aleuts and Eskimos. In 1970 there were 100 American Indian females to every 97 males (50.8% of the total).[142] This was a shift from 109 males for every 100 females in 1950.[161] Although educational attainment, and subsequently employment, has risen among Native Americans since 1950,[161] the population is still characteristically poor and has health problems associated with poverty. In addition, alcoholism and related conditions such as cirrhosis of the liver, trauma (e.g., car accidents), anemia, poor nutrition, and tuberculosis are common problems.

Native American women also experience a maternal mortality rate per

100,000 live births from 1.4 to 2.7 times higher than does the general maternal population of the United States.[122]

Asian-Pacific American women

This category of women includes those of East Asian, Southeast Asian, South Asian, and Pacific Island origins. The 1970 census determined that this racial group comprised 0.75% of the population with 1.5 million persons;[142] because of rapid immigration in the 1970s, mid-decade estimates are 2.5 million.[100]

The Asian-Pacific American is generally categorized as "other" in the United States data, hence accurate statistics are lacking. Even when data on Asians as a group are presented, they do not allow for differences among the different subgroups (e.g., Korean, Japanese, Filipino, Vietnamese) or for varied socioeconomic statuses.

Because many Asian-Pacific Americans are poor, particularly recent immigrants, and live in crowded substandard housing, health problems are again those associated with poverty. Tuberculosis, eye failure from working in poorly lit conditions, poor nutritional status, trauma, and wife abuse are known health problems in Asian-Pacific communities.[100] The high crime in the crowded Chinatowns of San Francisco and New York also affects health. Pian reports that "according to a 1977 San Francisco Chinatown family planning study, only 12 out of 632 cases of sexual assault reported at the Clinic had been reported to the police. The Sex Crime Detail of the San Francisco Police had no bilingual staff."[100] Alcoholism is also a health problem in the Asian-Pacific Community.[71]

• • •

The diversity of women's health status and needs is the result of numerous variables, including age, race, occupation, marital status, education, and economic resources. This diversity is reflected in women's varying utilization of the health system, including hospitalization, frequency and type of surgery, chronic disease incidence and activity limitation, mental health care, drug consumption, and nursing home occupancy.

When the individual differences are discounted and women are considered in the aggregate, data demonstrate that compared with men, women consume more drugs, are hospitalized and institutionalized more often, and experience more surgery. However, as this chapter indicates, aggregate data often obscure significant socioeconomic differences and their effects on women's health needs.

SUGGESTED TOPICS FOR DISCUSSION, FURTHER RESEARCH, AND FIELD PROJECTS

1. Select one disease and investigate its incidence among women. What ages of women are most susceptible? Why? Is incidence of this disease related to women's role? Could modifications be made in women's life-styles to lower the incidence of this disease?
2. Obtain a copy of the National Health Interview Survey and information on how the survey is conducted. Discuss ways in which the survey and interview process may produce results that may either overrepresent or underrepresent some groups of

women and therefore which may influence the reported health status of women.
3. Select a disease category typically thought of as "a man's disease" and investigate its incidence among women (e.g., cardiovascular disease, gout, alcoholism, lung cancer). What factors have led to an increased incidence among women? What is the incidence of this disease according to age and race characteristics?
4. How has the quality and quantity of prenatal care changed in the past decades? What factors have led to the change? How has/is prenatal care related to maternal and infant outcome?
5. What are the various methods of abortion? What are their relative outcomes? How is payment for abortion organized? Is abortion covered by health insurance plans? Research availability of abortion in your area.
6. What factors contribute to a higher fertility rate among black women? How does black fertility compare with fertility among other minority women? Why are more triplets and twins born to black women? Is this also true among other minority groups?
7. Select a surgical procedure that is non–sex specific. How does its incidence differ by sex, age, race, geographical area, and type of hospital?
8. What factors are causing increasing rates of women smokers, suicides, and alcoholics? Do these factors similarly affect men? What would be the important elements in a health program designed to reverse these increasing rates?
9. Research activities for the elderly in your community. What are the proportions of males to females in nursing homes in your area? What kinds of activities are available to these residents? What are their major health problems? How do these relate, if at all, to their social abilities?
10. Identify a minority population in your area. What are the age and sex characteristics of this population? What are the major health problems for women within this group? What is the source of care most frequently used by women in this group? Does this differ from that used by white women living within the same area? If so, what factors account for this difference?
11. At present, women have a longer life expectancy than do men. What factors are used to explain this difference? Do you think this difference will last? Why/why not? Identify what factors have led to women's longer life expectancy. Identify what factors may narrow the difference between men and women.

REFERENCES

1. Abortions and the poor: private morality, public responsibility, New York, 1979, Alan Guttmacher Institute.
2. Acevedo, Z.: Abortion in early America, Women & Health 4:159-166, Summer, 1979.
3. Ad Hoc Women's Studies Committee Against Sterilization Abuse: Workbook on sterilization and sterilization abuse, Bronxville, N.Y., 1978, Sarah Lawrence College.
4. An emerging issue: the female alcoholic, Miami, 1977, Health Communications, Inc.
5. Anderson, M. D.: Health needs of drug dependent clients: focus on women, Women & Health 5:23-33, Spring, 1980.
6. Anderson, W. W., and Kane, R. L.: Patterns of care given migrant workers in Utah by private physicians and clinics, Public Health Rep. 92:326-331, July/Aug., 1977.
7. Armitage, K. J., et al.: Response of physicians to medical complaints in men and women, J.A.M.A. 241:2186-2187, 1979.
8. Ash, M.: The changing attitudes of women: implications for psychology, J. Am. Med. Wom. Assoc. 29:411-413, 1974.
9. Bachrach, L. L.: Marital status and mental disorder: an analytical review, Series D, No. 3, Survey and Reports Branch, Division of Biometry, National Institute of Mental Health, no. (ADM)75-217, Washington, D.C., 1975, U.S. Government Printing Office.
10. Bardwick, J. M.: Readings on the psychology of women, New York, 1972, Harper & Row, Publishers.
11. Barker, M. G.: Psychiatric illness after hysterectomy: a critical review, Br. Med. J. 2:91, 1968.
12. Barker-Benfield, G. J. (Ben): Horrors of the half-known life, New York, 1975, Harper Torchbooks.

13. Beals, J.: Current issues facing the right to abortion, Women & Health **4:**107-109, Spring, 1979.
14. Berger, L.: Abortions in America: the effects of restrictive funding, N. Engl. J. Med. **298:**1475-1477, 1978.
15. Bonham, G. S.: Expected size of completed family among currently married women 15-44 years of age: United States, 1973, Advance Data, no. 10, National Center for Health Statistics, Washington, D.C., Aug. 12, 1977, U.S. Government Printing Office.
16. Broverman, I. K., et al.: Sex-role stereotypes and clinical judgements of mental health, J. Consult. Clin. Psychol. **34:**1-7, 1970.
17. Bullough, V. L., and Voght, M.: Women, menstruation and nineteenth century medicine, Bull. Hist. Med. **XLVII:**66-82, Jan/Feb., 1973.
18. Bunker, J. P.: Surgical manpower, N. Engl. J. Med. **282:**135-144, 1973.
19. Bunker, J. P.: Elective hysterectomy: pro and con, N. Engl. J. Med. **295:**264-268, 1976.
20. Cancer facts and figures, 1978, New York, 1977, American Cancer Society, Inc.
21. Cannon, M. S., and Redick, R. W.: Differential utilization of psychiatric facilities by men and women: United States 1970, Statistical Note No. 81, National Institute of Mental Health, Washington, D.C., June, 1973, U.S. Government Printing Office.
22. Carr, J. N.: Drug patterns among drug-addicted mothers: incidence, variance in use and effects on children, Pediatric Annals **4:**65-77, July, 1975.
23. Center for Disease Control: Adult and teenage cigarette smoking patterns — United States, Morbidity and Mortality Weekly Report, vol. 26, no. 19, May 13, 1977.
24. Center for Disease Control: National nosocomial infections study — United States, 1975-1976, Morbidity and Mortality Weekly Report, vol. 26, no. 46, Nov. 18, 1977.
25. Center for Disease Control: Abortion-related mortality — United States, 1977. Morbidity and Mortality Weekly Report, vol. 28, no. 26, July 6, 1979.
26. Chard, T., and Richards, M.: Benefits and hazards of the new obstetrics, Philadelphia, 1977, J. B. Lippincott Co. (See Chapter 3.)
27. Chesler, P.: Women and madness, New York, 1972, Doubleday & Co., Inc.
28. Cohn, V.: U.S. moves to curb unneeded surgery, Washington Post, Nov. 2, 1977.
29. Computerizing cuts prescribing of psychotropics, Medical World News, p. 11, Sept. 4, 1978.
30. Cooperstock, R.: Sex difference in the use of mood-modifying drugs: an explanatory model, J. Health Soc. Behav. **12:**238-244, Sept., 1971.
31. Cowan, B.: Women's health care: resources, writings and bibliographies, Ann Arbor, Mich., 1977, Anshen Publishing.
32. Davis, C.: Handicapped women's health concerns, Women and Health Roundtable Report, vol. II, no. 12, Dec., 1978.
33. Devereux, G.: A study of abortion in primitive societies, revised ed., New York, 1976, International Universities Press, Inc.
34. Devitt, N.: The statistical case for elimination of the midwife: fact versus prejudice, 1890-1935. I and II. Women & Health, **4:**81-96, 169-186, 1979.
35. Diamond, D. L., and Wilsnack, S. C.: Alcohol abuse among lesbians: a descriptive study, J. Homosexuality **4:**123-142, Winter, 1978.
36. Dreifus, C.: Sterilizing the poor. In Dreifus, C., editor: Seizing our bodies, New York, 1978, Vintage Books.
37. Dyck, F. J., et al.: Effect of surveillance on the number of hysterectomies in the province of Saskatchewan, N. Engl. J. Med. **296:**1326-1328, 1977.
38. Egbert, L. D., and Rothman, I. L.: Relation between the race and economic status of patients and who performs their surgery, N. Engl. J. Med. **297:**90-91, 1977.
39. Elliot, J.: 'Genocide' charged by Indian M.D. investigator, Medical Tribune, **11,** Aug. 24, 1977.
40. Faden, V. B.: Primary diagnosis of discharges from non-federal general hospital psychiatric inpatient units, U.S. 1975, Mental Health Statistical Note No. 137, National Institute of Mental Health, Washington, D. C., Aug. 1977, U.S. Government Printing Office.
41. Faden, V. B., and Taube, C. A.: Length of stay of discharges from non-federal general hospital psychiatric inpatient units, United States 1975, Mental Health Statistical Note No. 133, National Institute of Mental Health, Washington, D.C., May, 1977, U.S. Government Printing Office.
42. Fahy, T. J. : Depression after hysterectomy, Lancet (Letters) **2:**672-673, 1973.
43. For pill-poppers — Pills Anonymous, Medical World News, p. 81, Oct. 16, 1978.
44. Ford, K. : Contraceptive utilization in the

United States: 1973-1976. Advance Data, no. 36, National Center for Health Statistics, Washington, D.C., Aug. 18, 1978, U.S. Government Printing Office.

45. Ford, K.: Contraceptive utilization among widowed, divorced and separated women in the United States: 1973 and 1976, Advance Data, no. 40, National Center for Health Statistics, Washington, D.C., Sept. 22, 1978, U.S. Government Printing Office.

46. Forrest, J. D., et al.: Abortion in the United States, 1976-1977, Fam. Plann. Perspect. **10:**271-279, Sept/Oct., 1978.

47. Franks, V., and Burtle, V., editors: Women in psychotherapy: new psychotherapies for a changing society, New York, 1974, Brunner/Mazel Publishers.

48. Garraway, W. M.: The declining incidence of stroke, N. Engl. J. Med. **300:**449-452, 1979.

49. Gelles, R.: The violent home, Beverly Hills, Calif., 1972, Sage Publications, Inc.

50. Gough, H. G., and Hall, W. B.: Number of children wanted and expected by American physicians, J. Psychol. **96:**45-53, 1977.

51. Gray, N.: Chemical use/abuse and the female reproductive system, Phoenix, April, 1976, Do It Now Foundation, Institute for Chemical Survival.

52. Hansen, L. S., and Rapoza, R. S.: Career development and counseling of women, Springfield, Ill., 1978, Charles C Thomas, Publisher.

53. Haupt, B. J.: Utilization of short-stay hospitals: annual summary of the United States, 1977 Vital and Health Statistics, series 13, no. 41, National Center for Health Statistics, Washington, D.C., March, 1979, U.S. Government Printing Office.

54. Hays, H. R.: The dangerous sex: The myth of feminine evil, New York, 1964, G. P. Putnam's Sons.

55. Heart facts, 1978, Dallas, 1979. American Heart Association, Inc.

56. Hendershot, G.E.: Pregnant workers in the United States, Advance Data, no. 11, National Center for Health Statistics, Washington, D.C., Sept. 15, 1977, U.S. Government Printing Office.

57. Hibbard, L.: Despite higher risks, some doctors still prefer hysterectomy to tubal ligation, Fam. Plann. Perspect. (digest) vol. 2, Jan., 1973.

58. Hing, E., and Zappolo, A.: A comparison of nursing home residents and discharges from the 1977 National Nursing Home Survey: United States, Advance Data, no. 29, National Center for Health Statistics, Washington, D.C., May 17, 1978, U.S. Government Printing Office.

59. Hoffman, L. W.: The value of children to parents—a national sample survey, presented at the American Public Health Association Annual Meeting, Oct. 17, 1978, Los Angeles.

60. Hollister, L. E.: Valium: a discussion of current issues, Psychosomatics **18:** 44-58, 1977.

61. Hurd-Mead, K. C.: A history of women in medicine from the earliest times to the beginning of the nineteenth century, Conn., 1938, The Haddam Press.

62. Joffe, J.: Program for elective surgical second opinion. Evaluation report: Preliminary findings Jan., 1976-Aug., 1977, New York, June, 1978, Blue Cross and Blue Shield of Greater New York.

63. Keith, L., et al.: Drug-dependent obstetric patients: A study of 104 admissions to the Cook County Hospital, J. Obstet., Gynecol. Neonatal Nurs., **3:**17-20, 1974.

64. Kinzer, N. S.: Stress and the American woman, New York, 1979, Doubleday and Co., Inc.

65. Kobrin, F. E.: The American midwife controversy: a crisis of professionalization, Bull. Hist. Med. **40:**350-363, 1966.

66. Kovar, M. G.: Data from the Health Interview Survey, personal communication, May, 1979.

67. Laurent, A., et al.: Reporting health events in household interviews, Vital and Health Statistics, series 2, no. 49, National Center for Health Statistics, Washington, D.C., 1972, U.S. Government Printing Office.

68. Lembcke, P. A.: Medical auditing by scientific methods illustrated by major female pelvic surgery. J.A.M.A. **162:**646-655, 1956.

69. Lennane, K. J., and Lennane, R. J.: Alleged psychogenic disorders in women—a possible manifestation of sexual prejudice, N. Engl. J. Med. **288:**288-292, 1973.

70. Martin, D.: Battered wives, San Francisco, 1976, Glide Publications.

71. Matsushima, B., et al.: Alcoholism/alcohol abuse "needs assessment" study of the Pacific/Asian community, Asian American Drug Abuse Program, Inc., April, 1978, 5318 S. Crenshaw Blvd., Los Angeles, Calif. 90043.

72. Mausner, J. S., and Steppacher, R. C.: Suicide in professionals: a study of male and female psychologists, Am. J. Epidemiol. **98**:436-445, 1973.

73. Meigs, C.: Woman: her diseases and remedies, Philadelphia, 1851, Blanchard & Lee.

74. Meigs, J. W.: Epidemic lung cancer in women, J.A.M.A. **238**:1055, 1977.

75. Mellinger, G. D., et al.: Psychic distress, life crisis, use of psychotherapeutic medications: National Household Survey data, Arch. Gen. Psychiatry, **35**:1045-1052, 1978.

76. Metropolitan Life Insurance Company: Mortality from alcoholism, Stat. Bull. **58**:2-5, Dec., 1977.

77. Metropolitan Life Insurance Company: Survival and the life cycle, Stat. Bull. **59**:5-7, Oct.-Dec., 1978.

78. Meyer, N. G.: Diagnostic Distribution of Admissions to Inpatient Services of State and County Mental Hospitals, United States, 1975, Mental Health Statistical Note no. 138, National Institute of Mental Health, Washington, D.C., Aug., 1977, U.S. Government Printing Office.

79. Miller, J. B.: Towards a new psychology of women, Boston, 1976, Beacon Press.

80. Moore, L. M.: Health concerns of black women, Washington, D.C., Nov. 13, 1978, Division of Black American Affairs, Department of Health, Education and Welfare.

81. Morehead, M., and Trussell, R.: The quantity, quality and costs of medical care secured by a sample of teamster families in the New York area, New York, 1962, Columbia University School of Public Health and Administrative Medicine.

82. Morgan, S.: Sexuality after hysterectomy and castration, Women & Health **3**:5-10, Jan./Feb., 1978.

83. Mosher, E. H.: Portrayal of women in drug advertising: a medical betrayal, J. Drug Issues **6**:72-78, Winter, 1976.

84. Moss, J. E., chairperson, Subcommittee on Oversight and Investigations, 95th Congress, 1st Session: Background report on surgery in state Medicaid programs, print no. 95-20. Washington, D.C., July, 1977, U.S. Government Printing Office.

85. Moy, C. S., and Wilder, C. S.: Health characteristics of minority groups, United States, 1976, Advance Data, no. 27, National Center for Health Statistics, Washington, D.C., April 14, 1978, U.S. Government Printing Office.

86. Muller, C.: The over medicated society: forces in the marketplace for medical care, Science **17**:488-492, 1972.

87. Muller, C.: Women and health statistics: areas of deficient data collection and integration, Women & Health, **4**:37-59, Spring, 1979.

88. Munsen, M. L.: Wanted and unwanted births reported by mothers 15-44 years of age: United States, 1973, Advance Data, no. 9, National Center for Health Statistics, Washington, D.C., Aug. 10, 1977, U.S. Government Printing Office.

89. Nathanson, C., and Becker, M. H.: Physician behavior as a determinant of utilization patterns: the case of abortion, Am. J. Public Health **68**:1104-1114, Nov., 1978.

90. National Institute on Drug Abuse (NIDA): Women and drugs: information from the client oriented data acquisition process (CODAP), Program for Women's Concerns, Rockville, Md., Feb., 1978, National Institute on Drug Abuse.

91. National Institute on Drug Abuse (NIDA): Women and drugs: information from the drug abuse warning network (DAWN), Program for Women's Concerns, Rockville, Md., Feb., 1978, National Institute on Drug Abuse.

92. National Institute on Drug Abuse (NIDA): Women and prescription drugs, NIDA, Capsules, April, 1978.

93. Nellis, M., et al.: Final report on drugs, alcohol and women's health: an alliance of regional coalitions. Contract no. 271-77-1208, Washington, D.C., 1978, National Institute on Drug Abuse.

94. Ortemayer, L.: Females' natural advantage? or, the Unhealthy environment of Males? Women & Health, **4**:121-132, Summer, 1979.

95. Pappenfort, D. M.: Journey to labor, Chicago, 1964. Aldine Publishing Co.

96. Parker, B., and Schumacher, D. N.: The battered wife syndrome and violence in the nuclear family of origin: a controlled pilot study, Am. J. Public Health **67**:760-761, Aug., 1977.

97. Parry, H. S., et al.: National patterns of psychotropic drug use, Arch. Gen. Psychiatry **28**:769-783, 1973.

98. Petitti, D. B.: Abortion in California 1968-1976. Sacramento, Calif., 1979, Maternal and Child Health Branch, Office of Family Planning, Department of Health Services.

99. Petitti, D. B., and Cates, W.: Restricting Medicaid funds for abortions: projections of excess mortality for women of childbearing age, Am. J. Public Health **67**:860-862, Sept., 1977.

100. Pian, C.: Asian Pacific American women's health concerns, presented to Women & Health Roundtable, Sept. 14, 1978, Washington, D.C.

101. Polivy, J.: Psychological reactions to hysterectomy: a critical review. Am. J. Obstet. Gynecol. **118**:417-426, 1974.

102. Prather, J. E., and Fidell, L. S.: Sex differences in the content and style of medical advertising, Soc. Sci. Med. **9**:23-26, Jan. 1975.

103. Radloff, L.: Sex differences in depression. The effects of occupation and marital status, Sex Roles **1**:249-265, 1975.

104. Rawlings, S., Bureau of the Census: personal communication, July, 1979.

105. Ricci, J. V.: The geneology of gynecology. History of development of gynecology throughout the ages 2000 B.C. – 1800 A.D. Philadelphia, 1950, The Blakiston Co.

106. Rice, J., and Rice, D.: Implications of the women's liberation movement for psychotherapy, Am. J. Psychiatry **30**:191-196, Feb. 1973.

107. Richmond, J. B., U.S. Surgeon General: Smoking and health, U.S. Public Health Service, No. 017-000-00218-0, Washington, D.C., 1979, U.S. Government Printing office. (See p. A-18, Table 8.)

108. Robe, L. B.: Just so it's healthy, Minneapolis, 1977, Comp-Care Publications.

109. Rodriguez-Triaz, H.: Sterilization abuse, The Women's Center Reid Lectureship, Nov. 10 and 11, 1976, New York, 1978, Barnard College.

110. Sablosky, A.: Health care and women in the Mississippi delta, Women & Health **1**:21-23, July/Aug., 1976.

111. Sandmaier, M.: Alcohol abuse and women. A guide to getting help, National Institute on Alcohol Abuse and Alcoholism, no. 017-024-00514-2, Washington, D.C., 1977, U.S. Government Printing Office.

112. Saunders, D. G.: Marital violence: dimensions of the problem and modes of intervention, J. Marriage Family Counseling **3**:43-52, Jan., 1977.

113. Scott, G.: Prevalence of chronic conditions of the genitourinary, nervous, endocrine, metabolic, and blood and blood-forming systems and of other selected chronic conditions, United States, 1973, Vital and Health Statistics, series 10, no. 109, National Center for Health Statistics, no. (HRA) 77-1536, Washington, D.C., March, 1977, U.S. Government Printing Office.

114. Scott, P. D.: Battered wives, Br. J. Psychiatry **125**:433-441, 1974.

115. Second opinion before hysterctomy is advised, Seattle Times, E3, Jan. 19, 1978.

116. Shaul, S.: Within reach: providing family planning services to physically disabled women, New York, 1978, Human Sciences Press.

117. Shaul, S., et al.: Toward intimacy: family planning and sexuality concerns of physically disabled women, New York, 1978, Human Sciences Press.

118. Sherman, J. A.: On the psychology of women: a survey of empirical studies, Springfield, Ill., 1971, Charles C Thomas, Publisher.

119. Silverman, M.: The drugging of the Americas: how multinational drug companies say one thing about their products, in the United States and another thing to physicians in Latin America, Berkeley, 1976, University of California Press.

120. Sims, J. M.: Clinical notes on uterine surgery, New York, 1866, William Wood.

121. Sinai, N., and Anderson, O. W.: Emergency maternity and infant care: a study of administrative experience, New York, 1974, Arno Press.

122. Slocumb, J. C., and Kunitz, S. J.: Factors affecting maternal mortality and morbidity among American Indians, Public Health Rep. **92**:349-356, July-Aug., 1977.

123. Smith-Rosenberg, C.: The hysterical woman: sex roles in nineteenth century America, Social Research **39**:652-678, Winter, 1972.

124. Soranus: Gynecology, cited by Bullough, V. L.: Medieval medical and scientific views of women, Viator **4**:485-501, 1973.

125. Spake, A.: The pushers, The Progressive, pp. 17-20, April, 1976.

126. Steppacher, R. C., and Mausner, J. S.: Suicide in male and female physicians, J.A.M.A. **228**:323-328, 1974.

127. Stolley, P. D.: Lung cancer: unwanted equality for women, N. Engl. J. Med. **297**:886-887, 1977.

128. Straus, M. A.: Leveling, civility – violence

in the family, J. Marriage and Family **36:** 13-29, Feb., 1974.

129. Straus, M. A., et al.: Report of national survey of a representative sample of 2,143 families, presented at the American Association for Advancement of Science Annual Meeting, Feb. 25, 1977, Denver.

130. Streissguth, A. P.: Fetal alcohol syndrome: where are we in 1978? Women & Health **4:**223-237, Fall, 1979.

131. Student Association for the Study of Hallucinogens (STASH): Methadone and pregnancy — bibliographies, no. 1, National Institute on Drug Abuse, no. HSM-42-73-216, Washington, D.C., Sept., 1974, U.S. Government Printing Office.

132. Sutton, J. F.: Utilization of nursing homes, United States, National Nursing Home Survey, Aug., 1973-April, 1975, Vital and Health Statistics, series 13, no. 28, National Center for Health Statistics, no. (HRA) 77-1779, Washington, D.C., July, 1977, U.S. Government Printing Office.

133. Taffel, S.: Prenatal care in the United States 1969-1975, Vital and Health Statistics, series 21, no. 33, National Center for Health Statistics, Washington, D.C., 1978, U.S. Government Printing Office.

134. Tasto, D. L.: Health Consequences of Shift Work, Washington, D.C., March, Shift Work, contract no. 210-75-0072, Washington, D.C., March, 1978, National Institute of Occupational Safety and Health.

135. Taube, C. A., et al.: Mental disorders. In U.S. Department of Health, Education and Welfare: Health, United States 1978, Washington, D.C., 1978, U.S. Government Printing Office.

136. Tennov, D. Psychotherapy: the hazardous cure, London, 1975, Abelard-Schuman.

137. United Nations: Demographic year book 1975, Statistical Office, Department of International, Economic and Social Affairs, New York, 1975, United Nations.

138. United Nations: Demographic year book, 1977, Statistical Office, Department of International, Economic and Social Affairs, New York, 1977, United Nations: Additional data from Statistical Office of the United Nations, New York, personal communication, July, 1979.

139. United Nations Economic and Social Council, Statistical Commission: Draft principles and recommendations for population and housing census. Report of the secretary-general, E/CN.3/515, June, 14, 1978, United Nations.

140. U.S. Bureau of the Census: Current Population Reports, series P-25, no. 800, April, 1979, U.S. Department of Commerce.

141. U.S. Bureau of the Census: Population profile of the United States: 1978, Current Population Reports, series P-20, no. 336, Washington, D.C., 1979, U.S. Government Printing Office.

142. U.S. Department of Health, Education and Welfare: Health of the disadvantaged. Chartbook, Health Resources Administration, no. (HRA) 77-628, Washington, D.C., 1977, U.S. Government Printing Office.

143. U.S. Department of Health, Education and Welfare: Health United States, 1978, Washington, D.C., 1978, U.S. Government Printing Office, no. (PHS) 78-1232.

144. U.S. Department of Health, Education and Welfare: Professional standards review organization hospital discharge data sets. Jan.-Dec., 1977, Office of Professional Standards Review Organization, HCFA, Washington, D.C., 1978-1979, U.S. Government Printing Office.

145. U.S. Department of Health, Education, and Welfare, Office for Handicapped Individuals: personal communication, July, 1979. Data from Rehabilitation Act of 1973, P.L.93-112, and President's Committee on Employment of the Handicapped: One in eleven. Handicapped adults in America, Department of Labor, Washington, D.C., 1975, U.S. Government Printing Office. (Data from 1970.)

146. U.S. Department of Health, Education and Welfare: Sterilization and abortions. Federal financial participation, Federal Register, vol. 43, no. 217, Paragraph 441.255 42 CFR, Nov. 8, 1978.

147. Vasquez, P.M., and Estrada, C. A.: Chicanas: women's health issues, San Francisco, Oct., 1978, Mexican-American Legal Defense and Educational Fund.

148. Verbrugge, L. M.: Sex differentials in morbidity and mortality in the United States, Social Biology **23:**275-296, Winter, 1976.

149. Verbrugge, L. M.: Recent trends in sex mortality differentials in the United States, Women & Health **5,** Fall, 1980.

150. Verbrugge, L.: Marital status and health, J. Marriage and Family **7:**267-285, May, 1979.

151. Verbrugge, L. M.: Female illness rates and illness behavior: testing hypotheses about sex differences in health, Women & Health **4:**61-79, Spring, 1979.
152. Waldron, I.: Why do women live longer than men? Social Science and Medicine, **10:**349-362, 1976.
153. Warrior, B.: Working on wife abuse, 1978, Betsy Warrior, 46 Pleasant Street, Cambridge, Mass. 02139.
154. Weisstein, N.: Psychology constructs the female, or, the fantasy life of the male psychologist. In Garskoff, M. H., editor: Roles women play: readings toward women's liberation, Belmont, Calif., 1971, Brooks/Cole Publishing Co.
155. West, D. W., et al.: Five year follow-up of a smoking withdrawal clinic population, Am. J. Public Health **67:**536-544, 1977.
156. Westoff, C. F., and McCarthy, J.: Sterilization in the United States, Fam. Plann. Perspect. **II:**147-152, May/June, 1979.
157. Wilder, C. S.: Prevalence of chronic circulatory conditions, United States, 1972. Vital and Health Statistics, series 10, no. 94, National Center for Health Statistics, no. (HRA) 75-1521, Washington, D.C., Sept., 1974, U.S. Government Printing Office.
158. Willson, J. R.: Recruitment into obstetrics and gynecology, Obstet. Gynecol. **40:**432-437, 1972.
159. Wolcott, I.: Women and psychoactive drug use. Women & Health **4:**199-202, Summer, 1979.
160. Women's Bureau: Women of Spanish origin in the United States, U.S. Department of Labor, Washington, D.C., 1976, U.S. Government Printing Office.
161. Women's Bureau: American Indian women, U.S. Department of Labor, Washington, D.C., June, 1977, U.S. Government Printing Office.
162. Women's Bureau: Working mothers and their children, U.S. Department of Labor, Washington, D.C., 1977, U.S. Government Printing Office.
163. World Health Organization: International classifications of diseases, ninth revision (see definitions and recommendations), Geneva, 1977, World Health Organization.
164. Yanochek-Owen, A., and White, M.: Nutrition surveillance in Arizona: selected anthropometric and laboratory observations among Mexican-American children, Am. J. Public Health **67:**151-154, 1977.

ADDITIONAL READINGS

Aho, W. R.: Relationship of wives' preventive health orientation to their beliefs about heart disease in husbands, Public Health Rep. **92:**65-71, Jan.-Feb., 1977.
Alpert, L. I.: Approaches to breast cancer: a pathologist's perspective, Women & Health **4:**269-286, 1979.
American Public Health Association: Minority health chart book, contract no. (HRA) 106-74, Washington, D.C., 1974, U.S. Government Printing Office.
Balamuth, E.: Health interview responses compared with medical records. Vital and Health Statistics series 2, no. 7. National Center for Health Statistics, Washington, D.C., 1965, U.S. Government Printing Office.
Balter, M. B., et al.: Cross-national study of the extent of anti-anxiety/sedative drug use, N. Engl. J. Med. **290:**769-774, 1974.
Barlow, S.: Women and drugs, Guy's Hosp. Gazette (England), June 24, 1978.
Bould, S.: Female-headed families: personal fate control and the provider role, J. Marriage, and Family **39:**339-349, May, 1977.
Bracken, M. B., and Freeman, D. H.: Hospitalization for complications of abortion and association with legal induced abortion in the United States 1971-1975, presented at the American Public Health Association Annual Meeting, Oct. 15, 1978, Los Angeles.
Brody, J. E.: Hysterectomies reduced sharply under monitoring plan in Canada, N.Y. Times **12:**40, June 9, 1977.
Burchell, R. C.: Hysterectomy: functional versus anatomical indications, CA **27:**241-242, 1977.
Cannon, M. S.: Halfway houses serving the mentally ill and alcoholics, United States, 1973. series A, no. 16, Survey and Reports Branch Division of Biometry, National Institute of Mental Health, no. (ADM) 76-264, Washington, D.C., 1975, U.S. Government Printing Office.
Cates, W.: Abortion attitudes of black women, Women & Health **2:**3-9, Nov./Dec., 1977.
Cates, W., and Grimes, D. A.: Abortion and penicillin—treatments for social diseases, Women & Health **3:**3-5, Jan./Feb., 1978.
Center for Disease Control: Abortion surveillance 1976, Atlanta, Aug., 1978, Center for Disease Control.
Daling, J. R.: Effects of abortion on subsequent pregnancy outcome, presented at the American, Public Health Association Annual Meeting, Oct. 17, 1978, Los Angeles.
DeJong, G. F., and Sell, R. R.: Changes in child-

lessness in the United States: a demographic path analysis, Population Studies, **31:**129-141, 1977.

Dohrenwend, B. P., and Dohrenwend, B. S.: Sex difference and psychiatric disorders, Am. J. Sociol. **81:**1447-1454, 1976.

Dowsling, J., and Maclennan, A., editors: The chemically dependent woman, Toronto, Canada, 1978, Addiction Research Foundation, 33 Russell St., Toronto, Ontario, Canada M5S 2S1.

Freeman, E. W.: Influence of personality attributes on abortion experiences, Am. J. Orthopsychiatry **47:**503-513, 1977.

Freeman, E. W.: Abortion: subjective attitudes and feelings, Fam. Plann. Perspect. **10:**150-155, May/June, 1978.

Frederick, L.: How much unnecessary surgery? Medical World News, pp. 50-66, May 3, 1976. The unnecessary surgery debate (continued), Medical World News, pp. 13-16, May 31, 1976.

Gove, W. R., and Hughes, M.: Possible cause of the apparent sex differences in physical health: an empirical investigation, Am. Sociol. Rev. **44:**126-146, Feb., 1979.

Gray, J.: Use of tranquilizers in PAS hospitals, PAS Reporter **II:**1-2, Feb. 9, 1973.

Gust, D.: Career woman/going up fast: alcoholic/going down fast, Minneapolis, 1977, Comp-Care Publications.

Hellman, L. M., et al.: The use of health manpower in obstetric-gynecologic care in the United States, Int. J. Gynaecol. Obstet. II. **8:**732-738, 1970.

Horowitz, A.: The pathways into psychiatric treatment: some differences between men and women, J. Health Soc. Behav. **18:**169-178, June, 1977.

Kent, P.: An American woman and alcohol, New York, 1974, Holt, Rinehart & Winston, Inc.

Kent, S.: Urinary tract problems in women are linked to sexual activity, Geriatrics **30:**145-146, July, 1975.

Kirkpatrick, J.: Turnabout: help for a new life, New York, 1978, Doubleday & Co., Inc.

Klebba, A. J., et al.: Mortality trends: age, color and sex, United States 1950-1969, National Center for Health Statistics, PB 271 358, Washington, D.C., Nov., 1973, U.S. Government Printing Office.

Krassner, M., and Muller, C.: Manpower in obstetrics-gynecology in a period of declining birth rate, Med. Care **12:**1031-1037, 1974.

Lazar, J. B., editor: The report by the Task Panel on Women and Mental Health from the President's Commission on Mental Health, Washington, D.C., Jan. 1, 1978, U.S. Government Printing Office.

Lewis, C. E., and Lewis, M. A.: The potential impact of sexual equality on health, N. Eng. J. Med. **297:**863-869, 1977.

Linn, L. S., and Davis, M. S. The use of psychotherapeutic drugs by middle-aged women, J. Health Soc. Behav. **12:**331-339, 1971.

Lopata, H. Z.: Widows as a minority group. II. Gerontologist **II:**67-77, Spring, 1971.

Ludcke, A.: What's a nice girl like you doing with an illness like this? Minneapolis, 1977, Comp-Care Publications.

McCarthy, J., and Menken, J.: Marriage, remarriage, marital disruption and age at first birth, Fam. Plann. Perspect. **II:**21-30, Jan/Feb., 1979.

Mellinger, G. D.: Psychotherapeutic drug use among adults: a model for young drug users? J. Drug Issues, **1:**274-285, Oct., 1971.

Mendelson, M. A.: Tender loving greed, New York, 1974, Vintage Books.

Metropolitan Life Insurance Company: Longevity of first ladies of the United States, Stat. Bull., **58:**2-4, Jan., 1977.

Metropolitan Life Insurance Company: Socioeconomic mortality differentials by leading causes of death, Stat. Bull. **58:**5-8, Jan., 1977.

Metropolitan Life Insurance Company: Trends in average weights and heights among insured men and women, Stat. Bull. **58:**3-6, Oct., 1977.

Metropolitan Life Insurance Company: Longevity of prominent women, Stat. Bull. **60:**3-9, Jan.-March, 1979.

Moghissi, K. S., and Evans, T. N., editors: Nutritional impacts on women throughout life with emphasis on reproduction, New York, 1977, Harper & Row, Publishers.

Mohr, J. C.: Abortion in America, New York, 1978, Oxford University Press.

Montague, A.: The natural superiority of women, London, 1970, Collier-Macmillan Ltd.

Morgan, S.: Hysterectomy, Feminist history research project, California, 1978, and Boston Women's Health Book Collective, Inc., Boston, 1978.

Morton, W. E.: Socioeconomic status effect on incidence of three sexually transmitted diseases, presented at the American Public Health Association Annual Meeting, Oct. 16, 1978, Los Angeles.

Muller, C.: Methodological issues in health economics research relevant to women, Women & Health **1:**3-9, Jan/Feb., 1976.

Nathanson, C. A.: Sex, illness and medical care:

a review of data, theory and method, Soc. Sci. Med. **11**:13-25, Jan., 1977.

Nathanson, C. A., and Becker, M. H.: The influence of physicians' attitudes on abortion performance, patient management and professional fees, Fam. Plann. Perspect. **9**:158-163, July/Aug., 1977.

Pandolfi, J.: That 51% plus (a Ford Foundation report), New York, 1979, Ford Foundation, 320 E. 43rd St., New York, N.Y., 10017.

Placek, P. J.: The relationship of maternal health factors to sterilization following delivery of legitimate live births in hospitals: United States, Vital Statistics Report, vol. 26, no. 3, supp. 2, National Center for Health Statistics, Washington, D.C., June 20, 1977, U.S. Government Printing Office.

Placek, P. J.: The incidence of sterilization following delivery of legitimate live births in hospitals: United States, Vital Statistics Report, vol. 26, no. 3, supp. National Center for Health Statistics. Washington, D.C., June 17, 1977, U.S. Government Printing Office.

Polansky, E.: Take him home, Mrs. Smith, HealthRight **II**:1, Winter, 1975-1976.

Pomerleau, C.: Cardiovascular disease as a women's health problem, Women & Health **1**:12-15, Nov./Dec., 1976.

Prince, E. O.: Welfare status, illness and subjective health definition, Am. J. Public Health **68**:865-870, 1978.

Quick, J. D.: Liberalized abortion in Oregon: effects on fertility, prematurity, fetal death and infant death, Am. J. Public Health **68**:1003-1008, 1978.

Retherford, R. D.: The changing sex differential in mortality, Westport, Conn., 1975, Greenwood Press.

Sackett, D. L., et al.: The development and application of indices of health: general methods and a summary of results, Am. J. Public Health **67**:423-428, 1977.

Santa Cruz Women's Health Center: Herpes, Santa Cruz, Calif., 1977, Santa Cruz Women's Health Collective, 250 Locust St., Santa Cruz, Calif. 95060.

Saver, H. I., et al.: Geographic and other factors associated with differences in death rates, age 65-74, presented at the American Public Health Association Meeting, Los Angeles, Calif., Oct. 18, 1978.

Schnall, P.: Economic and social causes of cancer. In The social etiology of disease: HMO packet #2, Health/PAC, 17 Murray St., New York, N.Y. 10007.

Seidenberg, R.: Drug advertising and perception of mental illness, Mental Hygiene **55**:21-31, 1971.

Smith, H.: Gynecology and ideology in seventeenth century England. In Carroll, B., editor: Liberating women's history: theoretical and critical essays, Urbana, Ill., 1976, University of Illinois Press.

Swigar, M. E., et al.: Abortion applicants: characteristics distinguishing dropouts remaining pregnant and those having abortion, Am. J. Public Health **67**:142-146, Feb., 1977.

Thompson, B.: Problems of abortion in Britain-Aberdeen, a case study, Population Studies **31**:143-154, March, 1977.

Tietze, C.: Repeat abortions—why more? Fam. Plann. Perspect. **10**:286-288, Sept/Oct., 1978.

Tietze, C.: Induced abortion: 1979, New York, 1979, The Population Council.

Warrior, B.: Battered lives, Somerville, Maine, 1975, New England Free Press.

Weaver, J. L.: National health policy and the underserved: ethnic minorities, women and the elderly, St. Louis, 1976, The C. V. Mosby Co.

Wilder, M. H.: Prevalence of chronic skin and musculoskeletal conditions, United States, 1969, Vital and Health Statistics, series 10, no. 92, National Center for Health Statistics, no. (HRA) 75-1519, Washington, D.C., Aug., 1974, U.S. Government Printing Office.

Women's Bureau: Women with low incomes, Washington, D.C., Nov., 1977, U.S. Department of Labor.

Women's Bureau: Minority women workers: a statistical overview, Washington, D.C., 1977, U.S. Department of Labor.

Young, J. L., et al., editors: SEER program: cancer incidence and mortality in the United States, 1973-1976. Biometry Branch, Division of Cancer Cause and Prevention, National Cancer Institute, (NIH) 78-1837, Washington, D.C., U.S. Government Printing Office and Welfare.

Zink, M.: For silent sippers—a way out of hiding, Minneapolis, 1977, CompCare Publications.

Chapter 2

Obtaining ambulatory health care

The growth of the medical profession at the turn of the century and its growing respectability following the Flexner Report of 1910,[26] encouraged increasing numbers of women to seek its services. The upper classes particularly, mainly because they could afford the fees, turned to organized medicine. The lower classes continued to rely on themselves and home remedies, midwives, and local healers. Patent medicines,[37] many of which contained large amounts of opium or alcohol, were in widespread use by both classes until the Harrison Act[34] (Narcotics Control, 1914) and Volstead Act[4] (Prohibition, 1919) curtailed the availability of opium and alcohol and therefore their medicinal use. The fashion of female invalidism, or at least feminine frailty and delicacy among the upper classes,[22] was well supported by the medical profession through either sexual surgery (see Chapter 1) or therapies of inactivity and prolonged bed rest. Women were increasingly established as a patient class, and physicians promised cures. Commenting on this emerging trend, Dr. Mary Putnam Jacobi (1842-1906) stated in 1895: "I think, finally, it is in the increased attention paid to women, and especially in their new function as lucrative patients, scarcely imagined 100 years ago, that we find explanation for much of the ill-health among women, freshly discovered today."[22]

The shift of births to hospitals, the development of physician-managed contraception, government programs providing prenatal care, thereby facilitating use of physicians (see Chapter 3), the advent of third party payment, and the tremendous growth of the medical-industrial complex with its promotion of female symptoms and positive cures all were factors contributing to not only defining female morbidity but to establishing patterns of how and where health care could be obtained.

CHARACTERISTICS OF WOMEN'S HEALTH CARE UTILIZATION
Frequency of visits to physicians

Today women of all ages make 22% more visits to the physician than do men; this doubles if visits to accompany children are counted. Except for females under 17 years, women within each age-group also make more visits, rising to almost double men's visits in the 17 to 24 year age-group (see Table 2-1). On the average, women made 5.4 visits to a physician in 1977 as compared with 4.2 made by men;[41] the number of visits made by individual women in a year ranged from 0 to 53 or more. Women in families with lower incomes averaged more

Table 2-1. Number of physician visits by age and sex, United States, 1977*

Sex	All ages	Under 17 years	17 to 24 years	25 to 44 years	45 to 64 years	65 to 74 years	75 years and over
Number of physician visits							
Both sexes	1,020,397	245,108	135,663	260,850	233,509	93,194	52,073
Male	425,932	127,750	45,814	94,391	99,055	39,831	19,091
Female	594,465	117,358	89,849	166,459	134,453	53,364	32,982
Number of physician visits per person per year							
Both sexes	4.8	4.1	4.3	4.7	5.4	6.5	6.5
Male	4.2	4.2	3.0	3.5	4.8	6.4	6.4
Female	5.4	4.0	5.6	5.8	5.9	6.6	6.6

*From Howie, L. J., and Drury, T. F: Vital and Health Statistics, series 10, no. 126. National Center for Health Statistics, no. (PHS) 78-1554. Washington, D.C., Sept., 1978. U.S. Government Printing Office. Data are based on household interviews of the civilian noninstitutionalized population.

visits per year than did high-income women (a reversal of the 1960s pattern), and women who thought their health was poor or fair also made more visits.[73]

Data from the 1977 National Ambulatory Medical Care Survey, which measures strictly defined physician office-based ambulatory visits only, indicate that of women over age 15 who made physician visits in that year, 90.5% were white and 9.5% were included in the "all other" category. Of these women 19% were aged 15 to 24, 33% were between 25 and 44 years, 29% were 45 to 65 years of age, and 19% were 65 or older. Most women (64%) were previous patients of the physician visited, and they presented with old problems, 22% were previous patients who came with new problems, and 14% were new patients. These problems were most frequently rated as not serious (52%), with almost one third (30%) classed as slightly serious, and 18% regarded as serious or very serious.

For many women the visit lasted from 6 to 10 minutes (28.2%); other duration data show that 13.4% of visits lasted 1 to 5 minutes, 27.3% were from 11 to 15 minutes, 22.5% were from 16 to 30 minutes, 5.8% were from 31 to 60 minutes, and 0.5% lasted over 1 hour. Slightly over 2% of visits did not involve any time with the physician, but the patient was seen by an office nurse, for example, for an allergy shot or immunization.

From the time of onset of their particular health complaint, only 2.4% of women waited less than 1 day for a physician visit, 17.3% waited from 1 to 6 days, 13.7% waited from 1 to 3 weeks, 13.3% waited from 1 to 3 months, 34.9% waited 3 months or more, with the waiting time not specified for 18.4% of women.[25]

In 1977, minority women reported a lower rate of physician visits than did white women. From the Health Interview Survey, in which physician visits include all types of physician-patient encounters, black females averaged 5.0 visits (males, 3.8), white females averaged 5.5 (males, 4.2) while among "all others", females averaged 4.4 visits and males, 3.0. According to the Health Interview Survey, the number of visits for both sexes (4.8) was less in 1977 than

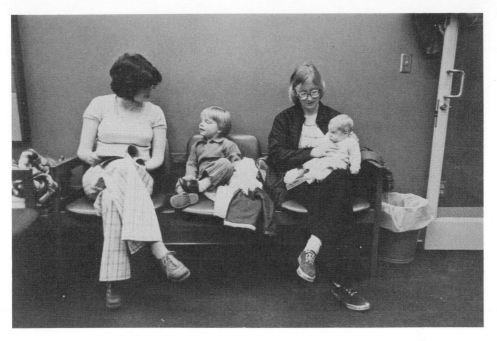

Fig. 2-1. Mothers and children waiting for the physician. (Courtesy Health Sciences Information Service, University of Washington, Seattle.)

in the 2 preceding years, when the averages were 4.9 and 5.1 in 1976 and 1975, respectively. The highest rate of visits per person in 1977 was in the West, and utilization of physicians was higher in metropolitan areas. In all, 75.1% of the population made a physician visit in 1977.

Many theories have been advanced for the sex differences in utilization and apparently therefore in morbidity. These include explanations that women report more illnesses than men because it is more culturally acceptable to do so, that women's social role is more compatible with also adopting a sick role, that women actually are sicker than men because their assigned roles are more stressful,[59,74,75] that women experience a greater sense of personal failure and use illness to justify this,[66] that women are more anxious,[1] and that the differences are the result of mild forms of physical illness which "can be primarily attributed to women confronting more nurturant role demands and generally being in poorer mental health."[29] The "captive population" nature of some of women's health needs, for example, contraception, prepartum and postpartum care, and relief of menopausal symptoms, for all of which women are encouraged to seek medical care, may also contribute to women's increased utilization. Similarly, advertising by the medical-industrial complex and assumptions by physicians that numerous conditions are both morbid and demanding of medical attention may also be contributory.

Reimbursement mechanisms may also affect women's greater health care utilization. Japan has the world's only insurance system to show a lower volume of medical care being sought by women than by men; in that country reimbursement of the medical care of dependents, who are usually female, is only about 66%, whereas for the usually male primary workers it is 100% (unlike the more equitable reimbursement in the United States).[70]

Paying for health care

In 1976 an estimated 79.2% of females (80.1% of males) had some form of private insurance and/or Medicare, 6.6% (4.8% of males) had Medicaid, 2.5% were covered through other programs (2.3% of males), and 10.5% had no insurance (11.6% of males). Most women, as most men, were covered through fee-for-service plans.[73] Although the percentage of covered individuals appears high, these data do not provide information on the extent of coverage that individuals have; many persons, for example, have coverage only for hospitalization, either in full or in part. Ongoing data analysis on this topic will eventually provide this information.

In 1974 a special supplement to the Health Interview Survey asked additional related questions, many of which were analyzed by sex. Regarding payment for health care, it was found that 80.1% of both females and males of all ages reported having some out-of-pocket health expenses, which included the purchase of insurance coverage.[20] Of women who had expenses, the average amount spent was $293 ($244 for men), and in almost all categories, women averaged a higher out-of-pocket expense than did men (see Table 2-2). This difference may be related to women's greater utilization, their greater participation in the part-time work force and therefore less access to jobs that include full health benefits, or the fact that their coverage obtained through their husbands may have terminated with death or divorce. It may also reflect maternity expenses, which until recently were poorly covered in many programs (see Chapter 3). For 1974, all of women's methods of payment for ambulatory care are displayed by age groups in Table 2-3. This is not a percent distribution, since many women used more than one source of payment.

Problems of access

Despite their greater utilization, many women still face substantial barriers preventing optimal access to health services. In 1974 over 12% of women of all ages reported problems ranging from one to three or more in obtaining health care; most (8.5%) reported only one problem (see Table 2-4).

Cost of health care was indicated by 3.1% of women as a problem in obtaining health care (see Table 2-5) and was indicated as a reason for not having a regular source of care by 2% of women in the same survey (see Table 2-13). Cost also was cited as a cause by 49.5% of those who reported having unmet health needs (see Tables 2-6 and 2-7).

Language and cultural beliefs and practices may present another barrier to access, particularly among non-English-speaking minority groups, who frequently use hospital clinics or emergency rooms for primary care. When these are staffed by foreign medical graduates with an inadequate command of English and no knowledge of the patient's language, the turmoil of overcrowded, impersonal facilities is exacerbated and not conducive to attempting comprehension

Table 2-2. Average out-of-pocket health expenses for persons with such expense, United States, 1974*

Sex and age	All types of health expenses†		Health expenses†						
	Including insurance premiums	Excluding insurance premiums	Hospital	Doctor	Dental	Prescription medicine	Optical	Health insurance premiums	Other
Both sexes									
All ages	270	226	225	99	97	57	62	97	154
Under 17 years	152	123	99	55	75	28	51	64	79
17 to 44 years	246	211	195	99	95	41	65	84	135
45 to 64 years	386	321	352	128	125	83	64	130	127
65 years and over	425	350	293	143	105	109	62	138	259
Male									
All ages	244	203	211	90	98	52	61	95	169
Under 17 years	150	122	103	54	74	28	49	63	88
17 to 44 years	207	172	164	84	94	37	62	85	185
45 to 64 years	357	299	359	121	130	76	63	125	181
65 years and over	430	356	298	148	121	110	67	139	182
Female									
All ages	293	246	236	106	97	60	63	99	142
Under 17 years	153	123	95	56	77	28	53	65	68
17 to 44 years	280	243	212	109	96	44	67	82	92
45 to 64 years	412	340	347	133	122	89	65	134	87
65 years and over	422	347	289	140	94	108	58	137	307

*From Drury, T. F.: Vital and Health Statistics, series 10, no. 115, National Center for Health Statistics, no. (HRA) 77-1543, Washington. D.C., March, 1977, U. S. Government Printing Office.
†Average expense in dollars for persons with expense.

Table 2-3. Females' sources of payment for ambulatory care, United States, 1974 (%)*

Payment sources†	All ages	Under 20 years	20 to 44 years	45 to 64 years	65 years and over
Direct payment	83.5	79.6	85.4	86.8	82.3
Private health insurance	30.8	25.4	35.4	34.9	24.1
Public payment	17.3	15.7	11.5	10.2	52.9
Other public sources	9.5	4.1	4.7	4.4	49.0
Medicaid or welfare	8.4	11.7	7.0	6.1	8.1
Other or unknown	3.7	5.0	2.9	3.3	3.2

*Based on unpublished data provided by T. F. Drury from the 1974 Health Interview Survey, Division of Health Interview Statitics, National Center for Health Statistics, Washington, D.C.
†More than one source possible per woman.

Table 2-4. Percent distribution of females of all ages who reported problems obtaining health care, United States, 1974*

Number of problems	Number who experienced problems	Number of times problems delayed obtaining care	Number of times problems prevented getting care
None	87.7	91.1	96.1
1	8.5	5.9	2.6
2	2.5	2.0	0.8
3+	1.3	1.0	0.5
TOTAL	100.0	100.0	100.0

*Based on unpublished data provided by T. F. Drury from the 1974 Health Interview Survey, Division of Health Interview Statistics, National Center for Health Statistics, Washington, D.C.

Table 2-5. Percent of females who experienced problems obtaining health care, United States, 1974*

Reported problem†	All ages	Under 20 years	20 to 44 years	45 to 64 years	65 years and over
Total reporting problem†	12.3	8.8	17.1	12.1	9.4
Getting appointments	6.2	4.0	10.10	5.3	2.8
Physician availability	3.1	2.4	4.3	3.1	2.2
Cost too high	3.1	2.1	3.8	3.9	2.0
Office hours inconvenient	1.8	1.4	2.9	1.3	0.8
Difficulties with transportation	1.6	1.3	1.6	1.3	3.3
Did not know where to go	1.2	0.6	2.1	1.0	1.0
Other problems	1.0	0.7	1.1	1.1	1.3

*Based on unpublished data provided by T. F. Drury from the 1974 Health Interview Survey, Division of Health Interview Statistics, National Center for Health Statistics, Washington, D.C.
†More than one problem possible per woman.

Table 2-6. Percent distribution of females who reported unmet health needs, United States, 1974*

Age	Percent reporting unmet needs	Unknown
All ages	6.4	0.4
Under 20 years	7.4	0.5
20 to 44 years	7.6	0.4
45 to 65 years	8.0	0.4
65 years and over	6.0	0.8

*Based on unpublished data provided by T. F. Drury from the 1974 Health Interview Survey, Division of Health Interview Statistics, National Center for Health Statistics, Washington, D.C.

Table 2-7. Percent of females who reported unmet health needs, United States, 1974*

Reasons for unmet health needs†	All ages	Under 20 years	20 to 44 years	45 to 64 years	65 years and over
Cost too high	49.5	49.5	48.7	52.9	44.2
Physician spends inadequate time	15.1	7.5	18.7	16.7	16.7
Difficulty getting appointment	14.3	13.6	17.2	10.6	14.1
Difficulties with transportation	9.6	10.3	5.4	9.2	25.1
Office hours inconvenient	6.3	7.8	6.5	6.6	1.5
Other	25.4	21.1	28.8	25.0	23.5
Unknown reason	9.5	14.8	7.3	7.6	10.2

*Based on unpublished data provided by T. F. Drury from the 1974 Health Interview Survey, Division of Health Interview Statistics, National Center for Health Statistics, Washington, D.C.
†More than one unmet health need possible per woman.

of the patient's problems. For many women, cultural modesty may further complicate such encounters, with sometimes tragic consequences.[77]

For women with families, and especially working women with families, access to health care may be severely curtailed by a physician's office hours. Inconvenient office hours were cited in 1974 by 1.8% of females who experienced problems in obtaining health care and as a cause by 6.3% of females who reported unmet needs (see Table 2-7).

Lesbian women have also reported that their sexual preference is a barrier to obtaining health care. Reporting feelings of humiliation and anger at judgmental treatment, implications of mental instability, and the insensitivity of a hetero-sexually-oriented approach, many lesbians have preferred to use the generally more empathetic services of women's clinics.[40,62]

Other barriers to access evidenced by Table 2-7 indicate that transportation difficulties (again particularly pertinent for women with young children and no baby-sitter), difficulties in obtaining appointments, and a sense that the physician was too rushed all inhibit satisfactory encounters with the health care system.

PRINCIPAL REASONS FOR OBTAINING CARE

In 1977, women over age 15 initiated visits to the physician mainly for medical or special examinations such as annual physicals, Pap tests, and breast and

Table 2-8. Principal reason for visit to physician by females aged 15 and over, United States, 1977*

Reason	Percent
General, special, and administrative examinations (e.g., annual examination, psychological testing, prenatal checkups, breast and pelvic examinations, school, employment and extracurricular activity examinations)	16.7
Symptoms referable to and diseases of musculoskeletal system and connective tissue (e.g., neck, back, and knee pain or weakness, bone pain, arthritis, bursitis, tenosynovitis, lupus erythematosus)	10.1
Symptoms referable to and diseases of the genitourinary system (e.g., abnormalities of urine, kidney trouble, menstrual disorders, menopausal symptoms, cystitis, complications of pregnancy, cervicitis, pelvic inflammatory disease, vaginitis, breast disease [excluding cancer])	8.9
Symptoms referable to and diseases of respiratory system (e.g., nasal congestion, sinus problems, flu, shortness of breath, tonsillitis, bronchitis, emphysema)	8.8
General symptoms (e.g., chills, fever, pain, weight loss, malaise)	6.9
Diagnostic tests, screening and preventive procedures, test results (e.g., allergy test, glucose level determination, blood tests, mammography, EKG, Pap test, vaccinations, cytology findings)	5.9
Symptoms referable to and diseases of skin, nails, hair, and subcutaneous tissue (e.g., acne, skin infection, rash, hair loss, boils, cellulitis, dandruff, psoriasis, allergic skin reaction)	5.5
Preoperative and postoperative care, progress visits, specific types of therapy, therapeutic procedures (e.g., discussion of cosmetic surgery, suture removal, follow-up visits, physical or respiratory therapy, psychotherapy, tube insertion, cauterization)	5.4
Symptoms referable to and diseases of digestive system (e.g., bleeding gums, difficulty in swallowing, nausea, stomach pain, flatulence, worms, peptic ulcer, appendicitis)	5.3
Symptoms referable to and diseases of eyes and ears (e.g., infection, discharge, hearing dysfunctions, conjunctivitis, otitis media)	5.0
Symptoms referable to and diseases of nervous system (excluding sense organs); congenital anomalies (e.g., convulsions, headaches, multiple sclerosis, epilepsy)	4.4
Symptoms referable to psychological and mental disorders and mental diseases (e.g., anxiety, fears, phobias, depression, alcoholism and drug dependence, sleep disorders, psychoses)	3.2
Medications, family planning (e.g., allergy shots, hormones, renew prescriptions, contraceptive counseling, birth control pills)	3.2
Symptoms referable to cardiovascular and lymphatic systems and diseases of circulatory system (e.g., abnormal pulsations, sore glands, rheumatic fever, hypertension, ischemic heart disease)	3.1
Injury, poisoning, adverse drug effects (e.g., fractures, dislocations, lacerations, puncture wounds, foreign body in eye, burns, motor vehicle accidents, dead on arrival, rape, food poisoning, intoxication)	2.5
Endocrine, nutritional, and metabolic diseases (e.g., goiter, hyperthyroidism, hypoglycemia, ovarian dysfunction)	1.3
Medical and special-problem counseling (e.g., counseling in nutrition or marital, parent-child, money, or work problems)	1.3
Neoplasms (e.g., cancer, benign neoplasms)	0.8
Infective and parasitic diseases (e.g., gastroenteritis, cholera, streptococcal, herpes, or fungus infections, hepatitis)	0.3
Diseases of blood and blood-forming organs (e.g., anemias) etc.	0.2
Uncodable reasons	1.2

*Based on unpublished data provided by T. Ezzati from the National Ambulatory Medical Survey, 1977, Ambulatory Care Statistics Branch, Division of Health Resources Utilization Statistics, National Center for Health Statistics, Washington, D.C.

Table 2-9. Reasons for office visits to physicians by females aged 15 and over according to principal diagnoses and ICDA code, United States, 1977*†

Principal diagnoses and codes	Percent
Special conditions and examinations without sickness (Y00-Y13)	19.0
Diseases of circulatory system (390-458)	10.4
Diseases of respiratory system (460-519)	10.2
Diseases of genitourinary system (580-629)	9.4
Diseases of nervous system (320-389)	7.2
Diseases of musculoskeletal system and connective tissue (710-738)	6.3
Endocrine, nutritional, and metabolic diseases (240-279)	5.5
Accidents, poisonings, and violence (800-999)	5.3
Diseases of skin and subcutaneous tissue (680-709)	5.2
Symptoms and ill-defined conditions (780-796)	4.8
Mental disorders (290-315)	4.8
Diseases of digestive system (520-577)	3.3
Infective and parasitic disease (001-136)	3.1
Neoplasms (140-239)	3.1
Other	1.4
No diagnosis	0.7
Unknown diagnosis	0.3

*Based on unpublished data provided by T. Ezzati from the National Ambulatory Medical Care Survey, 1977, Ambulatory Care Statisitics Branch, Division of Health Resources Utilization Statistics, National Center for Health Statistics, Washington, D.C.
†Diagnostic groupings and code number inclusions are based on the *Eighth Revision International Classification of Diseases, Adapted for Use in the United States.*

pelvic examinations (see Table 2-8). Data on office visits by women over 15 years according to the principal diagnosis made by the physician also show medical or special examinations as the physician's principal assessment of the reason for the visit (see Table 2-9). This is true for both men and women, although obviously the examinations were for different reasons. Women over age 15 who made office visits were next most frequently diagnosed as having diseases (in descending frequency) of the circulatory, respiratory, and genitourinary systems (see Table 2-9).

More detailed data on patient visits in 1975 and 1976 are displayed in Table 2-10. In that year men also made the same number of visits to the physician for upper respiratory infections as they did for medical or special examinations, but the former were the third leading diagnosis for women. In 1977 for every 100 women, 232.2 acute conditions were reported (204.4 for men); the highest number of acute conditions was reported in males (369.0) and females (402.8) under 6 years. Females aged 6 to 16 had 292.2 acute conditions per 100 persons (283.6 males), those aged 17 to 44 reported 245.9 (190.5 males), and women 45 years and over reported 137.8 (116.0 males).[41]

Therapies, services, and disposition

In 1977, according to data reported by the National Ambulatory Medical Care Survey, the morbidity that motivated women over 15 years of age to visit

Table 2-10. Office visits to physicians, United States, 1975 to 1976*†

Sex, most common principal diagnosis, and ICDA code‡	Office visits per 1000 population					
	All ages	Under 15 years	15 to 24 years	25 to 44 years	45 to 64 years	65 years and over
Both sexes§	2,770.7	1,982.1	2,259.0	2,794.2	3,377.2	4,356.6
Female	3,231.5	1,903.7	2,907.4	3,557.3	3,881.5	4,590.8
Medical or special examination (Y00)	241.7	366.5	256.4	253.9	166.9	69.9
Prenatal care (Y06)	195.4	9.8‖	530.1	376.9	3.1‖	NA
Acute upper respiratory infection, except influenza (460-465)	184.5	326.8	153.9	149.2	144.2	89.1
Medical and surgical aftercare (Y10)	142.0	62.5	89.8	183.2	206.1	183.0
Hypertension (400, 401, 403)	136.1	2.2	5.1	53.9	312.0	478.8
Neuroses and nonpsychotic disorders (300-309)	121.8	17.4	83.5	224.7	153.9	115.6
Arthritis and rheumatism (710-718)	111.1	5.6‖	21.9	64.2	206.2	398.1
Heart disease (390-398, 402, 404, 410-414, 420-429)	97.8	5.7	6.8	22.6	143.4	509.6
Ischemic heart disease (410-414)	68.7	1.2‖	1.5	9.0	100.5	383.8
Infections and inflammations of skin (680-698)	90.9	84.4	94.2	89.6	88.6	105.5
Diseases of ear and mastoid process (380-389)	86.0	163.7	50.3	58.1	66.7	78.0
Bronchitis, emphysema, asthma (490-493)	77.3	71.6	42.3	62.8	120.2	98.4
Eye diseases, except refractive (360-369, 371-379)	77.2	34.5	28.4	37.3	99.5	287.2

Sprains and strains (840-848)	60.6	16.2	61.2	87.0	85.3	49.2
Obesity (277)	58.6	6.6‖	62.2	112.6	71.2	19.9‖
Diabetes mellitus (250)	53.6	4.8‖	7.2	19.1	103.6	211.1
Refractive errors (370)	49.5	26.3	53.7	49.3	71.8	50.9
Hay fever (507)	44.4	38.4	40.8	60.1	47.1	23.3‖
Diseases of sebaceous glands (acne) (706)	41.7	16.4	114.3	50.3	13.5	11.3‖
Cystitis (595)	37.4	8.7‖	44.2	45.2	50.6	44.9
Malignant neoplasms (140-209)	36.1	3.9‖	7.2	17.9	78.3	111.8
Disorders of menstruation (626)	35.8	3.9‖	64.3	64.6	30.7	3.3
Menopausal symptoms (627)	35.4	NA	3.2	27.5	121.6	21.7‖
Observation without need for further medical care (793)	35.3	25.0	37.7	50.7	33.1	23.2‖
Synovitis, bursitis, tenosynovitis (731)	29.8	3.2‖	11.1	30.8	65.8	46.8
Fracture (800-829)	28.1	24.9	14.8	17.2	39.6	58.3
Diseases of breast (610-611)	25.6	2.2‖	22.9	48.3	32.6	16.1‖

*From Division of Health Resources Utilization Statistics, National Center for Health Statistics: Data from the National Ambulatory Medical Care Survey. Rates are based on the average annual civilian noninstitutionalized population, excluding Alaska and Hawaii.

†Data are based on reporting by a sample of office-based physicians.

‡Diagnostic groupings and code number inclusions are based on the *Eighth Revision International Classification of Diseases, Adapted for Use in the United States.*

§Includes office visits to physicians for the most common and all other principal diagnoses.

‖Figure does not meet standards of reliability or precision.

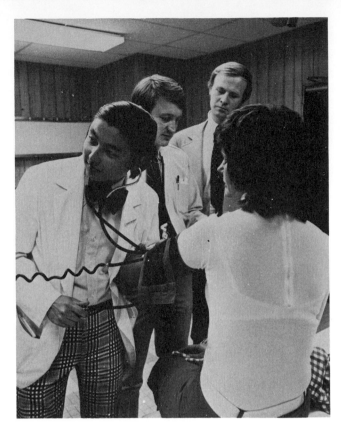

Fig. 2-2. Annual physical. (Courtesy Health Sciences Information Service, University of Washington, Seattle.)

physicians (only 4.9% of women were referred to the physician visited) and the primary diagnoses which physicians made of these conditions were primarily treated with drugs. Fifty-five percent of women received medications for their conditions; many received other therapies in addition. Almost 21% of women received medical counseling, 7.6% received diet counseling, 7.1% experienced a minor surgical procedure performed in the office, 6.4% received psychotherapy or "therapeutic listening," 3.5% were immunized or received desensitization shots, 3.2% received physiotherapy, 2.8% received other types of therapy, 2.5% received family planning services, and 20% received no services.[25]

Some of these same women also experienced diagnostic services at their visit. About 58% received a limited physical examination, 43.9% had their blood pressure checked, 24.4% had a clinical laboratory test, 20.9% had a general examination, 10.3% had a Pap test. 7.1% had an x-ray examination, 3.7% had a vision test, 2.8% had an EKG, 1.5% had an endoscopy examination (examination of any body cavity, except ear, nose, and throat), 4.5% had some other diagnostic examination, and 11.3% had no diagnostic service performed.

Most women over age 15 who visited the doctor in 1977 were told to return at a specified time (66.2%), 20.7% were told to return if necessary, 2.9% were checked with a follow-up telephone call, 2.5% were referred on to another practitioner, 2% were admitted to hospital, 0.9% were told to return at an unspecified time, 1.3% received some other disposition and 8.2% had no follow-up care planned.[25]

Minority women

Most black women who visited a physician in 1975 and 1976 received, as did all women, a limited examination as the main service; blood pressure readings were taken more often among black women, however. The most common reasons for visiting the physician among black women were for diseases of the respiratory system, for special conditions and examinations without illness, for diseases of the circulatory system, for accidents, for poisonings and violence, and for diseases of the genitourinary system.

Most conditions presented by black women were judged by the physician as not serious in about the same proportion as were visits by all women. Most black women patients received drugs (54%), and most were told to return at specified times (58%). More black than all women were told to return if necessary.[44]

Women aged 45 and over. Disproportion in the number of visits women make to physicians in comparison with men begins to decrease after age 45. In 1975 and 1976, about 80% of women 45 years of age and over had some contact with physicians, as did 72% of men. In 1974, 70% of women aged 45 to 64 visited a private physician's office, but only 54% of men did so. There was no difference in rates between the 16.2% of men and women over 45 years who used hospital outpatient departments, however. With eligibility for Medicare at age 65, men's health care utilization increases; there is no marked increase in older women's utilization.[45]

Respiratory infections were the most common conditions to affect women 45 years of age and older in 1977; for every 100 women, 64.4 were affected. Injuries affected 24.3 per 100 women, infective and parasitic diseases affected 15.9, and 7.4 were affected by digestive system conditions. About 26 were affected by other acute conditions.[41]

The most common diagnoses per 1000 population for women 45 to 64 years of age who made office visits in 1975 and 1976, were hypertension (312.0), arthritis and rheumatism (206.2), medical and surgical aftercare (206.1), medical or special examinations (166.9), neuroses and nonpsychotic disorders (153.9), acute upper respiratory infections except influenza (144.2), heart disease (143.4), menopausal symptoms (121.6, see Chapter 7 for discussion of estrogen replacement therapy), bronchitis, emphysema, asthma (120.2), and diabetes mellitus (103.6).[73, p. 277] For women aged 65 and over in 1975-1976, the most common diagnoses per 1000 population were heart disease (509.6), hypertension (478.8), arthritis and rheumatism (398.1), ischemic heart disease (383.8), eye diseases except refractive (287.2), diabetes mellitus (211.1), medical and surgical aftercare (183.0), neuroses and nonpsychotic disorders (115.6), malignant neoplasms (111.8), and infections and inflammations of the skin (105.5).[73]

For most conditions, women over age 45 who visited physicians in 1975 and 1976 were told to return at a specific time or to return if needed. This was the disposition for 96.5% of women in this age-group who visited the physician for hypertension, 93.9% who visited for ischemic heart disease, 91.7% who visited for menopausal symptoms, 90.3% who visited for bronchitis, emphysema, or asthma, and 90% of women who visited for neuroses or nonpsychotic disorders.[73, p. 287]

Loneliness and feelings of being useless have been frequently reported by older women[5] and have been specifically listed as a primary reason black women seek physician aid during menopause.[76] How much older women's morbidity is affected by these social needs is unknown, but it is estimated to be substantial. Unless social roles can be developed to compensate, with women's greater

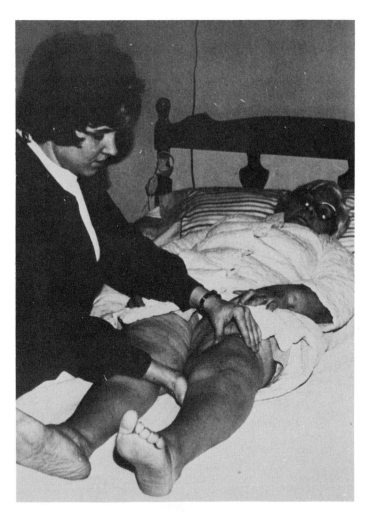

Fig. 2-3. Home health care nurse. (Courtesy Community Home Health Care, Seattle.)

longevity and the lower social value placed on aging women, this poor self-esteem, sense of isolation, and the effects of both on morbidity, are likely to remain.

Disability

The Health Interview Survey reports that morbidity for all acute conditions caused every 100 females to have 1047.4 days of restricted activity in 1977; by contrast there were 826.6 days of restricted activity among every 100 males. Respiratory conditions and injuries caused most restricted activity in both sexes. Women also experienced more days of bed disability in 1977 than did men. For all acute conditions every 100 women had 478.5 days of bed disability compared with 351.6 days per 100 men. Again, respiratory conditions and injuries were the cause of most days of bed disability.[41]

Disability data on acute conditions by age and sex show that males under 6 years of age had the most days of restricted activity and of bed disability in 1977. From age 6 years on, females report higher numbers. Of those over 6 years of age, women aged 45 to 64 averaged 26.5 days of restricted activity and those 65 years and over averaged 38.9 days in 1977. These same age-groups experienced most bed disability in 1977, 9.0 and 15.8 days, respectively.[41] Both

Table 2-11. Days of disability per person per year, United States, 1977*†

Sex and age	Number of days		
Both sexes			
All ages	17.8	6.9	5.0
Under 17 years	11.2	5.2	NA‡
17 to 24 years	11.5	4.5	4.3
25 to 44 years	15.8	5.9	4.7
45 to 64 years	24.4	8.2	5.9
65 years and over	36.5	14.5	4.2
Male			
All ages	15.8	5.8	4.7
Under 17 years	11.1	5.1	NA
17 to 24 years	10.5	3.4	4.1
25 to 44 years	13.5	4.3	4.4
45 to 64 years	22.0	7.2	5.5
65 years and over	33.0	12.7	5.0
Female			
All ages	19.6	7.9	5.3
Under 17 years	11.4	5.3	NA
17 to 24 years	12.5	5.6	4.5
25 to 44 years	17.9	7.4	5.2
45 to 64 years	26.5	9.0	6.4
65 years and over	38.9	15.8	§

*From Howie, L. J., and Drury, T. F.: Vital and Health Statistics, series 10, no. 126, National Center for Health Statistics, no. (PHS) 78-1554, Washington, D.C., Sept., 1978.
†Data are based on household interviews of the civilian noninstitutionalized population. *Note:* Work loss reported for currently employed persons aged 17 and over.
‡*NA* = Not applicable.
§Figure does not meet standards of reliability or precision.

types of disability caused more work-loss days among women than men (see Table 2-11). Women in the labor force report fewer bed-disability days (4.3) than do women not in the labor force (5.6), however.[69]

Other employment-related disability data also suggest that women's higher disability does not hold constant through all professions. Among Metropolitan Life Insurance employees, for example, male office personnel aged 55 to 64 reported higher disability than did female office personnel. This was also true for male sales personnel aged 45 to 64.[54] Disability of all types, restricted activity, bed disability, work-loss days, and school-loss days caused by acute conditions increased among women in recent years, but these have been offset by a decline in disability caused by chronic conditions.[55] Some of women's reported increased work-loss days may also be a reflection of "sick" women staying home from work because of sick children.

PRINCIPAL SOURCES OF CARE
Type of care

According to the 1974 Health Interview Survey, most women (86.7%) had a regular source of care (see Table 2-12). Most women who did not have a regular source of care reported that this was because they felt no need of one; this was particularly true among women 65 years and older (see Table 2-13).[21]

Table 2-12. Percent of females who had a regular source of health care, United States, 1974*

Age	Percent with regular source of health care	Percent unknown
All ages	86.7	0.8
Under 20 years	88.2	0.9
20 to 44 years	84.5	0.7
45 to 64 years	87.0	0.5
65 years and over	88.5	0.8

*Based on unpublished data provided by T. F. Drury from the 1974 Health Interview Survey, Division of Health Interview Statistics, National Center for Health Statistics, Washington, D.C.

Table 2-13. Percent distribution of females who had reasons for not having a regular source of care, United States, 1974*

Reason	All ages	Under 20 years	20 to 44 years	45 to 64 years	65 years and over
No perceived need	48.2	53.7	43.9	44.7	55.4
See different physicians	21.0	17.6	26.9	19.1	12.4
Old or right physician unavailable	17.8	15.8	18.8	19.3	17.1
Other, including too expensive†	10.5	9.5	8.7	13.5	13.9
Unknown reason	2.5	3.4	1.7	3.4	1.2

*Based on unpublished data provided by T. F. Drury from the 1974 Health Interview Survey, Division of Health Interview Statistics, National Center for Health Statistics, Washington, D.C.
†Also includes health care facility available (e.g., company clinic, armed services facility) and physicians used only for serious illnesses.

In 1974 women utilized a variety of health services, although physician services were the most frequently used (see Table 2-14). A small percentage of women of all ages received care at home (1.9%), but this increased to 5.3% for women 65 years and over. Unknown numbers of women also received selected services from women's clinics and other alternative services, although their overall numbers are still relatively small (see Chapter 8).

Site of care

The site for most women's care in 1977 was the private physician's office (see Table 2-15); the physician was most likely to be in solo practice.[25] The

Table 2-14. Percent of females who used one or more of various types of health care services, United States, 1974*

Service	All ages	Under 20 years	20 to 44 years	45 to 64 years	65 years and over
Physician	71.1	63.7	77.8	71.9	72.0
Dental	50.9	53.2	57.5	48.6	29.0
Telephone consultation	20.1	22.5	22.9	15.4	13.2
Outpatient department	19.8	20.3	22.4	17.4	15.0
Short hospital stay	12.9	7.4	17.8	12.7	15.8
Neighborhood health center	5.4	5.6	7.2	4.0	1.5
Chiropractic	3.5	1.1	4.4	6.1	3.7
Podiatric	3.2	1.0	1.8	5.8	9.1
Home	1.9	1.4	1.2	1.8	5.3
Physical therapy	1.6	0.6	1.6	2.6	2.6

*Based on unpublished data provided by T. F. Drury from the 1974 Health Interview Survey, Division of Health Interview Statistics, National Center for Health Statistics, Washington, D.C.

Table 2-15. Percent distribution of usual site of health care of females, United States, 1974*

Site	All ages	Under 20 years	20 to 44 years	45 to 64 years	65 years and over
Private physician's office	60.9	57.8	58.6	65.4	68.2
Group practice	27.3	28.4	28.7	25.7	22.8
Hospital outpatient clinic	4.7	5.8	4.7	4.0	2.7
Physicians' clinic	2.2	2.4	2.5	1.7	1.8
Hospital emergency room	0.4	0.5	0.5	0.1	0.3
Home	0.3	0.1	0.1	0.1	1.4
Company or industry clinic	0.2	0.2	0.2	0.4	0.1
Other	2.6	3.1	3.6	1.2	0.9
Unknown	1.4	1.7	1.1	1.4	1.8

*Based on unpublished data provided by T. F. Drury from the 1974 Health Interview Survey, Division of Health Interview Statistics, National Center for Health Statistics, Washington, D.C.

Table 2-16. Percent of females with a particular physician at usual source of care, United States, 1974*

Usual source	All ages	Under 20 years	20 to 44 years	45 to 64 years	65 years and over
Females with particular					
physician	91.0	88.0	90.4	93.8	96.2
General practitioner	61.2	53.8	60.7	67.7	72.9
Specialty status unknown	0.5	0.3	0.5	0.4	1.1
Specialist	29.3	33.9	29.2	25.7	22.2
Pediatrican	10.3	28.7	0.5	0.2	†
Internist	8.0	1.6	8.1	14.7	14.8
Obstetrician gynecologist	6.9	1.0	16.6	5.3	0.7
General surgeon	2.0	1.0	1.9	3.1	3.8
Osteopath	0.6	0.5	0.6	0.7	0.8
Orthopedist	0.2	0.1	0.2	0.2	0.2
Urologist	0.2	0.1	0.1	0.2	0.08
Neurologist	0.2	0.1	0.2	0.2	0.3
Otolaryngologist	0.1	0.2	0.2	0.05	†
Dermatologist	0.08	0.1	0.08	†	0.1
Psychiatrist	0.06	†	0.1	0.08	0.1
Ophthalmologist	0.04	0.04	†	0.03	0.1
Radiologist	0.04	0.02	0.02	0.1	†
Other specialist	0.6	0.4	0.6	0.8	1.2

*Based on unpublished data provided by T. F. Drury from the 1974 Health Interview Survey, Division of Health Interview Statistics, National Center for Health Statistics, Washington, D.C.
†This specialty not identified as usual physician at usual source of care by women in this age group.

majority of women (63.5%) in 1977 saw the physician in less than 6 months after a previous visit; this was also true for men. A substantial number of women aged 45 to 64 (8.5%) had not seen a physician for 1 year, and 8.8% had not seen one for 2 to 4 years. Of women 65 years and over, 6.4% and 7.1% had not seen a physician for 1 year or 2 to 4 years, respectively.[41]

Physician characteristics

In 1974, of those women who saw a physician regularly, most (61.2%) visited a general practitioner or family practice physician. Of the 29.3% who saw a specialist, most women aged 20 to 44 saw an obstetrician−gynecologist; of those over 45 years, most saw an internist (see Table 2-16).

Data from the 1977 National Ambulatory Medical Care Survey confirm the above. Most physician visits by women over age 15 were made in that year to general practitioners or family practice physicians (39.7%). Other visits in order of frequency for women over age 15 were 16.5% to obstetrician-gynecologists, 12.8% to surgical specialists other than general surgeons, 12.7% to internists, 6.6% to general surgeons, 6.4% to other medical specialists, 3.1% to psychiatrists, 0.9% to pediatricians, and 1.3% to other specialists.[25]

Current organization of obstetrical and gynecological services

The specialty of obstetrics and gynecology has traditionally been thought of as the specialty for most of women's health needs. Although it is the most fre-

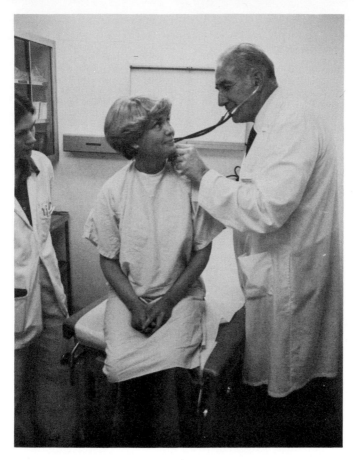

Fig. 2-4. The physician's office. (Courtesy Health Sciences Information Service, University of Washington, Seattle.)

quently used specialty for women aged 20 to 44 (the childbearing years), with the exception of maternity-related care, the specialty would not necessarily seem the most appropriate to treat the reasons perceived by women for physician visits nor the principal diagnoses attributed to these women (see Tables 8 to 10). Studies of practice patterns and the widespread use of this specialty by at least this one age cohort of women have suggested, as discussed later, a need to expand the training of the obstetrician-gynecologist to more appropriately respond to women's actual health needs. Alternatively women might be appropriately encouraged to seek care from internists or general practitioners, who are more relevantly prepared (see Chapter 9).

Contemporary practice patterns of obstetrician-gynecologists were extensively studied in the early 1970s; some other more recent data from a federally-funded study conducted under sponsorship of the American College of Obstetricians and Gynecologists (ACOG) and the University of Southern California

Division of Research and Medical Education are already published, with more to be available in the early 1980s.*[48]

ACOG reported in 1972 that the average practicing obstetrician-gynecologist spent a median of 27.5 hours per week in his/her office (exclusive of time spent at the hospital or in other activities) seeing 90 to 100 patients. About half of these were women who were seeking prepartum or postpartum care, and the majority of the remainder were well women who were returning for periodic examinations.[78] Data from 1977 show that obstetricians and gynecologists worked a median of 50.09 professional hours per week, but these hours comprised "all hours related to medicine, including continuing education, travel time, completing forms, attending committee meetings, and so on." These hours also include "vacation, so that data are applicable to the 52-week year." Per weekday, obstetrician-gynecologists worked a median number of 9.05 hours.[53]

In surveying the average obstetrician-gynecologist's practice, Dr. Alfred Yankauer reported in 1971 and 1972 that 90% of the respondents were engaged in private practice and of these, 44% were in solo practice, 43% were members of small (two or three persons) specialty groupings, and 13% were in multispecialty groups. Most commonly, solo practitioners were located in the Northeast, small specialties in the South, and multispecialties in the West.[82] Forty-three percent of the solo practitioners reported employing a registered nurse (RN) as did 82% of the multispecialty group physicians.[81] One out of every three to four solo practitioners reported using the RN to see the patient if the physician were called in an emergency.

Data from 1977 discuss physician practice characteristics by age. Preference for solo practice increased with age; of persons 55 to 64-years-old, 43.8% were in solo practice, contrasted with 6.2% of those under 35. Most solo practices were in the Northeast, closely followed by the South. Older obstetrician-gynecologists (65 and over) were excluded from this study because the sample was too small, but they might reasonably have been expected to continue to show the pattern of increased preference with age for solo practice.[53]

Thirty practices in 22 states were surveyed in 1977, and the data show a total employment of 66 nonphysician professionals (NPPs) in those practices. Most of those employed were nurse practitioners, closely followed by nurses with additional on-the-job training and certified nurse-midwives. Patients and providers in general accepted the NPPs, who provided a range of services, including annual examinations, contraceptive services, and complete maternity care.[63]

Physician productivity in 1971, by number of patient visits per week, was higher in the South and North Central regions, where there were fewer physicians than in the Northeast and West. This held true for all types of practice arrangements. The group practitioners in small specialties appeared to be consistently

---

*Much of this information is taken from Marieskind, H. I.: Gynecological services: their historical relationship to the women's movement with recent experience of self-help clinics and other delivery modes, doctoral dissertation, UCLA School of Public Health, 1976, University Microfilms, Ann Arbor, Mich., No. 762-5222-01500.

the most productive, attending to 4.0 patient visits per hour and from 100 to 110 patients visits per week.[83] This compared favorably with the findings of the *National Disease and Therapeutic Index* in 1974 that the obstetrician-gynecologist specialist averaged 19.5 patients per day based on a 7-day week, compared with the national average for all physicians of 19.9.[60]

The data from 1977 also showed that physicians in the South and North Central regions had more patient encounters per week (126.5 and 133.0 respectively). The median time spent per patient encounter (defined as office visits, hospital visits, which included "obstetric delivery or an abdominal hysterectomy," and telephone calls) was 9.82 minutes with a mean of 13.87 minutes. By contrast, a similar survey found a median of 14 minutes in internal medicine. Most (34.5%) obstetrician-gynecologist patient encounters were in the 1 to 5–minute range, with 29.5% taking 6 to 10 minutes. Only 1.9% took 61 or more minutes.[53]

The respondents to Yankauer's survey estimated that 50% of their practice time was spent in obstetrical care, 40% in gynecological care, 7% in family planning care, and 3% in other types of care. On the basis of this, three broad classifications were established: 58% of obstetrician-gynecologists could be said to have a mixed obstetrical-gynecological practice, 23% a primarily gynecological practice, and 19% a primarily obstetrical practice. Solo practitioners usually had practices in the latter two classifications, with gynecological practices being more common in all types of settings in the West.[82]

Preventive care accounted for the bulk (70%) of the obstetrical-gynecological office visits; of the 40% of the visit spent in gynecological care, 50% of that was spent in nonobstetrical health check-ups. Excluding obstetrical procedures other than cesarean sections, the average obstetrician-gynecologist performed 60 to 65 major gynecological operations and 75 to 80 minor surgical operations per year, an average of about three surgical procedures per week. About 160 babies per specialist were delivered each year; by 1975 annual average deliveries were 144.9 (see Chapter 7).

Fifty-seven percent of all respondents reported predominantly upper and upper-middle income group patients, and half of the respondents who practiced in large specialty groups (three or more obstetrician-gynecologists) reported serving predominantly upper income patients.

About 40% of all respondents in private practice reported that at least 50% of their patients relied on them as primary physicians. In the Northeast they were less likely to perceive themselves in this role. This was true there among those whose practices were primarily gynecological and who were also more likely to perceive themselves as primary providers.[82]

As have other specialists, obstetrician-gynecologists have begun to include lower level health professionals in their practices. Obstetrician-gynecologists vary in terms of task delegation, especially as to the amount of delegating they endorse in theory as opposed to what they practice in fact.[81] In Yankauer's survey, respondents were presented with 19 specific services carried out in ambulatory obstetrical-gynecological practice. The vast majority (95%) of the practitioners reported that they "virtually never delegated eight of the nineteen tasks

even though they all involved relatively simple technical skills." The nondelegated services listed were as follows: check fetal size/position, check fetal heart,
perform pelvic examination, take internal measurements, take vaginal smear for
infection, take Pap smear, fit diaphragm, insert IUD.

Some of the tasks that were nondelegated in ambulatory settings were reported delegated in a hospital environment. For example, "90 percent of respondents reported that nursing staff regularly checked fetal hearts and 35 percent
reported that nurses regularly performed vaginal examinations."[81]

Services that were delegated in an ambulatory setting are ranked as follows
in order of their frequency of performance by all types of auxiliary personnel:
urinalysis, blood pressure measurement, giving telephone advice, giving advice
in the office, taking past history, taking internal history, taking present illness
history, giving contraceptive advice. Drawing venous blood — another delegated
task — was preferably assigned to a laboratory technician when one was employed.
Of the last two delegated tasks — home visiting for prenatal or postnatal care, and
group classes for parents — the former was reported as not performed at all by
88% of the physicians and the latter was not performed by 76%. Home visiting,
when done, was almost always carried out by the physician, and educational
classes were usually conducted by an RN. RNs were similarly preferred over all
other health workers by the physician to assist him in performing a vaginal
examination. Any task construed as "laying-on-of-hands" (e.g., vaginal examinations), although delegated to nurses in a hospital setting, was reserved for only
the physician in office practice. Commented Yankauer:

These observations of office practice contrast sharply with the nature of the tasks delegated
in hospitals where vaginal examinations and labor monitoring are frequently performed by
nurses. Delegation of tasks carries a variety of relationships to the hospital care of the
patient. It would be unwarranted to conclude that care in labor is inadequate when much
of the patient monitoring is delegated to non-physicians. However, there is rarely a time in
pregnancy when the need for skillful observation is greater. It is a strange reflection upon
the priorities of obstetric care that so much of this responsibility is delegated to nurses who
play so small a role in the bulk of ambulatory obstetric and gynecologic care.[83]

The National Disease and Therapeutic Index (1974) provided data on
obstetrician-gynecologists and their patient constituency. Not surprisingly,
almost all the obstetrician-gynecologist's patients were female and 70% were in
the childbearing range, defined by them as from 20 to 40 years. Seventeen percent
of the obstetrician-gynecologist's patients were in the menopausal and post-
menopausal age-group (40 to 60 years), and only 3% of patients were aged 60 or
older. Of the 10% under 20, nearly all of these were over 12 years of age.[60]

There is considerable emphasis on defining obstetrician-gynecologists as
primary care providers for women.[64,68,79,80] To support this claim — or perhaps in
acknowledgement of their lack of adequate preparation for the role — the American Board of Obstetrics and Gynecology decided to reinstitute a basic "foundation year" before the 3 years of specialty training. Notes Dr. Jack Pearson:

This fundamental decision indicates that the specialty has recognized that the obstetrician
and gynecologist must be further trained as a *primary physician* [emphasis in original] to

diagnose, treat, or refer the many patients with diseases not traditionally in the purview of obstetrics and gynecology.[64]

Methods of reimbursement, development of family medicine programs, national health insurance, and women's preferences will determine the outcome of the primary provider role of the obstetrician-gynecologist.

UTILIZATION OF SELECTED SERVICES
Birthing sites

Since 1940 most babies in the United States have been born in hospitals. When the data are examined by race, however, they show that in that year, 59.9% of white babies were born in hospitals with a physician in attendance but only 26.7% of "all others" were. Among the latter group, most babies (49.2%) were born out-of-hospital with a midwife or other nonphysician such as a friend or family member in attendance. By 1974 the overwhelming majority of babies of all races were born in hospitals — 99.2% of all babies, 99.3% of whites, and 98.4% of "all others."

Since 1974, however, there has been a small but steady decline in the number of hospital births. In 1977, for example, 98.5% of all babies were born in hospitals with a physician or midwife in attendance, as were 98.6% of white babies and 98.3% of babies of all other ethnicities. The steady decrease in hospital births has been countermatched by a steady increase in the number of physician-, midwife-, or "other"-attended births, with the most significant change between 1974 and 1977 occurring among white births in this latter group (see Table 2-17).

Consumer dissatisfaction with the hospital birthing process and desire for recognition of birth as a normal family-centered event have led not only to the growth of in-hospital birthing rooms (see Chapter 7), but also to free-standing birth centers, for example, the Maternity Center Association in New York City,[3,47] and home delivery services usually staffed by lay midwives or, in still rare instances, by physicians or certified nurse-midwives.[23,24,61]

The issue of out-of-hospital birth is emotionally charged, but there is scant data to support arguments for or against it. Many of the data that have been published by the prohospital birthing forces have tended to be invalid for purposes of assessing comparative birth risks. They have often used infant mortality rates[16] (infant deaths up to 1 year of age), which include many deaths totally unrelated to the birth event, for example, deaths from sudden infant death syndrome (SIDS). Other morbidity and mortality rates cited for home births have not distinguished between planned and unplanned out-of-hospital births, been controlled for prenatal care, considered whether the births were attended or unattended, had the degree of skill and training of attendants controlled, nor analyzed death rates by birth weight or for presence of congenital anomalies incompatible with life.[36,38] In addition, charges like those of Dr. Warren Pearse, the executive director of the American College of Obstetricians and Gynecologists, that "home delivery is maternal trauma" and "child abuse" have done little to develop a rational approach to developing safe birthing settings.[39]

Table 2-17. Number and percent distribution of live births by attendant and place of delivery, United States, selected years 1940 to 1977*†

Year	Total live births	All races (%)			White (%)			All races other than white (%)		
		Physician in hospital‡	Not in hospital		Physician in hospital‡	Not in hospital		Physician in hospital‡	Not in hospital	
			Physician	Midwife, other, and not specified		Physician	Midwife, other, and not specified		Physician	Midwife, other, and not specified
1940	2,360,399	55.8	35.0	9.3	59.9	36.5	3.6	26.7	24.1	49.2
1945	2,735,456	78.8	14.7	6.5	84.3	13.7	2.0	40.2	21.7	38.1
1950	3,554,149	88.0	7.1	5.0	92.8	5.9	1.3	57.9	14.3	27.8
1955	4,047,295	94.4	2.5	3.2	97.5	1.8	0.8	76.0	6.8	17.2
1960§	4,257,850	96.6	1.2	2.2	98.8	0.7	0.5	85.0	3.5	11.5
1965§	3,760,358	97.4	0.9	1.8	98.9	0.6	0.5	89.8	2.1	8.2
1966§	3,606,274	98.0	0.5	1.5	99.3	0.3	0.4	91.6	1.4	7.1
1967¶	3,520,959	98.3	0.4	1.3	99.4	0.3	0.4	92.9	1.1	6.0
1968§	3,501,564	98.5	0.4	1.2	99.4	0.3	0.3	94.0	0.9	5.0
1969§	3,600,206	99.1	0.2	0.7	99.6	0.1	0.2	96.3	0.5	3.2
1970§	3,731,386	99.4	0.1	0.5	99.7	0.1	0.2	97.8	0.2	1.9
1971§	3,555,970	99.1	0.3	0.6	99.5	0.2	0.3	97.1	0.6	2.3
1972‖	3,258,411	99.2	0.2	0.5	99.5	0.2	0.3	98.0	0.4	1.6
1973‖	3,136,965	99.3	0.2	0.5	99.5	0.2	0.3	98.3	0.3	1.4
1974‖	3,159,958	99.2	0.3	0.5	99.3	0.3	0.4	98.4	0.4	1.1
1975‖	3,144,198	98.7	0.4	0.9	98.9	0.3	0.8	98.1	0.6	1.3
1976‖	3,167,788	98.6	0.4	1.0	98.7	0.3	1.0	98.3	0.5	1.2
1977‖	3,326,632	98.5	0.4	1.1	98.6	0.3	1.1	98.3	0.5	1.2

*Based on data from Vital Statistics of the United States, 1974, vol. I, Natality, and from National Center for Health Statistics, Washington, D.C.
†Beginning in 1970, excludes births to nonresidents of the United States.
‡Includes all births in hospitals or institutions and births attended by physicians in clinics. Almost 99% of all hospital births are physician attended.
§Based on a 50% sample of births.
¶Based on a 20% to 50% sample of births.
‖Based on 100% of births in selected states and on a 50% sample of births in all other states.

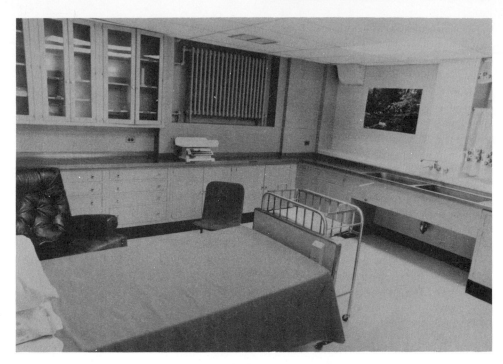

Fig. 2-5. Maternity Center Association, New York. (Courtesy Maternity Center Association, New York.)

Similarly, there are problems with data presented by advocates of out-of-hospital birthing, mainly that the populations studied tend to be middle class, comparatively well educated, and, as evidenced by the data in Table 2-17, white, a group with traditionally lower morbidity.[35,50-52,71] Advocates also cite supportive data from the Frontier Nursing Service in Kentucky and from other countries.

Although the Frontier Nursing Service did provide birthing at home to a socioeconomically deprived, and therefore more risk-prone, population, achieving perinatal and maternal outcomes superior to the rest of the state, the providers of care—the midwives—were uniformly well trained and highly skilled, and their results were being compared with data from all areas of a relatively poor, inadequately served state.[43] Midwives in many European countries, most notably the Netherlands, also achieve superior maternal and perinatal statistics, but they work within a supportive health care service with a formalized emergency backup system.[31] Such home birth situations are rare in the United States today.

To date, Oregon is one of the few states that has rigorously analyzed its out-of-hospital births. When Oregon published data on out-of-hospital births for 1976, these comprised 2.7% of total Oregon births;[18] by 1977, the 1492 infants born out-of-hospital comprised 3.9% of total births. Oregon notes that the number of births indicate that they represent planned, as opposed to accidental, out-of-hospital births. Between 1976 and 1977 the percentages of births in the home

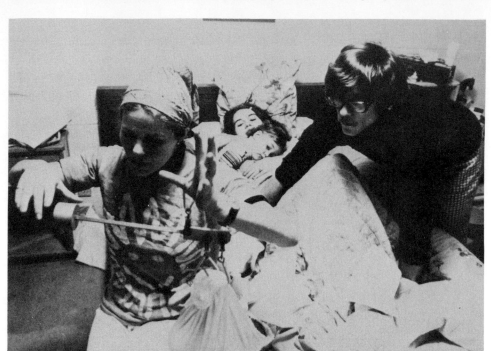

Fig. 2-6. Weighing the baby after a home birth. (Courtesy Tom Salyer.)

and clinics changed. In 1976, 74% of out-of-hospital deliveries occurred at the woman's home and 18% in free-standing birth clinics; by 1977, 60% occurred at home and 32% were clinic deliveries.

In 1977 the neonatal death rate was 7.8 per 1000 live births for all of Oregon, and the infant death rate (up to age 1) was 12.1; for the out-of-hospital births, the rates were 3.4 and 10.1, respectively. Dingley[19] notes that the average number of deaths for out-of-hospital infants over the past 5 years had been 15 and therefore the 16 deaths in 1977 were comparable. However, as the denominator of the rates, the number of out-of-hospital births, has increased dramatically, the death rate has dropped. Over the past 5 years the leading causes of death of infants born out of hospitals were SIDS, followed by anoxic and hypoxic conditions and congenital anomalies. When death rates for full-term infants were compared, the rates were 3.0 per 1000 live births for total births and 6.0 per 1000 for out-of-hospital births.[19]

In Oregon a person can be a midwife and assist in the normal delivery of children without first being licensed as an RN and certified as a nurse-practitioner or midwife. Furthermore, provided that a lay midwife does not administer medications or perform an episiotomy, it is legal for the midwife to attend a birth in Oregon; in effect, if this restriction is observed, anyone may attend a birth in Oregon.[67] In 1977 out-of-hospital births were attended by physicians, osteopaths,

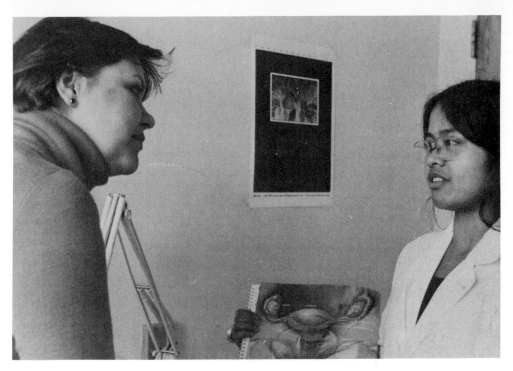

Fig. 2-7. Women's health care specialist in family planning clinic. (Courtesy Health Sciences Information Service, University of Washington, Seattle.)

naturopaths, lay midwives, certified nurse-midwives, RNs, friends, "helpers," parents, chiropractors, and members of a religious community. In 1976, 20% of the attendants were licensed with some type of medical training and attended 58% of the deliveries; in 1977, 22% of the attendants were licensed and attended 61% of the births; of the 78% (387) unlicensed attendants in 1977, 345 attended the delivery of only one child.[19] Further research is needed however, to determine if there is a relationship between skill of the attendant and outcome. Resolution of this question would provide a rational basis on which women could make choices of birthing sites and also for developing maternity services.

Contraceptive services

According to a recent survey, an estimated 4.1 million women received contraceptive services through organized programs in 1976. These were provided through health departments (1.7 million women), Planned Parenthood (1.1 million), hospital clinic programs (563,000) and other agencies such as free clinics, neighborhood health centers, and community action agencies (689,000). Most women who obtained contraception through organized programs had low or marginal incomes, most were young with low parity, and most had at least graduated from high school.[72]

The Alan Guttmacher Institute estimates that 9.9 million low-income women

Table 2-18. Number of dental visits, United States, 1977*†

Sex	All ages	Under 17 years	17 to 24 years	25 to 44 years	45 to 64 years	65 years and over
Number of dental visits						
Both sexes	342,766	91,819	51,648	93,909	76,248	29,142
Male	154,090	44,088	21,382	42,870	33,577	12,172
Female	188,676	47,731	30,265	51,039	42,671	16,970
Number of dental visits per person per year						
Both sexes	1.6	1.5	1.6	1.7	1.8	1.3
Male	1.5	1.4	1.4	1.6	1.6	1.3
Female	1.7	1.6	1.9	1.8	1.9	1.3

*Based on data from Howie, L. J., and Drury, T. F.: Vital and Health Statistics, series 10, no. 126, National Center for Health Statistics, no. (PHS) 78-1554, Washington, D.C., Sept., 1978, U.S. Government Printing Office.
†Data are based on household interview of the civilian noninstitutionalized population.

were in need of contraceptive services in 1976. Of these women, 3.6 million (37%) received services through the organized programs and 2.2 million (22%) received services through private physicians. An estimated 41% did not receive services from either source, although some may have received services and be using contraception, but did not make annual visits to a clinic or private physician. Types of contraceptives used are discussed in Chapters 1 and 7.

Dental services

In 1977 women of all ages made an average of 1.7 visits to the dentist. Women ages 17 to 24 years had the highest rate of visits (1.9) and women 65 years and over the lowest (1.3) (see Table 2-18). A higher rate of visits was reported by families with the highest income, and more visits per 1000 population were made in the West.[73]

For most women, less than 6 months had elapsed since their last dental visit. Among women 65 years and over, however, 44.9% had not seen a dentist for at least 5 years, and the time lapse since last dental visit for at least 30% of women aged 17 to 44 was from 1 to 4 years.[41]

Emergency services

In 1975 the Health Interview Survey reported that 26.6 million women (31.2 million men) sustained injuries that were medically attended. Of these, 36.7% were treated in a physician's office, 36.0% were treated in a hospital outpatient department, 17.1% were treated through telephone consultation, and 9.5% were treated by other sources, which included treatment at home, company or industry clinic, other, or unknown place of first medical attention.[41, p. 294]

In 1977, 31.6 million women were injured (42.3 million men). The highest rates of injuries occurred at home, at work, (see Chapter 5), or with a moving motor vehicle, in descending order of frequency. For every 100 women of all

ages, 311.9 days of restricted activity and 91.1 days of bed disability were incurred as the result of an injury.[41] Of product-related injuries treated in hospital
emergency rooms, most occurred to women aged 25 to 44 years. The most common sources of injuries in this age-group were knives and cutlery, kitchen appliances, home workshop apparatus, and yard and garden equipment.[73, p. 296]

Other utilization of emergency services by women is described in Chapter 1
in the discussion of drug usage.

SELECTED SOCIALLY INDUCED MORBIDITY

Many, if not most, diseases are caused in part by a social component. Wom-
en's social role and socialization make them particularly vulnerable to the
socially-induced morbidity discussed here.

Venereal disease (VD)

Increased sexual contacts, both tolerated and encouraged by social forces,
including the media, have led to an increased incidence of sexually transmitted,
or venereal, diseases. In 1978, 415,797 cases of gonorrhea and 5,331 cases of
primary and secondary syphilis were reported among women of all ages.[12] For
gonorrhea, this was a 499% increase since 1956 and for syphilis a 127% increase
since that year (see Tables 2-19 and 2-20) (for women under age 20, see Chapter 6).
Since the Center for Disease Control estimates that only about half of all cases
are reported, these numbers probably substantially underrepresent true incidence.
The center also notes that the decline since 1975 in both syphilis and gonorrhea
may indicate that the diseases have plateaued, although 1978 data again indicate
a rise.[11] Congenital syphilis in infants has not risen.[13]

Of particular concern to women is the increasing incidence of herpes II,
cited as one of the most rapidly increasing venereal diseases.[10] Estimates on the
incidence and prevalence of herpes II vary widely, since it is not included in the
national reporting system and there are only a few states which require that the
disease be reported. Nationally the prevalence of the herpes II antibody is estimated at 8% to 12% in the sexually active population, although depending on the
geographic area and the socioeconomic characteristics of the population studied,
prevalence may be substantially higher, ranging from 20% to 50% of those sexually active. The number of women who come to term with active cervical herpes
is estimated to be from 0.5% to 1.5%.[15]

Herpes II is hazardous to the pregnant woman. Infants infected by herpes II
can suffer from brain, kidney, and lung damage or can die.[27,33] To avoid this possibility, which affects about 85% of newborns of mothers with active herpes, the
child is delivered by cesarean section. Although there is some discussion as to the
appropriate management of patients with a history of herpes II, it is generally
agreed that (1) if cultures in late pregnancy (about 30 to 32 weeks) are negative
for active herpes II, and/or (2) if during labor a cervical smear shows no shedding,
and/or (3) if during labor no lesions are present in the vagina, then a vaginal
delivery is appropriate.[14,15]

Also of concern to women is the incidence of asymptomatic gonorrhea in
men. Prior to the early 1970s it was believed that gonorrhea was only asympto-

Table 2-19 Gonorrhea morbidity and rates per 100,000 population aged 20 years and over, United States, selected years, 1956 to 1977*†

Age	Year	Total morbidity			Rates per 100,000 population		
		Female	Male	Total	Female	Male	Total
20 to 24 years	1956	21,724	52,969	74,693	406.8	1255.8	781.8
	1960	24,668	63,155	87,823	443.7	1354.4	359.2
	1973	127,928	205,495	333,423	1406.7	2479.4	1918.2
	1974	141,304	215,523	356,827	1522.5	2515.2	1999.0
	1975	155,196	236,561	391,757	1631.4	2659.8	2128.3
	1978	158,155	229,829	387,984	1568.7	2409.9	1977.6
25 to 29 years	1956	11,660	36,964	48,624	198.6	692.6	434.2
	1960	12,023	39,190	51,213	217.8	779.1	485.5
	1973	44,203	107,852	152,055	565.8	1461.6	1000.9
	1974	48,926	117,821	166,747	601.1	1528.0	1052.0
	1975	57,424	135,132	192,556	676.1	1674.7	1162.6
	1978	60,434	141,940	202,374	669.3	1648.0	1147.0
30 to 34 years	1956	6,165	21,443	27,603	97.6	369.0	227.6
	1960	6,547	23,198	29,747	107.8	412.7	254.4
	1973	15,498	43,640	59,138	235.1	703.8	462.3
	1974	16,440	47,270	63,710	240.1	732.1	478.8
	1975	18,971	53,920	72,891	268.3	806.9	530.0
	1978	20,614	63,642	84,256	257.4	833.8	538.7
35 years	1956	6,060	18,917	25,002	16.4	55.2	35.1
and over	1960	6,794	24,829	31,621	17.0	67.8	41.3
	1973	12,495	41,702	54,197	26.8	103.8	62.4
	1974	13,533	43,642	57,175	28.7	107.8	65.3
	1975	14,041	49,657	63,698	29.5	121.6	72.0
	1978	14,268	57,638	71,906	28.8	127.0	78.3
TOTALS	1956	69,418	155,265	224,683	81.7	192.4	135.7
	1960	76,372	182,561	258,933	83.6	210.2	145.3
	1973	332,800	509,821	842,621	309.4	507.2	404.9
	1974	367,011	539,110	906,121	338.6	532.2	432.1
	1975	406,183	593,754	999,937	371.6	581.3	472.9
	1976	405,381	596,613	1,001,994	368.2	579.9	470.5
	1977	403,381	596,796	1,000,177	363.4	575.6	465.9
	1978	415,797	597,639	1,103,436	371.5	571.8	468.3

*Based on data provided by Kathy Dry, Statistical Assistant, Venereal Disease Control Division, Center for Disease Control, Atlanta, from the V.D. statistical letter, form CDC 9.2638, HEW: PHS:CDC:BSS:VDCD:ESSS.

†Cases not reported by age have been included on the basis of the known age distribution. Rates are based on population estimates of the Bureau of the Census. Cases include Alaska and Hawaii for 1956, 1960, 1973, and 1975 to 1978. Rates based on cases excluding Alaska and Hawaii for 1956. Rates based on cases including Alaska and Hawaii for 1960, 1973, and 1975 to 1978.

Table 2-20. Primary and secondary syphilis morbidity and rates per 100,000 population aged 20 years and over, United States, selected years, 1956 to 1977*†

Age	Year	Total morbidity			Rates per 100,000 population		
		Female	Male	Total	Female	Male	Total
20 to 24 years	1956	620	1,138	1,758	11.6	27.0	18.4
	1960	1,566	3,126	4,692	28.2	67.0	45.9
	1973	2,513	4,662	7,175	27.6	6.3	41.3
	1974	2,328	4,972	7,300	25.1	58.0	40.9
	1975	2,263	5,063	7,326	23.8	56.9	39.8
	1978	1,656	4,388	6,044	16.4	46.0	30.8
25 to 29 years	1956	405	858	1,263	6.9	16.1	11.3
	1960	907	2,478	3,385	16.4	49.3	32.1
	1973	1,374	3,977	5,351	17.6	53.9	35.2
	1974	1,349	4,148	5,497	16.6	53.8	34.7
	1975	1,272	4,341	5,613	15.0	53.8	33.9
	1978	1,088	4,037	5,125	12.0	46.9	29.0
30 to 34 years	1956	278	611	889	4.4	10.5	7.3
	1960	546	1,862	2,409	9.0	33.1	20.6
	1973	817	2,511	3,328	12.4	40.5	26.0
	1974	656	2,711	3,367	9.6	42.0	25.3
	1975	720	2,863	3,583	10.2	42.9	26.1
	1978	544	2,512	3,056	6.8	32.9	19.5
35 years and over	1956	342	902	1,244	.9	2.6	1.8
	1960	595	2,329	2,923	1.5	6.4	3.8
	1973	1,072	3,768	4,840	2.3	9.4	5.6
	1974	993	3,966	4,959	2.1	9.8	5.7
	1975	880	4,194	5,074	1.9	10.3	5.7
	1978	631	3,614	4,245	1.3	3.5	4.6
TOTALS	1956	2,342	4,053	6,395	2.8	5.0	3.4
	1960	5,009	11,136	16,145	5.5	12.8	9.1
	1973	7,937	16,888	24,825	7.4	16.8	11.9
	1974	7,482	17,903	25,385	6.9	17.7	12.1
	1975	7,132	18,429	25,561	6.5	18.0	12.1
	1976	6,430	17,301	23,731	5.8	16.8	11.1
	1977	5,155	15,207	20,362	4.6	14.7	9.5
	1978	5,331	16,325	21,656	4.8	15.6	10.0

*Based on data provided by Kathy Dry, Statistical Assistant, Venereal Disease Control Division, Center for Disease Control, Atlanta, from the V.D. statistical letter, form CDC 9.2638, HEW:PHS: CDC:BSS:VDCD:ESSS.

†Cases not reported by age have been included on the basis of the known age distribution. Rates are based on population estimates of the Bureau of the Census. Cases include Alaska and Hawaii for 1956, 1960, 1973, 1975-1978. Rates based on cases excluding Alaska and Hawaii for 1956. Rates based on cases including Alaska and Hawaii for 1960, 1973, 1975-1978.

matic in women, and hence routine screening was for women only. Asymptomatic gonorrhea in men varies from 0.95% to 5.6%, depending on the study population and the inclusion of males who have a history of exposure to gonorrhea but no symptoms, as opposed to those with no history and no symptoms.[6,17,32] Nonetheless, the advisability for women to insist on use of condoms and other venereal disease prophylactic techniques[7,65] is obvious.

Cosmetic surgery

The youth cult in the United States has led to the performance of an estimated 1 million plastic surgeries annually to tuck tummies, augment breasts, and tighten sagging eyelids, chins, cheeks, and almost any other part of the anatomy.[28] This does not include reconstructive surgery to correct deformities or rehabilitate accident victims. Most of the cosmetic surgery (estimates are at least 60%) is performed on women, although an increasing but unknown percentage of cosmetic surgery is performed on men. Data is particularly scarce in this field because a large proportion of the surgeries are performed in offices and clinics not subject to any reporting system.

Costs of cosmetic surgery can be high, both in financial and physiological terms. The most common procedure, the face lift (rhytidectomy) costs from $2000 to $3000.[56] Complications include hematomas, hair loss, sensory loss, hemorrhage, and severance of the facial nerve.[49]

Breast augmentation, which costs $1500 to $2000, is estimated to be requested by 75% of women who seek plastic surgery. It is generally achieved by inserting liquid silicone contained in a thin plastic bag between the breast tissue and the chest muscles. Sales of silicone for injection directly into the breast tissue have been prohibited by the Food and Drug Administration (FDA),[57] but reputedly the highly dangerous practice continues, particularly in offices and clinics not subject to quality control; it has resulted in several lawsuits. Even with the silicone insert, complications can include fluid retention, hematoma, wrinkling of the implant, firmness or hardness of breast tissue, pain, discomfort, sensory loss, scarring, and lactation problems.[30,56]

Liquid protein diets

As with cosmetic surgery, liquid protein diets offered a quick opportunity to attain a socially determined standard of beauty. The Center for Disease Control (CDC) describes the diets as generally consisting of liquid-based protein hydrolysates, made largely from cowhides, collagen, and/or gelatin to which saccharin and artificial flavoring have been added. The proteins included in such diets are nutritionally of low biological quality, indicating that they do not contain the full complement of essential amino acids.[8]

Although the diets had only become highly popular in the United States in 1976[46] (used by an estimated 4 million persons),[42] by November, 1977, the CDC and the FDA were investigating reports of cardiac irregularities and deaths associated with liquid protein diet use.[8] Subsequent investigation of 40 deaths showed that 15 were in women without serious underlying disease who died from cardiac arrhythmias after prolonged and exclusive use of liquid protein products for weight reduction.[9] Three other deaths in individuals without underlying disease occurred to a "woman who died of a perforated stomach after starting to eat again" and to a man and a woman who both died of pancreatitis.[9] As a result, the FDA is proposing a warning to be used on weight loss products.

Cosmetics

Each year billions of dollars are spent in the United States on cosmetics. According to an FDA survey, the most commonly used cosmetic is soap, although ironically this is excluded from the Food, Drug, and Cosmetic Act. Toothpaste, shampoos, mouthwash, talcum, and hand lotion followed in volume consumed.

Although the FDA is only beginning to require ingredient labeling and warnings on cosmetics, another FDA survey in 1974 showed that many cosmetics do in fact harm people. The 10 categories of products showing the highest rate of adverse reactions were deoderants/antiperspirants, depilatories (chemical hair removers), moisturizers/lotions, hair sprays/lacquers, mascara, bubble bath, eye creams, hair color/dye lighteners, facial skin creams/cleaners, and nail polish.[58]

These are all products primarily used by women; the social conditioning which leads to the belief that cosmetic use will enhance their appeal has made most women oblivious to the health risks of unregulated cosmetics. In the interests of public health, stronger regulation of the cosmetics industry is acutely needed.

•   •   •

Women's use of ambulatory health services is principally to receive examinations for specific purposes. These are usually obtained from general practitioners in an office setting. As reported, most women do not have problems of access to health care, although for those who do, availability of appointments, cost, and lack of time spent with the physician are sources of concern.

Factors that determine women's use of ambulatory health care include self-diagnosed morbidity, socially accepted or required patterns of care, for example, prenatal checkups, employment or insurance examinations, and socially induced morbidity. Women's consumption of ambulatory services is greater than men's, although much of this difference is due to obtaining contraceptive and maternity care.

SUGGESTED TOPICS FOR DISCUSSION, FURTHER RESEARCH, AND FIELD PROJECTS

1. How common is out-of-hospital birth in your area? Who attends the mother? Who utilizes out-of-hospital birth? What, if any, legal restraints exist? What is the local medical society's attitude? How does out-of-hospital birth interface with institutionalized medicine, for example, through hospital backup, prenatal care, and emergency transportation?
2. How do days of work loss for disability compare between men and women in a sample of your local industries and offices? Does disability of women differ when they enter predominantly male fields? Compare the causes of disability between men and women.

(Suggested reference: Final report. Evaluation of women in the Army, United States Army Administration Center, Fort Benjamin, Harrison, Ind., 46216.)

3. If alternative situations for labor and delivery are available in your area, consider the following topics for comparing the different methods:
   a. Comparison of attitudes of staff in different birthing sites
   b. Cost differences among different birthing sites for deliveries of comparable risk levels
   c. Comparison of staffing differences

4. Would a national health insurance program affect women's utilization of ambulatory health services? If so, how? Would any of women's unmet needs and problems in obtaining health care as discussed in this chapter be addressed by a national health insurance program? If so, how?

5. Research federal cosmetics regulation laws. What are the basic purposes of these laws? Are they adequately protecting the public? If not, how would you improve them? What has been the history of attempts to pass laws regulating cosmetics? Who have been the groups opposed to the laws?

6. Compare two health insurance plans and coverage under a health maintenance organization. What are the differences in coverage? What benefits that are typically for women, for example, maternity, abortion, contraceptive coverage, are offered?

7. Select two specialties that are not primarily used by one sex and compare their utilization by men and women. Does it differ? If so, what are the characteristics of this difference? Interview both a male and female practitioner of each specialty. What are the characteristics of their patient populations?

8. Research women's consumption of over-the-counter (OTC) drugs. Does their consumption pattern differ from men's? If so, why? What are the effects of women's OTC drug usage?

9. Research the incidence of venereal disease in your community. What age-groups are most affected? Where is treatment most often obtained? How would you organize a venereal disease educational campaign to reach women under 20, over 20?

10. Select two examples of socially induced morbidity other than those discussed here. What are the causes of these morbidities? What age-groups of women are most affected? Are men similarly affected? What steps could be taken to curtail incidence of these morbidities?

11. Interview four women of diverse ages, ethnic groups, and socioeconomic groups and, most important, who obtain their health care from different sources (e.g., private physician, prepaid health plan, Medicaid or Medicare, community health clinic). Cover the following questions in your interviews:

Basic data

1-4. What is your age, ethnic group, income (give a range choice), and education in years?
  5. What types of health providers do you have?
  6. How do you pay them?
  7. What is their specialty?
  8. How often do you use your health services/go to the doctor?
9a. Do you have a man or a woman physician?
9b. Are you happy with this?
10. Do you always see the same physician?
11. For what types of health problems do you go to the doctor?
12. Do you ever treat yourself (e.g., with OTC drugs)?
13. Who pays for the prescription drugs?

14. If you have to go to a hospital, who pays for this?
15. If you have been to a hospital in the last 2 years, how much did it cost, what was it for, and how long did you stay? Did you have out-of-pocket expenses?
16. What are the major difficulties (if any) with your health care services?
17. What opportunities are there for presenting your complaints about the service?
18. How would you describe the provider of your health service?
19. How many health personnel are you in contact with at the time of each visit?
20. What types of health personnel are they?
21. What is their scope of function?
22. What is the most expensive part of your health care?
23. If you obtain health care in a manner other than fee for service, what kinds of health expenses are not paid for?
24. Do other members of your family use the same health service?
25. How long do you wait to get an appointment with your physician?
26. How long do you wait to see the physician when you get there?
27. Do you ask the physician questions? Are they answered?
28. How would you rate yourself in terms of health status?
29. How would you rate yourself in terms of being an "informed health consumer?"
30. How satisfied are you with your health service?

REFERENCES

1. Banks, M. H., et al.: Factors influencing demand for primary medical care in women aged 20-44 years: a preliminary report, Int. J. Epidemiol. **4:**189-195, 1975.
2. Barker-Benfield, G. J.: Horrors of the half-known life, New York, 1975, Torchbooks.
3. Bean, M. A.: The nurse-midwife at work, Am. J. Nurs. **71:**949-952, 1971.
4. Blakemore, A. W.: National prohibition. The Volstead Act annotated, Albany, N.Y., 1923, Mathew Bender and Co. Inc., (Volstead Act 41 Stat. 305, Oct. 28, 1919.)
5. Block, M. R.: Uncharted territory: issues and concerns of women over 40, College Park, Md., 1978, Center for Aging, University of Maryland.
6. Braff, E. H., and Wibbelsman, C. J.: Asymptomatic gonococcal urethritis in selected males, Am. J. Public Health **68:**779-780, 1978.
7. Brecher, E. M.: Prevention of the sexually transmitted diseases, J. Sex Res. **2:**318-323, Nov., 1975.
8. Center for Disease Control: Deaths associated with liquid protein diets, Morbidity and Mortality Weekly Report **26:**383, Nov. 18, 1977.
9. Center for Disease Control: Follow-up on deaths in persons on liquid protein diets, Morbidity and Mortality Weekly Report **26:**443, Dec. 30, 1977.
10. Center for Disease Control: Personal communication, Atlanta, June, 1978.
11. Center for Disease Control: Results of culture testing for gonorrhea — United States, 1978, Morbidity and Mortality Weekly Report **28:**290-291, June 29, 1979.
12. Center for Disease Control: Data from V.D. statistical letter, provided by Dry, K.: Personal communication, June, 1979.
13. Center for Disease Control: Congenital syphilis — United States, 1978-1979, Morbidity and Mortality Weekly Report **28:** 433-434, Sept. 14, 1979.
14. Chang, T. W., and O'Keefe, P.: Cesarean section and genital herpes, N. Engl. J. Med. **296:**573, 1977.
15. Corey, L., Head of Virology, University of Washington, Seattle, Wash.: Personal communication, July, 1978.
16. Data on home birth risk mounts, ACOG Newsletter, **21,** Nov., 1977.
17. Dexter, D. D., et al.: Asymptomatic urethral gonorrhea among men in public New York City social hygiene clinics, J. Am. Vener. Dis. Assoc. **2:**7-11, June, 1976.
18. Dingley, E.: Birth place alternatives, Oregon Health Bull. **55:**1-4, 1977.
19. Dingley, E.: Birth place and attendants: Oregon's alternative experience, 1977, Women & Health **4:**239-253, Fall, 1979.
20. Drury, T. F.: Current estimates from the Health Interview Survey, U.S. 1975, Vital

and Health Statistics, series 10, no. 115, National Center for Health Statistics, no. (HRA) 77-1543, Washington, D.C., March, 1977, U.S. Government Printing Office.

21. Drury, T. F.: Unpublished data from the 1974 Health Interview Survey, Division of Health Interview Statistics, National Center for Health Statistics, Washington, D.C., 1979.

22. Ehrenreich, B., and English, D.: Complaints and disorders: the sexual politics of sickness, Old Westbury, N.Y., 1973, The Feminist Press.

23. Epstein, J. E., and McCartney, M.: A home delivery service that works, Women & Health **3:**10-12, Jan./Feb., 1978.

24. Estes, M. N.: A home obstetric service with expert consultation and back-up, Birth & The Family Journal, **5:**151-157, Fall, 1978.

25. Ezzati, T.: Unpublished data from the National Ambulatory Medical Care Survey, Ambulatory Care Statistics Branch, Division of Health Resources Utilization Statistics, National Center for Health Statistics, Washington, D.C., 1979.

26. Flexner, A.: Medical education in the United States and Canada, New York, 1910, The Carnegie Foundation.

27. Florman, A. C., et al.: Intrauterine infection with herpes simplex virus: resultant congenital malformations, J.A.M.A. **225:**129-132, 1973.

28. Garrick, R., Public Relations Consultant, American Society of Plastic and Reconstructive Surgeons: Personal communication, July 23, 1979.

29. Gove, W. R., and Hughes, M.: Possible causes of the apparent sex differences in physical health: an empirical investigation, Am. Sociol. Rev. **44:**126-146, 1979.

30. Grossman, A. R.: The current status of augmentation mamaplasty, Plast. Reconstr. Surg. **52:**1-7, July, 1973.

31. Haire, D.: The cultural warping of childbirth, special report, Seattle, 1972, International Childbirth Education Association, 1414 N.W. 85th St., Seattle, Wash. 98117.

32. Handsfield, H. H., et al.: Asymptomatic gonorrhea in men, N. Engl. J. Med. **290:**117-123, 1974.

33. Hanshaw, J. B.: Herpes virus hominis infections in the fetus and the newborn, Am. J. Dis. Child. **126:**546-555, 1973.

34. Harrison Act 38 Stat. 785, Dec. 17, 1914.

35. Hazell, L.: A study of 300 elective home births, Birth & The Family Journal **2:**11, Spring, 1975.

36. Health department data shows danger of home births, press release, Chicago, Jan. 4, 1978, American College of Obstetricians and Gynecologists.

37. Hechtlinger, A.: The great patent medicine era, New York, 1970, Galahad Books.

38. Higher mortality rate found in home births, ACOG Newsletter, **22,** Feb., 1978.

39. Home delivery: "maternal trauma, child abuse," OB Gynecol. News, Oct. 1, 1977.

40. Hornstein, F.: Lesbian health issues, Los Angeles, 1976, The Los Angeles Feminist Women's Health Center.

41. Howie, L. J., and Drury, T. F.: Current estimates from the Health Interview Survey, U.S. 1977. Vital and Health Statistics, series 10, no. 126, National Center for Health Statistics, no. (PHS) 78;1554. Washington, D.C., 1978, U.S. Government Printing Office.

42. Keerdoja, E., and Lord, M.: Protein warning, Newsweek: 20, Feb. 26, 1979.

43. Kentucky vital statistics, Frankfort, Kentucky, 1974, Department of Human Resources.

44. Koch, H., and Gagnon, R. O.: Office visits by black patients, National Ambulatory Medical Care Survey: United States, 1975-1976. Advance data, no. 50, National Center for Health Statistics, Washington, D.C., July 23, 1979, U.S. Government Printing Office.

45. Kovar, M. G., and Drury, T. F.: Use of medical care services by men and women in their middle and later years, presented at the Gerontological Society annual meeting, Nov. 19, 1978, Dallas.

46. Linn, R.: The last chance diet, New York, 1976, Bantam Books, Inc. (Popularity of liquid protein diets soared with publication.)

47. Lubic, R. W.: Statement of Maternity Center Association, testimony before the Health Committee of the Legislature of the Commonwealth of Massachusetts, Feb. 28, 1977.

48. Manpower planning in obstetrics-gynecology, Chicago, 1977-1980, American College of Obstetrics and Gynecology. (Contact Judy Fielden, ACOG, 1 E. Wacker, Chicago, Ill. 60601.)

49. McGregor, M. W., and Greenberg, R. L., editors: Complications of face lifting. In Symposium on aesthetic surgery of the face, eyelid, and breast, St. Louis, 1972, The C. V. Mosby Co., p. 5864.

50. Mehl, L. E.: Options in maternity care, Women & Health **2**(2):29-42, Sept./Oct., 1977.

51. Mehl, L. E., et al.: Complications of home birth, Birth & The Family Journal **2**:110-123, Winter, 1975.

52. Mehl, L. E., et al.: Risk factors in low-risk-childbirth. I. Differences between home & hospital birth, paper presented to the American Public Health Association annual meeting, Oct. 31, 1977, Washington, D.C.

53. Mendenhall, R. C., et al.: Manpower for obstetrics-gynecology. I. Demographic considerations and practice work load, Am. J. Obstet. Gynecol. **130**:927-932, 1978.

54. Metropolitan Life Insurance Company: Incidence of disability—1978, Stat. Bull. **60**:16, 1979.

55. Metropolitan Life Insurance Company: Trends in disability among women, Stat. Bull. **60**:12, 1979.

56. Moore, K. H., and Thompson, S.: The surgical beauty racket, Port Washington, N.Y., 1978, Ashley Books, Inc.

57. Morrison, M.: In only four weeks, FDA Consumer, Washington, D.C., June, 1975, U.S. Government Printing Office.

58. Morrison, M.: Cosmetics: the substances beneath the form, revised, FDA Consumer, no. (FDA) 78-5007. Washington, D.C., 1978, U.S. Government Printing Office.

59. Nathanson, C. A.: Illness and the feminine role: a theoretical review, Soc. Sci. Med. **9**:57-62, 1975.

60. National Disease and Therapeutic Index (NDTI): Obstetrics gynecology specialty profile, Ambler, 1974, IMS America.

61. Neilsen, I.: Midwife-physician team in private practice, Am. J. Nurs. **75**:1693-1695, 1975.

62. O'Donnell, M.: Lesbian health care: issues and literature, Science for the People **10**:8-19, 1978.

63. Pearse, W. H.: ACOG studies status of non-physician professionals, Contemp. OB/Gyn **12**:119-121, Oct., 1978.

64. Pearson, J. W., The obstetrician and gynecologist: primary physician for women, J.A.M.A. **231**:815-816, 1975.

65. Population reports. Barrier methods, series H, no. 3, Washington, D.C., Jan., 1975, George Washington University Medical Center.

66. Prince, E. O.: Welfare status, illness and subjective health definition, Am. J. Public Health **68**:865-870, 1978.

67. Redden, J. A.: Legal status of a midwife in Oregon, attorney general opinion, Department of Justice (no. 7468), June, 1977, Oregon.

68. Report Z, American Medical Association Board of Trustees, Chicago, Ill., 1974, pp. 132-134.

69. Rice, D. P., and Cugliani, A.: Health status of American women, Women & Health **5**:5-22, Spring, 1980.

70. Roemer, M. I., University of California, Los Angeles: Personal communication, 1976.

71. Statistics for 882 births managed by farm midwives (10-8-70 to 6-30-78), Summertown, 1978, The Farm, 156 Drakes Lane, Summertown, Tenn. 38483.

72. Torres, A.: Organized family planning services in the United States, 1968-1976, Fam. Plann. Perspect. **10**:83-88, 1978

73. U.S. Department of Health, Education and Welfare: Health United States, 1978, no. (PHS) 78-1232, Washington, D.C., 1978, U.S. Government Printing Office, p. 261.

74. Verbrugge, L. M.: Females and illness: recent trends in the United States, J. Health Soc. Behav. **17**:387-403, 1976.

75. Verbrugge, L. M.: Sex differentials in morbidity and mortality in the United States, Soc. Biol. **23**:275-296, Winter, 1976.

76. Walls, B. E., and Jackson, J. J.: Factors affecting the use of physicians by menopausal black women, Urban Health **6**:53-56, March, 1977.

77. Weaver, J. L.: National health policy and the underserved: ethnic minorities, women, and the elderly, St. Louis, 1976, The C. V. Mosby Co.

78. Willson, J. R.: Recruitment into obstetrics & gynecology, Obstet. Gynecol. **40**:432-437, 1972.

79. Willson, J. R., and Burkons, D. M.: Obstetrician-gynecologists are primary physicians to women. I. Practice patterns of Michigan Obstetrician-gynecologists, Am. J. Obstet. Gynecol **126**:627-632, 1976.

80. Willson, J. R., and Burkons, D. M.: Obstetrician-gynecologists are primary physicians to women. II. Education for a new role, Am. J. Obstet. Gynecol. **26**:744-754, 1976.

81. Yankauer, A., et al.: Performance and delegation of patient services by physicians in obstetrics and gynecology, Am. J. Public Health **61**:1545-1555, 1971.

82. Yankauer, A., et al.: Practice of Obstetrics

and gynecology in the United States, Obstet. Gynecol. **38:**800-808, 1971.
83. Yankauer, A., et al.: Physician output, productivity and task delegation in obstetric-gyneologic practice in the United States, Obstet. Gynecol. **39:**151-161, 1972.

ADDITIONAL READING

Adkins, B. S.: Committment to a better life: national policy concerns for older women, Federal Council on the Aging, no. 052-003-00150-1, Washington, D.C., 1977. U.S. Government Printing Office.

Annas, G. J.: Are childbirth laws adequate? Women & Health **2:**23-28, Sept./Oct., 1977; response in: Sparer, E. V.: Inadequate childbirth care: a different perspective on law and lawyers, Library Bull., Feb., 1978, University of Pennsylvania.

Birth day at home: is it safe? Medical World News **20:**105-106, April 19, 1976.

Bredesen, N. B.: The granny midwife: her training, licensure, and practice in Georgia, Louisiana and Texas, no. PB-271 852, Washington, D.C., April 1970, National Center for Health Services Research.

Cherniak, D., and Feingold, A.: V.D. handbook, Box 1000, Station 9, Montreal, 130, Quebec, Canada.

Corder, L. S.: Health care coverage: United States, 1976, Advance Data, no. 44, National Center for Health Statistics, Washington, D.C., Sept, 20, 1979, U.S. Government Printing Office.

Fox, J. H.: Effects of retirement and former work life on women's adaptation in old age, J. Gerontol. **32:**196-202, March, 1977.

Gagnon, R. O.: Office visits involving x-rays, National Ambulatory Medical Care Survey: United States, 1977, Advance Data, no. 53, National Center for Health Statistics, Washington, D.C., Sept. 11, 1979, U.S. Government Printing Office.

Hinds, M. W.: Gonorrhea screening in family planning clinics: when should it become selective? Public Health Rep. **92:**361-364, July-Aug., 1977.

Judson, F. N., et al.: Screening for gonorrhea and syphilis in the gay baths—Denver, Colorado, Am. J. Public Health **67:**740-742, 1977.

Kitzinger, S., editor: The place of birth, Oxford, 1978, Oxford University Press.

Koch, H., et al.: 1976 Summary: National Ambulatory Medical Care Survey. Advance Data, no. 30, National Center for Health Statistics, Washington, D.C., July 13, 1978, U.S. Government Printing Office.

Kuhn, M. E.: The older woman in society, Keynote address presented at NIH and NIA Conference, Sept. 14, 1978, Bethesda, Md.

Metropolitan Life Insurance Company: Disability among males, Stat. Bull. **59:**14, July-Sept., 1978.

National Institute on Aging and National Institute of Mental Health: Final report of the Workshop on the Older Woman: Continuities and Discontinuities, Sept. 14-16, 1978, Bethesda, Md.

National Midwives Association: Newsletter, National Midwives Association, Box 163, Princeton, N.J. 08540.

Office practice patterns of OB-Gyns, Medical World News **19:**75, May 29, 1978.

Richwald, G.: Response to ACOG news release on home birth, NAPSAC News, **3,** Summer, 1978, NAPSAC, P.O. Box 267, Marble Hill, Mo. 63764.

Stewart, L., and Stewart, D., editors: Safe alternatives in childbirth NAPSAC, 1976, Box 1307, Chapel Hill, N.C. 27514.

Treas, J.: Family support systems for the aged, Gerontologist **17:**486-491, 1977.

Uhlenberg, P.: Changing structure of the older population of the USA during the twentieth century, Gerontologist **17:**197-202, 1977.

Verbrugge, L. M.: Health in Detroit study, Institute for Social Research and the Department of Brostatistics, School of Public Health, University of Michigan, Ann Arbor, 1977.

Yanover, M. J., et al.: Perinatal care of low-risk mothers and infants: early discharge with home care. N. Engl. J. Med. **294:**702-705, 1976.

Chapter 3

Governmental programs and women's health

HISTORICAL BACKGROUND

Prior to 1900, federal, state, and local legislative interest in the health of women (and men) focused on the establishment of mental hospitals (see the work of Dorothea Dix),[52] basic sanitation services, quarantine services, the development of local boards of health, hospital dispensaries for free medical care for the poor, and the provision of health services for seamen, veterans, and Native Americans.[14,45,82,83,90] By the late 1800s and early 1900s the tremendous immigration of Europe's poor to the crowded city ghettos had exacerbated all the health problems of poverty and squalid living conditions. Social experiments such as Jane Addams' Hull House[22] and Lillian Wald's Henry Street Settlement,[27] while providing valuable aid, could meet the needs of only relatively few. Other existing services and charity efforts, initially begun to ameliorate some of these conditions by "uplifting" immigrants or teaching them how to cope with their poverty were inadequate and frequently both racist and classist. Formal health programs for defined populations, accessible and acceptable, publicly supported, and in accordance with the designation of state and federal powers under the Constitution, had to be developed to meet public need.

Acceptability of organized programs to the expanding medical profession proved more difficult to achieve than acceptability to patients. In the early 1900s (ca. 1905), the National Association for the Study and Prevention of Tuberculosis was founded. Tuberculosis (TB) was the leading cause of death among women (see Chapter 1) but the agency, to avoid conflict with the private physician sector, could only study TB, provide health education, and advise people on how to be hospitalized. Similarly, health centers operated by local health departments faced strong opposition because they ventured into the curative rather than public prevention field;[83] even today organized medicine is still opposed to publicly organized maternal and child health services for people other than the poor (resolution passed by the American Medical Association's House of Delegates, 1962).

This organized opposition has effectively shaped public health programs and health legislation at all levels. Publicly supported health activities since 1900 have been essentially confined to establishing control and detection measures for communicable diseases (e.g., VD, TB); establishing a vital statistics system; providing health education; organizing surveillance and control of the quality of basic resources such as water, food, milk, and air; providing prenatal, well-baby, and family planning care to the poor; and providing general care to Native Americans, members of the armed services and their dependents, and veterans. Other public funds are used to support special programs, for example, for the elderly through Medicare, for end-stage renal disease patients, and for the medically indigent through Medicaid. In each case, however, the provision of care comes primarily through the private sector.

SELECTED EARLY PROGRAMS
Milk stations, 1873 to about 1917

Milk stations evolved in response to the high infant mortality at the turn of the century, particularly from infant diarrheal diseases believed to be caused by impure milk. Basically, they provided milk for infants of the poor, either free or at a nominal charge.

Mothers who were nursing their infants also attended milk stations for the child care lessons.[12] Although these stations were primarily designed to benefit children, women also greatly benefited by having healthy babies, learning positive patterns of child care, and learning sterilization techniques.

Initially begun in Europe in the mid-1800s, milk stations began independently in the United States, with the first opening in 1873 in affiliation with the

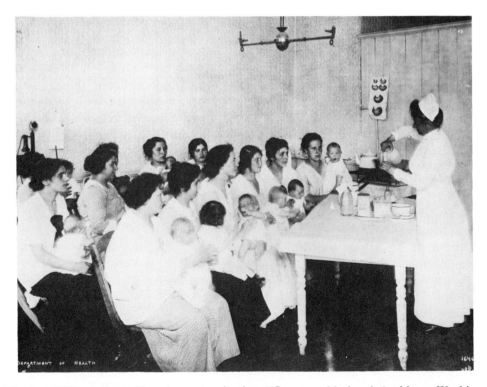

Fig. 3-1. Milk station. Class in pasteurization. (Courtesy National Archives, Washington, D.C.)

New York Diet Kitchen Association. Many voluntary efforts followed, most notably by Nathan Strauss, Wilbur C. Philipps, and Elsie Cole Philipps.[83] The first publicly funded station was opened in 1897 by the Rochester, New York, Health Department and followed an earlier French model by additionally offering well-baby checkups and lessons in child care.[12,35] The Rochester health officer, Dr. George W. Goler, soon developed (as had other milk stations, but to a greater extent) a commission and system for ensuring a pasteurized milk supply for the city; in 1900 Rochester became the first American city to set up a bacterial content standard for cleanliness of milk: 100,000 bacteria per cubic centimeter.[12] Other cities gradually followed.

In New York City the findings of health visitors who did follow-up studies on babies visiting the milk stations, as well as the demonstrated success of an edu-

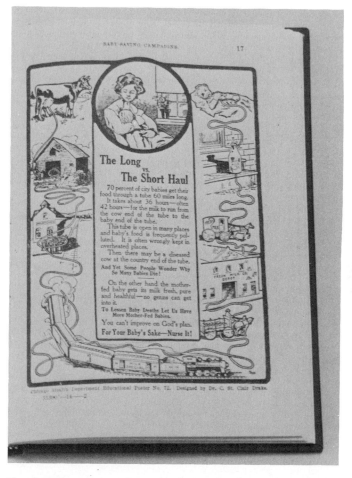

Fig. 3-2. Health education poster advocating breast-feeding. (From The health of women and children [baby-saving campaign, U.S. Department of Labor, 1914]. Reprinted by Arno Press, Inc., New York.)

cational program to provide instruction in tenements on reducing infant mortality, led to the establishment in 1908 of the first Division of Child Hygiene. Under the leadership of Dr. S. Josephine Baker, the New York milk stations increased and expanded in function; they were also used for "mothers' meetings, sewing classes, Little Mothers' League meetings (education of young girls in maternal care), neighborhood societies, and as general centers where the nurses through personal efforts, frequently provided food, clothing, medical care, shelter, employment, outings, excursions, etc., for the members of the baby's family"[11] (Fig. 3-1).

Breast-feeding was encouraged by the milk stations, and Blake notes the increasing numbers of breast-fed babies registered from 1912 on, with the "decline of the milk-dispensing feature into mere bait"[12] (Fig. 3-2). Other cities began to follow New York's example; in 1909 Detroit established a child hygiene division and by 1915, 20 cities were listed as having child hygiene divisions or bureaus as part of their health departments.[36] The numbers of milk stations continued to grow across the United States but were "gradually evolving into well-baby clinics with supervision by physicians, home visits by nurses, and lectures to mothers."[12,96] It is from these programs that federally supported maternal and child health services eventually emerged (see later).

Chamberlain-Kahn Act, 1918 to 1926

In 1917 the federal government with its newly acquired source of funds from income tax (the Sixteenth Constitutional Amendment was passed in 1913) began giving grants to the states for special projects. The Chamberlain-Kahn Act of 1918 awarded money annually to the states for venereal disease (VD) control programs. Money was available for testing, treatment, and education; by 1926 every state had a VD office with central coordination of the program through the U.S. Public Health Service (USPHS). Funding was withdrawn in 1926 but reestablished in 1947.

Interest in VD expanded rapidly as the social reform and public health movement of the early 1900s grew. The prospect of the United States' entry into World War I and the possibilities of the spread of VD from "camp followers" alarmed the public, especially since one report indicated that of 200,000 women identified as being in "the regular army of vice," 60% to 75% had VD.[108]

Sheppard-Towner Act, 1921 to 1929

With the establishment of the Children's Bureau in the Department of Labor on April 9, 1912, and under the energetic direction of its first chief, Julia Lathrop, maternal and child issues were pushed into national attention. Lathrop had organized data collection, surveys of child welfare, and the publication and distribution of educational pamphlets promoting maternal and infant well-being. By 1918, designated Children's Year, there was a concerted effort to establish federally supported health programs for mothers and children.

Many efforts, including those of Congresswoman Jeannette Rankin of Montana, culminated in the eventual passage in 1921 of the Sheppard-Towner Act (Morris Sheppard, Texas; Horace Mann Towner, Iowa), officially known as the Maternity and Infancy Act, which established a federal-state program for maternal and infant health. Opposition to the bill had been strong and sexist; those opposed were not aware of the need for education in good child care practices. Commented Senator James Reed of Missouri:

It seems to be the established doctrine of this bureau [the Children's Bureau] that the only people capable of caring for babies and mothers of babies are ladies who have never had babies [laughter]. . . . I cast no reflection on unmarried ladies. Perhaps some of them are too good to have husbands. But any woman who is too refined to have a husband should not undertake the care of another woman's baby when that other woman wants to take care of it herself. . . . Official meddling cannot take the place of mother love.[100]

The bill had also been branded as "socialistic, bolshevistic and radical."

Grace Abbott, the new Children's Bureau chief at the end of 1921, administered the Sheppard-Towner Act. It was the first federal formula grant program established in the field of health. (Formula grants are those in which money is allocated to the states on the basis of a formula—generally, population × per capita income × need.) Although the concept of public health care to pregnant women was new to many, Abbott stated the purposes of the act as: "First, to secure an appreciation among women of what constitutes good prenatal and obstetrical care. Second, how to make available adequate community resources so that the women may have the type of care which they need and should be asking for."

Each state was obligated to match the federal funds but then could use the money as it saw fit. By 1927, 45 states and the then territory of Hawaii had a Sheppard-Towner program. Fourteen states chose to license, inspect, supervise, and instruct midwives; one state expanded its fledgling prenatal clinic program; and others promoted maternal health by conferences with expectant mothers and establishment of maternity and child health centers in each county. The program also provided women with a checklist of adequate prenatal care that they could use to assess their own care. Abbott stated that, in general, there were five main areas of maternal and child health services being provided under the act: "promotion of birth registration, cooperation between health authorities and physicians, nurses, dentists, nutrition workers, and so forth, establishment of infant welfare centers, establishment of maternity centers, and educational classes for mothers, midwives, and household assistants or mother's helpers, and 'little mothers.' "

Despite even more vitriolic opposition, the Sheppard-Towner Act was renewed in 1927 for 2 more years. *The Women's Patriot,* a journal of the time, protested:

Children are now the best political graft in America. They furnish the best possible screen behind which to hide cold-blooded, calculated socialist feminist political schemes to raid the United Treasury to supply . . . "new, fat jobs" plus publicity, prominence and power, to childless bureaucrats and women politicians to "investigate and report" the hard-working, taxpaying, child-bearing mothers of America, under pretense of promoting "child welfare" and "saving mothers and babies."[100]

At the close of the program, Abbott noted its accomplishments, including that by 1929, 46 states and the District of Columbia (totaling 95% of the United

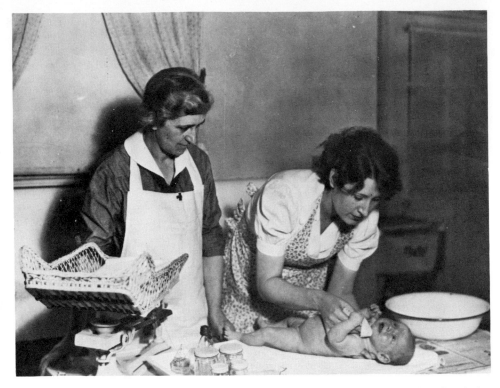

Fig. 3-3. The public health nurse teaches a young mother how to bathe her first baby. (Courtesy National Archives, Washington, D.C.)

States population) now had required registration of births. Furthermore, in 1920 there were child hygiene bureaus or divisions in 28 states, 16 of them created in 1919, and the act had brought the establishment of 19 additional divisions. The act had also sponsored the establishment of 1594 permanent local child health, prenatal, or combined prenatal and child health consultation centers between 1924 and 1929; public health nursing services for mothers and children had also expanded (see Fig. 3-3). Even after the act ended in 1929, the legislatures of 19 states and the Territory of Hawaii continued to appropriate for maternal and child health programs.

Preventing gonorrheal ophthalmia neonatorum

In 1879 Credé published an article discussing the benefits of dropping silver nitrate into newborn babies' eyes to prevent the spread of gonorrheal infections potentially contacted during birth and which could cause blindness.[20] Again, although not specifically oriented to women, the adoption of this practice, first in 1911 by South Dakota and by almost all states by the 1930s,[103] greatly benefited women through eliminating this cause of blindness in their babies.[85]

1935 AND AFTER
Social Security Act, 1935

The Social Security Act, which was passed on August 14, 1935, had four major social measures: social insurance for retirees and for the unemployed; income maintenance for indigent persons who fit the specific categories of Old Age Assistance, Aid for Dependent Children, and Aid to the Blind; the provision of funds for public health work; and the provision of funds for maternal and child health services.

The establishment of a maternal-child welfare program through Title V of the Social Security Act this time met with little opposition, since organized medicine had come to understand the mutual benefits of providing women the funds to seek maternity care. Title VI of the act additionally provided funds for public health departments, and all the states used these funds in part to establish bureaus or divisions of maternal and child health as major components of state health departments.

Title V. Over the years since 1935 several different programs have been established and funded under the authority of Title V of the Social Security Act. Previously administered through the Children's Bureau but generally administered today through the Bureau of Community Health Services within the Health Services Administration, USPHS, in the Department of Health, Education and Welfare, these programs have all aimed at promoting maternal and child well-being by providing maternity care, services for crippled children, intensive infant care, and well-child care for young children, and by funding research grants for related issues. (See Chapter 6 for discussion of children and youth program.) Funds for these programs are matched in full or in part by the states.

Projects for maternity and infant care (first funded in 1963) have as their goals the establishment of programs that offer

reasonable assurance of satisfactorily helping to reduce (1) the incidence of mental retardation and other handicapping conditions caused by complications associated with childbearing, and (2) infant and maternal morbidity and mortality through provision of necessary health care to prospective mothers (including, after childbirth health care to mothers and their infants) who have or are likely to have conditions associated with childbearing or who are in circumstances which increase the hazards to the health of mothers or their infants (including those which may cause physical or mental defects in the infants).[99]

The programs are to be established in areas "with concentrations of low-income families."[99]

Almost all maternal and infant care projects are essentially expanded versions of original maternal and well-baby services provided under Sheppard-Towner. Although providing effective prepartum, intrapartum, and postpartum care for the pregnant woman, these programs have been criticized as causing fragmentation because "the services are limited to a certain population group defined by its income level, by its age grouping, but most all, by its relation to a single event, pregnancy. As soon as a mother is past the event of pregnancy,

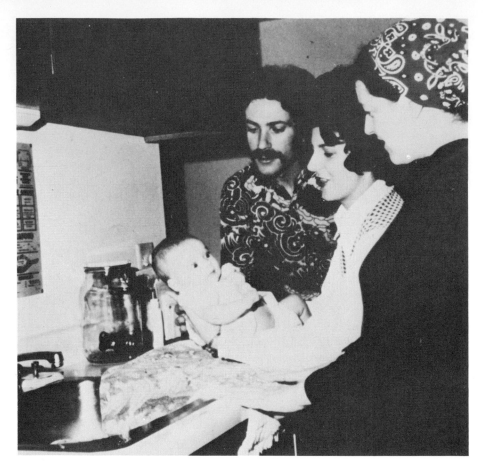

Fig. 3-4. Contemporary public health nurse teaching bathing techniques. (Courtesy Seattle-King County Department of Public Health, Seattle.)

achieves a higher income, or her child becomes older, this source of care is no longer available."[34,49] In both 1978 and 1979, approximately 740,500 women were served through these programs.

Projects for family planning services under Title V, again mandated to be located "in areas with concentrations of low-income families," have to offer reasonable assurance of satisfactorily helping to reduce "(1) the incidence of mental retardation and other handicapping conditions caused by complications associated with childbearing, and (2) infant and maternal morbidity and mortality, through the provision of family planning services."[99] Contraceptive counseling and services were provided through these projects, again frequently sponsored by health departments or hospital clinics, to over 2.5 million women in 1978 and to over an estimated 2.6 million women in 1979[70] (see Fig 3-4).

More general maternal and child health services for low-income families, including dental care and medical services to promote the health of preschool and school-age children, were provided to 398,980 persons in 1978 and an estimated 414,920 in 1979.[70] Additional programs provide training for personnel for "health care of and related services for mothers and children, particularly mentally retarded children and children with multiple handicaps."[29, p. 161]

Research programs funded under Title V state their objectives as "to provide research projects relating to maternal and child health services or crippled children's services which show promise of substantial contribution to the advancement of such services."[29, p. 160] Some projects funded under these project grants have been studies in obstetrical care, most notably Haverkamp's electronic fetal monitoring studies (see Chapter 7), and in determining variables affecting infant outcome measurements, including studies through the Pennsylvania and California State Health Departments.[69] In total, $429 million were allocated to these Title V programs and various infant and children's programs in fiscal year 1977. By fiscal year 1979 the allocation was $491 million.[53]

Emergency maternity and infant care

Although no longer functioning, the program relating to women's health that appeared chronologically after the 1935 Social Security Act was the Emergency Maternity and Infant Care program (EMIC). In August, 1941, military medical personnel at Fort Lewis, Washington, appealed to the Washington State Health Department to help them meet their obligations defined under the 1884 Military Dependents Act to provide maternity services for the wives of the growing U.S. Army. (Medical benefits had been provided for World War I servicemen and dependents under the 1917 War Risk Act.) Proposing to use monies from Fund B of Title V of the Social Security Act (special nonmatched project funds), the Washington State Health Department applied for and was granted approval by the Children's Bureau. Thus an emergency program for providing maternity services, including, significantly, coverage for delivery costs and hospitalization, was developed. From August, 1941, until July, 1942, 677 women in the area were registered for care.[88] The program drew much public attention because, although 160,000 mothers previously had received prenatal care under the maternal and child health program of Title V of the Social Security Act, the act had not, at that time, also covered delivery and hospitalization.

By March, 1942, many states were recommending similar programs be established for their service families; by July 1, 1942, 27 other states had received approval to use Fund B monies for an emergency program. By early 1943 Ms. Katharine F. Lenroot, chief of the Children's Bureau, and Dr. Martha M. Eliot, associate chief, justified to Congress requests for additional Fund B monies to support the rapidly expanding programs.

Although there was much debate about whether the Children's Bureau or the army should administer a formal program of emergency maternity and infant care for servicemen, whether there should be a means test, whether this was a new or continuation program, and whether the Children's Bureau could set standards for obsterical practice, the final outcome was that on July 12, 1943, H.R. 2935 became Public Law 135 with an initial 1944 fiscal year appropriation of $4.4 million. As soon as the program was widely announced, demand soared, and 6 weeks after the initial appropriation, the Children's Bureau was granted another $18.6 million. Despite fears that this was socialized medicine, Congress continued to appropriate funds for EMIC until November, 1946; in September, 1943, however, a means test was essentially applied by only allowing EMIC services for wives of servicemen in the lowest pay grades — 4 to 7 — about three fourths of the armed forces.[61,88,100]

The program basically appealed to Congress. One congressman noted: "The man at the front, receiving $50.00 a month with his wife in the family way, has a great easing of mind if he knows she is going to have proper care in her time of trouble."[97]

At the height of the program, EMIC covered the maternity services and baby care for one out of every seven births in the United States. By the end of the program, 1.2 million maternity cases had been covered, as had the care for 230,000 infants. In addition, EMIC had several long-range effects. Minimum standards were established for hospitals and maternity and newborn services, a growing trend to hospitalization for birth was reinforced, and the infant mortality rate dropped from 45.3 per 1000 live births in 1941 to 31.3 in 1949, the year the program finally ended.[100] Efforts to revive EMIC during the Korean War failed, but from the model of EMIC came CHAMPUS (Comprehensive Health and Medical Plan, United States), a health program for members of the armed forces and their dependents.

Public Health Service Act

The Public Health Service Act was originally passed on August 14, 1912, and established the U.S. Public Health Service; as with other major acts, subsequent amendments, particularly in the 1940s and 1960s, have expanded its original functions. Today some programs under the Public Health Service Act specifically benefit women, although most apply to both sexes.

Specifically of benefit to women are the grants for research for mothers and children, which "strive to improve the health and well-being of mothers, children and families as the key to assuring a healthy adult population."[29, p. 389]

Not solely for women, but of particular benefit to them, are the family planning projects funded in part under Title X of the Public Health Service Act. These projects are "to provide educational, comprehensive medical and social services necessary to enable individuals to freely determine the number and spacing of their children, to promote the health of mothers and children and to help reduce maternal and infant mortality." Priority is given to providing services in these projects to persons with low incomes.[29, p. 152] Related funds under Title X are for training programs "to improve utilization and career development of paraprofessional and paramedical manpower in family planning services,"[29, p. 175] for example, women's health care specialists. Population research funded under the Public Health Service Act "seeks solutions to the fundamental problems of the reproductive process and strives to develop and evaluate safer and more effective and convenient contraceptives . . ."[29, p. 388] (see Chapter 7 and Fig. 3-5).

Of more general benefit are programs to fund research on aging and to develop an improved health status in the elderly,[29, p. 391] project grants (funds for

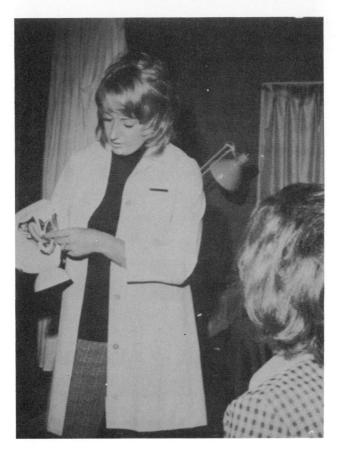

Fig. 3-5. Teaching family planning. (Courtesy Seattle-King County Department of Public Health, Seattle.)

a specific program) for venereal disease services,[29, p. 179] and immunization programs.

Several programs for mental health services are also funded under the Public Health Service Act. Hospital improvement grants are for state mental hospitals "for projects which will improve the quality of care, treatment, and rehabilitation of patients, encourage transition to open institutions; and develop more cooperative relationships with community programs for mental health."[29, p. 163] Mental health and hospital staff development grants are designed to "increase the effectiveness of staff in mental hospitals and to translate knowledge into more effective services to patients." These grants also provide help with "backup support for specific projects dealing with children, the elderly and drug and alcohol-related problems."[29, p. 164]

Research money for other aspects of mental health, several of which directly affect women, is also available under the Public Health Service Act, and the authorization section, Section 301 (c) of Public Law 78-410, cites that "areas of special interest include epidemiology, early child care, metropolitan mental health problems, crime and delinquency, minority group mental health problems, rape prevention and control and mental health programs of the aging."[29, p. 165] Other mental health funds must be matched by the states for the general provision of comprehensive public health services[29, p. 150] and the training of mental health specialists "to provide needed mental health services to targeted geographic areas and populations."[29, p. 166]

Since 1962, migrant health services have also been provided for in part by the Public Health Service Act, with the objective of supporting "the development and operation of migrant health centers and projects which provide primary health services, supplemental health services and environmental health services which are accessible to people as they move and work; to migrant agricultural farm workers, seasonal farm workers and their families."[29, p. 167]

Occupational health funds and monies for research and training grants with the objectives of encouraging research to detect and eliminate work place hazards[29, p. 176] and to develop specialized professional personnel[29, p. 176] are also budgeted under the USPHS, although the legislative authority is separate.

Medicare

As part of the Social Security Act Amendments of 1965, Title XVIII was passed, which introduced Medicare, a health insurance program for people 65 years of age and older; subsequent amendments in 1968 required Medicare beneficiaries to be at least 65 years of age and to have a requisite number of work quarters. Medicare has two parts: Part A (Medicare hospital insurance) provides basic protection by paying 80% of the costs of inpatient hospital care, posthospital extended care, and posthospital home health care. Part B (Medicare medical insurance) provides supplemental protection against costs of physicians' services, medical services and supplies, home health care services, outpatient hospital services and therapy, and other miscellaneous services (see Fig. 3-6).

The basic purpose of Medicare is to enable the elderly to have and maintain access to health care services. Although Medicare was initially opposed by organized medicine on the grounds of "creeping socialism", the benefits of it to both provider and consumer are readily acknowledged. After Medicare was initiated, hospitalization among the elderly increased, although use of ambulatory health services did not rise comparably.[24,33,91] A recent study of the 10 top surgical procedures among all the Medicare population found rates per 1000 Medicare population of 9.9 for cataract surgery, 6.8 for prostatectomy, 4.0 for inguinal hernia, 3.1 for cholecystectomy, 2.7 for resection of the small intestine or colon, 2.6 for hip replacement, 1.8 for mastectomy, 1.4 for dilation and curettage (D&C), 1.3 for hysterectomy, and 0.6 for hemorrhoidectomy.[71]

Although there are regional variations in the frequency and length of hospitalization of the Medicare population, there are no differences in benefits available. Because of the longevity and the particular economic vulnerability of the elderly woman, Medicare is an essential component in ensuring adequate health services for women.

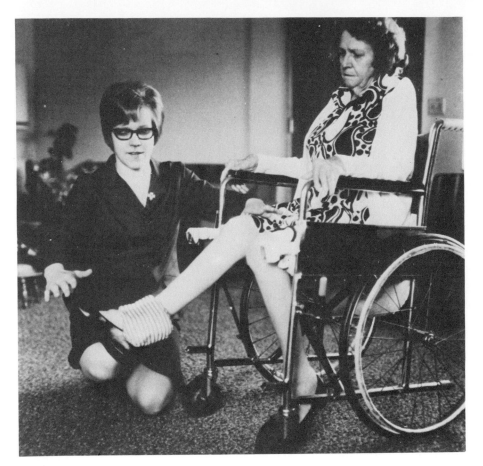

Fig. 3-6. Home health care. (Courtesy Seattle-King County Department of Public Health, Seattle.)

Medicaid

Title XIX, also passed in 1965, amended the Social Security Act to provide for the health care of the medically indigent through matching federal and state contributions. Because states design their own Medicaid programs within federal guidelines, there is wide variation in the various programs. However, all states at a minimum must provide inpatient hospital care, outpatient hospital services, other laboratory and x-ray services, skilled nursing home services, physicians' services, screening, diagnosis, and treatment of children, and home health care services. In many states, Medicaid (with matching federal contributions) also pays for dental care, prescribed drugs, eyeglasses, clinic services, and other diagnostic, screening, preventive, and rehabilitative services.

Medicaid is particularly important for women because it has enabled low-income women to seek needed obstetrical care, including, until recently (see

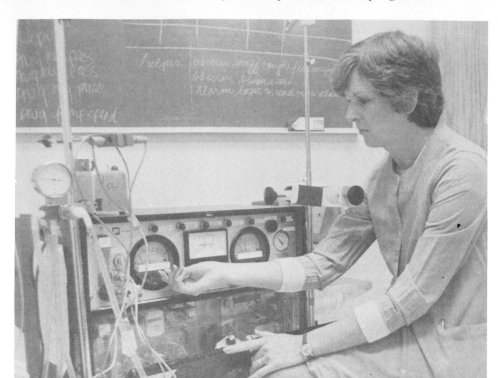

Fig. 3-7. End-stage renal disease dialysis technician. (Courtesy Bill Ransdell.)

later) funds for abortions. About 4.6 million women of reproductive age are eligible for Medicaid.

End-Stage Renal Disease Program

Another amendment to the Social Security Act, Public Law 92-603 of November, 1972, provided coverage for all persons "fully or currently insured under social security" who required kidney transplantation or dialysis."[39] This amendment is known as the End-Stage Renal Disease Program and is one of the few Medicare programs that is disease related rather than age related (see Fig. 3-7).

Costs and beneficiaries of the program have risen dramatically since 1973 when funding became available; by 1979 there were about 55,600 beneficiaries for a total cost to the federal government of almost $1 billion annually. As of June, 1979, 45.2% of ESRD beneficiaries were women, and among the women 72.9% were white, 24.4% were black, and 2.7% were of other races. The majority of women were aged 45 to 64, followed by those 65 and over and those aged 25 to 44.[58] Kidney disease appears to strike proportionately more blacks than whites and is among the 10 leading causes of death for black females (see Chapter 1).

OTHER GOVERNMENTAL AGENCIES AND PROGRAMS
Department of Agriculture

Although not directly related to health, the Department of Agriculture has several food-related programs that may significantly affect the health of eligible low-income women and their families. In fiscal year 1977-1978, the Women, Infants, and Children Program established under amendments to the Child Nutrition Act of 1966, provided "supplemental nutritious foods" to about 1.1 million participants "identified to be nutritional risks because of inadequate nutrition."[29, p. 47] About $382 million was spent on this program in fiscal year 1978, with an estimated expenditure of $550 million for fiscal year 1979.[56]

Through the Commodities Supplemental Food Program, also funded by the Department of Agriculture, needy families are provided bulk food products such as flour and grains; $13,642,174 was spent on food through this program in fiscal year 1979 and $2,046,326 was spent on administration.[56]

Food Stamps, authorized under Public Law 88-525 of August 30, 1964, are intended to "improve diets of low-income households by supplementing their food purchasing ability."[29, p. 42] In fiscal year 1978 an average of 16,043,861 persons participated and $8,310,918,211 was spent.[109] The Needy Family Program with similar goals, also funded by the Department of Agriculture, served an average of 89,731 persons in fiscal year 1978 and received $13,030,175 in funds.[109] Other food-related programs are the Food Donation Program, which specifically mentions "pregnant and lactating women" among its intended participants,[29, p. 41] the Child Care Food Program, which is designed to "maintain or expand non-profit food service programs for children in non-residential institutions providing child care,[29, p. 48] and numerous school food service programs.

Health-related programs for specific populations

The handicapped. The Rehabilitation Act of 1973 established the Office For Handicapped Individuals with the objective of serving

as the focal point within the Department of Health, Education and Welfare for advocacy, review, coordination, information and planning related to Department-wide policies, programs, procedures and activities relevant to the physically and mentally handicapped; and to operate for the Department a national information resource program known as the Clearinghouse on the Handicapped.[29, p. 312]

Although data on handicapped individuals and handicapped women in particular are sparse, the clearinghouse hopes to have expanded information after the 1980 census (see Chapter 1). An additional crucial program is the President's Committee on Employment of the Handicapped established by Executive Order 11840. Through promotional efforts, the committee "helps to create broader employment opportunities for the physically handicapped, mentally restored and mentally retarded."[29, p. 754]

The aging. Through the Older Americans Act of 1965 (Public Law 89-73) and subsequent amendments, numerous programs to address the needs of the elderly, most of whom are women, have been developed. Among these are the

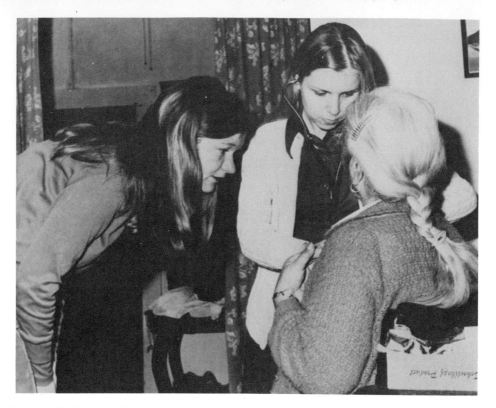

Fig. 3-8. Public health nurse visiting elderly patient in Ruby, Alaska. (Courtesy Health Sciences Information Service, University of Washington, Seattle.)

Nutrition Program for the Elderly, designed "to provide older Americans with low cost nutritious meals, with appropriate supportive services, including health services, education and counseling, outreach socialization and recreation,"[29, p. 325] and Model Projects on Aging whose purposes are "to demonstrate new approaches, techniques and methods which hold promise of contributing to improving the quality of life for older persons."[29, p. 324] Other funds are available for statewide planning of social services for the elderly,[29, p. 323] for research on "the needs and conditions of older persons,"[29, p. 326] for the establishment of new and support of existing multidisciplinary centers of gerontology[29, p. 327] and to "support activities that attract qualified persons to the field of aging. . . ."[29, p. 327] In addition, the Older Americans Act established Multipurpose Senior Centers "to provide a focal point in communities for the development and delivery of social services and nutritional services designed primarily for older persons."[29, p. 328]

Native Americans. The Indian Health Services–Health Management Development Program (Public Law 93-638) enabled tribal governments to assume operational responsibility for programs previously conducted by the Indian Health Service. The objective of the act was "to raise to the highest possible level the health of American Indians and Alaska Natives by providing a full range of curative, preventive, and rehabilitative health services that include public health nursing, maternal and child health care, dental and nutrition services, psychiatric care and health education. . . ."[29, p. 157] This act has particular significance for Native American women because of the funds made available to assist in lowering their markedly higher maternal mortality rates (see Chapter 1).

Another equally important health legislation for Native Americans is the Indian Sanitation Facilities Act, which aims "to alleviate unsanitary conditions, lack of safe water supplies and inadequate waste disposal facilities which contribute to infectious and gastroenteric diseases among Indians and Alaska Natives." Funds are also made available for the Indian Health Service to engage "in environmental health activities, including construction of sanitation facilities for individual homes and communities."[29, p. 158] The need for this act is an indication of the poverty and unsanitary conditions in which many Indians live. Through the Community Service Act of 1974, additional funds have been made available to assist Indians in developing services to promote individual and family self-sufficiency and economic development efforts[29, p. 313] — another program with potential impact on this population's health (see Fig. 3-8).

Appalachia. The intense poverty of the Appalachian region is addressed in part through the Appalachian Health Programs, a federally funded program "to provide a flexible, non-categorical approach to the development of health demonstration projects through community planning on a multicounty basis and implementation of that planning through service."[29] In fiscal year 1977, 262 service projects were funded and 38 facilities were approved for construction;[29, p. 632] together with the Appalachian Housing Project,[29, p. 633] these two projects are substantially contributing to improving the lives of this rural, isolated, and impoverished population.

Miscellaneous programs

Numerous other programs that may directly or indirectly affect health are also federally funded, including maintenance assistance, of which Aid to Families with Dependent Children is an example,[21] and Narcotic Addict Rehabilitation, which provides contracts for examination, treatment, rehabilitation, and aftercare services for addicts.[29, p. 165] Other programs are Women's Educational Equity,[29, p. 296] Occupational Safety and Health[29, p. 593] (see Chapter 5), drug abuse prevention formula grants,[29, p. 180] and telecommunications demonstrations, which are "to promote the development of non-broadcast telecommunications facilities and services for the transmission, distribution, and delivery of health education and social service information."[29, p. 341] Particularly important for women are such programs as child support enforcement,[29, p. 340] Comprehensive Employment Training, including programs for displaced homemakers,[18] Women and Mortgages, through the Department of Housing and Urban Development,[28] and the Women's Bureau of the Department of Labor. Other federally supported agencies and programs are Social Security, the numerous research programs through the National Institutes of Health, domestic violence programs through the Law Enforcement Assistance Administration Family Violence Program,[19] health career opportunity grants for the disadvantaged,[105] and the newly established office of

Health Technology.[75] These programs vary widely as to amount, specific source, and length of funding, and all are subject to political forces that may abruptly curtail or expand their potential.

Food and Drug Administration

The Food and Drug Act of 1906 established a watchdog agency with an oversight responsibility for the food produced and sold in the United States; in May, 1930, a subsequent act established the contemporary Food and Drug Administration (FDA). Other acts more closely defined the FDA's watchdog functions. Beginning in 1938 drug manufacturers had to test drugs for safety, at least on animals, prior to marketing, and after 1962, they had to prove both safety and that a proposed new drug will have the effect it is represented to have.

Despite the laws, however, the FDA appears relatively powerless to prevent harmful and/or ineffective drugs from proliferating in the marketplace. An investigative report in 1976 showed that although the "effectiveness law" was then 14 years old and 707 drugs were no longer marketed, only two fifths of the total drug formulations available were rated effective. Because of protracted legal challenges, 90 drugs rated ineffective were still on sale, as were 352 rated "possibly" effective, 99 "probably" effective, and 772 rated "effective for one or more, but not all, of the multiple uses for which they are approved."[59]

The FDA has acted to stem some of the tremendous influence exerted by manufacturers through drug advertising, however, and has forced companies to send "Dear Doctor" letters correcting false or misleading advertisements. Usually these letters come after drugs have already been widely distributed and used, having been released after positive findings from frequently inadequate studies performed by the manufacturers.

Much FDA attention has been focused recently on mandating the inclusion of patient package inserts in pharmaceutical products and medical devices. Basically the idea is to provide information to the consumer, who can then make an informed choice regarding use. The FDA requires physicians to give patients the opportunity to read the inserts and ask questions prior to making decisions regarding use. Inserts now required include those with intrauterine devices (as of November 7, 1977),[41] estrogenic drugs (as of October 18, 1977)[26] oral contraceptives (updated version; as of April 4, 1978)[66,68] and progestins (as of December 12, 1978)[30,77] Eventually the FDA hopes to have patient package inserts for almost all drugs.[31,32] Expanded labeling, another means of advising patients, has been mandated for aspirin,[5] alcoholic beverages, Valium (diazepam), and Librium (chlordiazepoxide). The FDA has also revised its approval for use of oxytocin in elective inductions (see Chapter 7).

Although patient package inserts and expanded labeling are positive steps toward responsible drug and device use, the FDA has no legal authority or mechanisms to ensure that physicians do in fact comply with the regulations. Opposition to package inserts, particularly estrogen package inserts, has been vocal. The American College of Obstetricians and Gynecologists filed suit[87] to stop their use and has generally accused the inserts of interfering with the physician-patient relationship, destroying patients' trust in their physicians, and increasing self-diagnosis and self-medication.

CURRENT LEGISLATIVE ISSUES
Sterilization

Sterilization guidelines were first proposed by the Department of Health, Education and Welfare (DHEW) in 1973 in response to blatant and tragic examples of sterilization abuse under federally funded programs, specifically the sterilization of the adolescent Relf sisters in Alabama[76] and cases of coerced sterilization in South Carolina.[89,94] Other examples of sterilization abuse that have been documented include cases at Los Angeles County–University of Southern California Women's Hospital,[25,50,93] cases among Native American women,[95,98] and cases in Puerto Rico, where in 1965 a Puerto Rican department of health study found that 34% of Puerto Rican women between the ages of 20 and 49 years were sterilized.[102] In addition, one study demonstrated that minority women in general had received a disproportionate number of sterilizations through federally financed family planning programs.[101]

After the initial guidelines were promulgated, which effectively established a moratorium on sterilization of people under 21 years of age and of those who

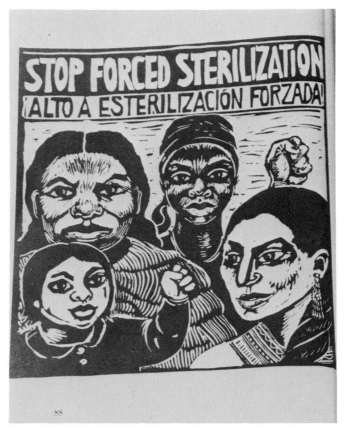

Fig. 3-9. Anti-sterilization abuse poster. (From RSP Collective: Getting stronger, Cambridge, Mass., 1978, Red Sun Press.)

could not legally consent, it was found in 1975, that only about 6% of the nation's teaching hospitals were in compliance.[44,55] Many organizations and physicians were in opposition to the guidelines. A group of six obstetricians in new York sued the Department of Health Education & Welfare (DHEW), New York State, and the New York City Health and Hospital Corporation to have the guidelines overturned.[37,79,80] A law establishing sterilization guidelines was nonetheless adopted in April, 1977, regulating sterilization of both women and men, and applying to both public and private facilities in New York City.

After other court challenges of the authority of DHEW to set regulations, DHEW prevailed and finally issued new regulations on November 8, 1978, to be effective February 6, 1979.[94] These regulations try to strike a balance between assuring access to sterilization and preventing coersion or abuse. They require that a consent form describing the risks, benefits, and contraceptive alternatives to sterilization must be presented orally and in writing in a language understood by the patient. Assurances also have to be included which state that no federal benefits will be lost if the patient refuses. Those receiving a federally funded sterilization must be at least 21 years old and mentally competent and have given consent voluntarily; consent may not have been obtained during labor or an abortion or when the patient was under the influence of alcohol or drugs. At least 30 days (previous regulations stipulated 72 hours), but not more than 180, must elapse between signing the consent and the performance of the operation; this may be reduced to a 72-hour time interval in cases of premature delivery or emergency abdominal surgery. Spousal consent is not required. Federal funding will not be allowed for sterilizations performed on persons in correctional facilities, mental hospitals, or other rehabilitative facilities, nor for hysterectomies performed solely for purposes of "rendering the person permanently incapable of reproduction." Adequate records of compliance must be maintained and in 3 years from the regulation taking effect DHEW will review the guidelines. DHEW states that a special monitoring program will be conducted to ensure compliance, but no sanctions for noncompliance are outlined in the regulations.[94,107]

Federal funding for abortion

The first anti-abortion legislation was passed in the United States in 1821 and by the 1860s antiabortion laws had been enacted by most of the states.[2,73,86] Although women continued to obtain abortions, the laws made abortion criminal. A few states struck down their restrictive abortion laws in the late 1960s and early 1970s, but it was not until the Supreme Court ruling of January 22, 1973,[23,81] that abortion became legally available throughout the United States. Medicaid funding was made available to cover abortions, and numerous needy women were served. In 1977, for example, nearly 295,000 Medicaid-eligible women obtained abortions, although another 133,000 eligible women who wanted them, did not, either because the services were unavailable to them or because the states had policies prohibiting such payments.[1]

In 1976, abortion opponents sought to further prohibit Medicaid payments. An amendment to the fiscal year 1977 Labor-DHEW appropriations bill was first introduced in June, 1976, by Representative Henry Hyde (Republican, Illinois) to prohibit the use of federal funds for abortion. After substantial debate, a compromise between Senate and House was passed, prohibiting the use of federal funds for abortion except in those cases in which "the life of the mother would be endangered if the fetus were carried to term." But the same day the bill went into effect, a temporary restraining order, followed by an injunction issued by Federal District Judge John F. Dooling, prevented the enforcement of Medicaid cutoffs until August 4, 1977.

Opponents of abortion gained support from the Hyde Amendment and organized, and some states began to pass restrictions on use of state Medicaid funds for abortion purposes. Suits were filed against two of these restrictive state policies, those in Connecticut and Pennsylvania. On June 20, 1977, the Supreme Court upheld the right of those states to withhold state Medicaid funds for abortion stating that: "The Equal Protection Clause [of the Constitution] does not require a state participating in the Medicaid program to pay the expenses incident to non-therapeutic abortion for indigent women simply because it has made a policy choice to pay expenses for childbirth."[7,51] The Court also decided that public hospitals were not required to provide nontherapeutic abortion services.[74] Dissenting, Justice Thurgood Marshall stated:

The impact of the regulations here [restricting public financing of abortions for the indigent] falls tragically upon those among us least able to help or defend themselves. As the Court well knows, these regulations inevitably will have the practical effect of preventing nearly all poor women from obtaining safe and legal abortions. . . . The enactments challenged here brutally coerce poor women to bear children whom society will scorn for every day of their lives. . . . I fear that the Court's decisions will be an invitation to public officials, already under extraordinary pressure from well-financed and carefully orchestrated lobbying campaigns, to approve more such restrictions. The effect will be to relegate millions of people to lives of poverty and despair. When elected leaders cower before public pressure, this Court, more than ever, must not shirk its duty to enforce the Constitution for the benefit of the poor and powerless.[54]

For fiscal year 1978, a similar amendment was proposed to the DHEW-Labor appropriations bill to curtail Medicaid funds, and again, after debate, a compromise was passed by Congress on December 7, 1977. It provided that

none of the funds contained in this paragraph [DHEW-Labor Appropriations] shall be used to perform abortions except where the life of the mother would be endangered if the fetus were carried to term; or except for such medical procedures necessary for the victims of rape or incest, when such rape or incest has been reported promptly to a law enforcement agency or public health service; or except in those instances where severe and long-lasting physical health damage to the mother would result if the pregnancy were carried to term when so determined by two physicians.[10]

Fiscal year 1979 saw the same amendment attempts, except in this year the House passed restrictions on Medicaid abortion funding that were even more severe: Medicaid funds were to be used only to fund abortions to save the woman's life. The first Hyde Amendment cut Medicaid funding for abortions by 99% (only 2421 abortions were performed in 1978 as compared with almost 300,000 in 1977). The last amendment whittles away at even the remaining 1%.

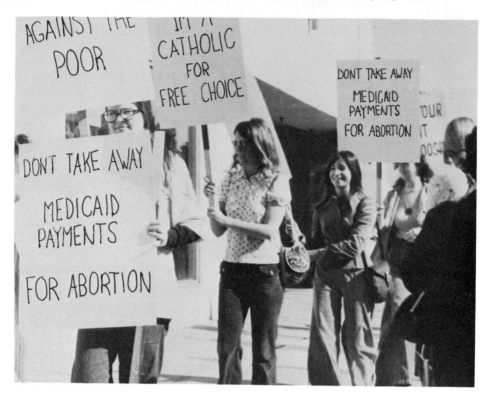

Fig. 3-10. Picketing for Medicaid funds for free choice in abortion. (Courtesy Anne Marie Deubl.)

Funding for abortions for military personnel and dependents through federal health plans was also abolished in 1978, and a similar amendment to the Defense Appropriations Bill was proposed for fiscal year 1979. As Congress becomes more conservative, even more restrictions can be anticipated.

In the face of congressional and Supreme Court support for restrictive Medicaid funding, most states have also limited the use of their Medicaid funds for abortions. As of February, 1979, 18 states still funded not only according to the federal criteria of 1978 for rape or incest victims, to save the woman's life, or to prevent long-lasting physical health damage to the woman. These states also funded abortions for women whose mental health would be endangered if the pregnancy were carried to term, for women who know their child will be born seriously deformed or diseased, for women who know their child is so deformed it will die soon after birth, and for older and young women who are outside appropriate childbearing years. Women in these latter categories are all prohibited by the Hyde Amendment from receiving federal Medicaid abortion funds.

The organized opposition to federal funding for abortions has not only had success in the Congress and in state legislatures but also has launched abortion clinic sit-ins,[84] arson and vandalism attacks on abortion clinics,[104] and harassment of abortion patients,[8] and has sought to publish names of physicians performing Medicaid abortions.[57] Most seriously, opponents and almost one third of the states have sought to call a Constitutional Convention for the purpose of amending the Constitution to outlaw abortion.[8]

Numerous organizations and groups who support a woman's right to choose abortion have launched massive drives for public prochoice affirmations but have been dogged by national apathy. Despite continued polls that show overwhelming national support for the 1973 abortion ruling,[60] apathy and incredulity that a Constitutional amendment prohibiting abortion could be passed prevail. Among the most active groups, and the largest single-issue lobbying group, is the National Abortion Rights Action League (NARAL), which works "to keep abortion safe, legal, and available for all women."[8] NARAL has filed amicus curiae briefs against several state and city ordinances that restrict abortion, publishes a newsletter monitoring antiabortion rights activities, and in addition to lobbying, provides expert testimony on the national need for safe, legal abortion.

Pregnancy disability

In 1976 the Supreme Court ruled that the authorization of maternity benefits under company-sponsored sickness disability plans was not the congressional intent of Title VII of the Civil Rights Act and referred the matter back to Congress for clarification.[47]

On October 31, 1978 an amendment to Title VII of the Civil Rights Act became effective, determining that employment discrimination includes pregnancy and requiring that employers with disability benefit plans must treat pregnancy in the same way as any other disability covered by the plan. The law also stipulated that women affected by pregnancy and related conditions be treated the same as any other employees on the basis of the ability or inability to work. Pregnant women cannot, therefore, be fired or forced to go on sick leave if they are able to go to work. Seniority benefits would also be retained during pregnancy-related absences.[15]

A compromise subamendment to the main amendment was also passed and gives employers discretion to exclude abortion coverage in their health and disability plans, except where the life of the mother would be endangered if the fetus were carried to term. The specific costs of the abortion can be excluded, but if a woman suffers complications from an abortion, medical payments and disability or sick leave benefits for the treatment of the complications would be covered.[9] However, in June, 1979, the United States Catholic Conference and the National Conference of Catholic Bishops filed a national class action suit on behalf of all employers who have objections to abortion on moral, religious, or ethical grounds. The suit's purpose is to restrain enforcement of this latter part of the pregnancy disability law and to disallow coverage for abortion-related disability.[106]

In essence, the pregnancy disability legislation reflects the reality that nearly half of the children in the United States have working mothers, and they are deprived of needed family income by denial of pregnancy-related benefits.

Equal Rights Amendment

The Equal Rights Amendment (ERA) reads as follows:

Section 1. Equality of rights under the law shall not be denied or abridged by the United States or any state on account of sex.

Section 2. The Congress shall have the power to enforce, by appropriate legislation the provisions of this article.

Section 3. This amendment shall take effect two years after the date of ratification.[38]

Equal rights amendments essentially identical to the current amendment have been introduced in nearly every Congress since 1923. Basically, ERA would stipulate that the law cannot treat men and women differently solely because of their sex.[13]

Women's health issues would be affected by passage of ERA, particularly regarding occupational health (see Chapter 5), athletic opportunities, and recognition of the equal obligations of both parents to support their children. Women will also be affected less directly, but nonetheless significantly, through revision of family laws, particularly those pertaining to women's economic rights within the family, revision of criminal laws, increased educational opportunities, and equal access to the armed forces and its benefits.

Opposition to ERA has used the spurious, yet emotionally charged, arguments that under the ERA homosexual marriage and coed toilets would be permitted. As a result, as of 1979, only 35 of the necessary 38 states had ratified this amendment. On August 15, 1978, the House of Representatives approved a 39-month ratification extension of the March 22, 1979, deadline, as did the Senate on October 6, 1978. The ERA is the stepping-stone for women's move from legislative equality to social equality.

National health insurance

Intermittently since the early 1900s, the subject of a national health insurance program has been aired. Since the advent of Medicaid and Medicare, and the continuously escalating health care costs of the 1970s, national health insurance has become a key issue.

There are currently several proposals before Congress,[46] and all but one are forms of health insurance plans that would not alter the delivery of health care services but would, to varying degrees, modify the current methods of payment. The Health Care Service Act[17] would essentially alter the mode of delivery by nationalizing health care facilities and by making providers employees of the National Health Service.

Issues of concern to women under any national health plan are coverage for complete maternity services, including contraception, abortion, genetic counseling, childbirth education, and those of alternative providers such as midwives and family practice physicians; coverage for home health services now generally provided by unpaid female relatives; recognition and coverage of women's use of two basic physicians, an internist and an obstetrician-gynecologist; adequate mental health services coverage, including support services for sexual assault victims and abused wives; and coverage for women that is independent of employment or marital or living arrangements.* At this time, despite much discussion and fanfare, no national health insurance program appears imminent.

Selected miscellaneous issues

Other health-related issues recently decided or still pending before federal or state bodies include a Massachusetts patients' rights bill, which, effective in August, 1979, permits civil suits for violations of a number of principles of good medical practice and informed consent. Provisions include the patient's right to know the attending physician's educational background, hospital affiliation, and financial interest in any medical facility, and—of special interest to women—the right for breast cancer patients to be fully informed about all alternative treatments that are medically viable.

Another right-to-be-informed bill became effective in New York State on September 1, 1978, and requires physicians and nurse-midwives attending the birth of a child to inform the expectant mother of the drugs they expect to administer during pregnancy and delivery, and to inform the mother of the possible effects.[92]

Other related actions in New York State include a decision by the New York Court of Appeals that failure to inform prospective parents of the possibility of their bearing defective children that they do subsequently bear is remediable through the courts,[63,67,72] and a bill mandating the State Commissioner of Health to launch a campaign to locate, screen, and assist in treatment of individuals exposed to diethylstilbestrol (DES).[64]

In Congress, Senate Bill 656, introduced by Daniel Inouye of Hawaii, would provide for the inclusion of certified nurse-midwifery services among those reimbursable by Medicare and Medicaid. Senate Bill 657, also by Inouye, would provide for access to a certified nurse-midwife without prior referral in the federal employee health benefits program.

A drug reform bill also pending in Congress has among its numerous provisions the requirement to make test data on new drugs available to the general public, prohibition of the exportation of drugs that have not received FDA approval, surveillance of approved drugs and their effects once they are on the market, inclusion of patient package inserts and improved patient information with all prescription drugs, improved patient informed consent procedures, improved regulatory powers to rapidly remove unsafe drugs from the market, public participation on drug advisory committees, controls on drug advertising and promotion, posting of comparative drug pricing, composition of a federal drug compendium, and establishment of a National Center for Clinical Pharmacology to independently test and research new and existing drugs.[43] Faced with strong lobbying from the pharmaceutical industry, Congress appears to be substantially amending this bill and limiting its progressive and public interest aspects. (An amended bill was voted out of Senator Edward Kennedy's health subcommittee in July, 1979.)

---

*References 3, 4, 40, 42, 46, 48, 62, 65.

One other health-related issue that received recent national attention is that of defining and prosecuting rape between a husband and wife.[78] The issue is beginning to be addressed by legislative actions in some states.[6,16]

• • •

The complexity, diversity, enormous costs, and incompleteness of federally funded programs and their related laws suggest that a comprehensive national health insurance program could more equitably and efficiently meet the nation's needs. Such a system would allow for a more rational distribution of the nation's resources; it is irrational, for example, to expend millions in a feeding program to ensure healthy mothers and children yet pay no attention to the early childhood and adolescent nutrition of girls and young women to ensure that they reach the childbearing years well nourished and able to produce healthy babies. Such a system would also alleviate the appearance of a two-class system of care frequently developed in response to the interests of organized medicine, (for example, maternal and child health services) but inevitably also fostered by government programs that serve the indigent as opposed to all citizens. Although the numerous programs discussed in this chapter have benefited millions, maintenance of a public and a private sector serves to divide a nation's health resources rather than rationally use them for the common good.

SUGGESTED TOPICS FOR DISCUSSION, FURTHER RESEARCH AND FIELD PROJECTS

1. What are the effects of lack of government support for abortion services? If funding has been cut in your area, investigate the effects. Has an illegal abortion market emerged? If funding has not been cut, what portion of the state budget is spent on abortion services?
2. Select a government program that benefits women. How does a woman qualify for the program? What are its benefits? Does the program contribute to maintaining the condition it attempts to alleviate? What factors contribute to the success/lack of success of the program? What, if any, similar services are provided by the private sector?
3. What are the differences between early Title V programs for mothers and children and present Title V programs? Whom do these programs mainly serve today? Does this population differ from that served previously? How has administration differed, if it has, in the two time periods?
4. What is the impact for women of the congressional decision that pregnancy is included under Title VII discrimination intent? How will this decision affect women's participation in the work force?
5. Research the lives of some early women pioneers in public health, for example, Dorothea Dix, Julia Lathrop, Martha Elliot, Jane Addams, and Josephine Baker. What contributions did these women make? How are their contributions incorporated into contemporary health programs?
6. What is the purpose of the 30-day waiting period in the sterilization guidelines? What are the pros and cons of this requirement? Is this waiting period in conflict with the concept of a woman's right to control her own body?
7. Research a selection of patient package inserts. Are these readable? What information can be learned from them? Do they need improvement? If so, what do you suggest? Research how widely distributed they are in your area.

8. Research a federally supported health-related program in your area. What is the target population for this program? Whom does it serve? What is its budget and what portions of this are spent on service delivery and administration? What are the political considerations of the program?
9. Compare several current national health insurance proposals. What benefits does each offer? What benefits does each offer from a women's health perspective? What effects do you anticipate these proposals will have on women's health?
10. How do a selection of the non–health-specific programs discussed in this chapter affect women's health? If you were organizing a national health system, how would you encompass the services these programs provide?

REFERENCES

1. Abortion and the poor: private morality, public responsibility, New York, 1979, Alan Guttmacher Institute.
2. Acevedo, Z.: Abortion in early America, Women & Health **4:**159-167, Summer, 1979.
3. American Public Health Association Standing Committee on Women's Rights: Women and health: some majority concerns, The Nation's Health, **9:**8-9, Aug., 1979.
4. American Public Health Association Task Force on National Health Insurance, Standing Committee on Women's Rights: Principles regarding women's issues and national health insurance, Washington, D.C., 1976, American Public Health Association.
5. Antonoff, M.: FDA to warn against aspirin's ill effects, Moneysworth **6,** March 14, 1977.
6. Associated Press: Man jailed in rape of wife, The Seattle Times, p. D5., Sept. 25, 1979.
7. *Beal* v. *Doe,* June 20, 1977.
8. Beals, J.: Current issues facing the right to abortion, Women & Health **4:**107-109, Spring, 1979.
9. Beard, E.: Beard Amendment, 1978.
10. Berger, L.: Abortions in America: the effect of restrictive funding, N. Engl. J. Med. **298:**1475-1477, 1978.
11. Blake, J. B.: Historical study of the New York City Department of Health, New York, 1951, published as Staff Report of the New York City Health Department with the permission of the Mayor's Committee on Management Survey, pp. 64-65.
12. Blake, J. B.: Origins of maternal and child health programs. In Rosenkrantz, B. G., editor: The health of women and children, New York, 1977, Arno Press.
13. Bonosaro, C., editor: Statement on the Equal Rights Amendment. Washington, D.C., 1978, United States Commission on Civil Rights, U.S. Government Printing Office (Clearinghouse publication 56).
14. Brieger, G. H.: The use and abuse of medical charities in late nineteenth century America, Am. J. Public Health **67:**264-267, March, 1977.
15. Bunch, P. L., et al.: The pregnant worker—who bears the burden? Women & Health **4:** 333-344, Winter, 1979.
16. City of Seattle: Proposed amendment to criminal code on sexual abuse, Aug. 15, 1979.
17. Committee for a National Health Service: A national health service—questions and answers, New York, 1975 (P.O. Box 2125, New York, N.Y. 10001).
18. Comprehensive Employment and Training Act, 1973.
19. Congressional Clearinghouse on Women's Rights: Domestic violence legislation **4:** 1-13, Washington, D.C., May 22, 1978.
20. Credé, K. S. F.: Die Verhutung der Augenentzundung der Neugeborenen, *Arch. Gynaekol.* **17:**50-53, 1881.
21. Datta, L.: Watchman, how is it with the child? Some aspects of child welfare policy from 1776 to 1976. In Grotberg, E. H., editor: Washington, D.C., 1977, Office of Child Development, Department of Health Education, and Welfare.
22. Davis, A.: American heroine: the life, and legend of Jane Addams, New York, 1973, Oxford University Press.
23. *Doe et al.* v. *Bolton,* no. 70-40, Jan. 22, 1973.
24. Donabedian, A., and Thorby, J. A.: The systemic impact of Medicare, Medical Care Review **26:**567-585, June, 1969.
25. Dreifus, C.: Sterilizing the poor. In Dreifus, C., editor: Seizing our bodies, New York, 1977, Vintage Books.
26. Drugs for human use: estrogens and other drugs, Federal Register **41:**43108, 1976.

27. Duffus, R. L.: Lillian Wald: neighbor and crusader, New York, 1938, Macmillan Publishing Co., Inc.

28. Equal Credit Opportunity Act, P.L. 93-495, Oct., 1974; Amended P.L. 94-239, 1976; and Section 808b, Housing and Community Development Amendments, 1978.

29. Executive Office of the President, Office of Management and Budget: 1978 catalog of federal domestic assistance, Washington, D.C., 1978, U.S. Government Printing Office.

30. FDA says doctors must give patients progestin warning, Medical World News **19:** 87-88, Nov. 13, 1978.

31. FDA wants birth defect warning on booze bottles and more PPIs, Medical World News, **18:**16, Nov. 14, 1977.

32. Food and Drug Administration: Press release on required patient package inserts, HEW News, June 29, 1979.

33. German, P. S., et al.: Health care of the elderly in medically disadvantaged populations, Gerontologist **18:**547-555, 1978.

34. Gold, E. M., and Stone, M. L.: Total maternal and infant care: a realistic appraisal, Am. J. Public Health **58:**1219-1229, 1968.

35. Goler, G. W.: Methods adopted by the Board of Health at Rochester, New York, to secure better milk for infants, Arch. Pediatr. **14:**845, 1897.

36. Goodwin, E. R.: A tabular statement of infant welfare work by public and private agencies in the United States, Infant Mortality Series, no. 5, U.S. Children's Bureau, Washington, D.C., 1916, U.S. Government Printing Office.

37. *Gordon W. Douglas, M.D., et al.* v. *John L. S. Holloman, Jr., et al.* Civil Action File No. 76, Cw 6 U.S. District Court, Jan. 5, 1976.

38. H.R.J. Res. 208, 92nd Congress, 1st Session, 86 Stat. 1523, 1971.

39. Implementation of coverage of suppliers of end stage services, Federal Register **41:** 22502-22522, June 3, 1976.

40. Insurance Commissioner's Advisory Task Force on Women's Insurance Problems: Final report and recommendations, Harrisburg, Pa., June, 1974, Pennsylvania Insurance Department.

41. Intrauterine contraceptive device: professional and patient labeling, Federal Register **40:**27796, 1975.

42. Kasper, A. S.: Women and national health insurance, The Spokeswoman **8:**7-8, Oct. 15, 1977

43. Kasper, A. S.: Major drug reform legislation now in congress. The Spokeswoman **9:**6, July 15, 1978.

44. Krauss, E.: Hospital survey on sterilization policies: Reproductive Freedom Project, ACLU Reports, March, 1975.

45. Leavitt, J. W., and Numbers, R. L.: Sickness and health in America: readings in the history of medicine and public health, Madison, Wis, 1978, University of Wisconsin Press.

46. Lewis, D.: Women and national health insurance: issues and solutions, Medical Care **14:**549-558, July, 1976.

47. Macfarlane, D. R.: Maternity and employment benefits in the United States—where are we now? Women & Health **1:**21-26, Jan/Feb., 1976.

48. Madar, O. M.: Discrimination against women in current health insurance programs, presented to the Women's Leadership Rally on National Health Insurance, March 9-10, 1976, Washington, D.C.

49. Madison, D. L.: Organized health care and the poor, Medical Care Review **26:**783-807, Aug., 1969.

50. *Madrigal* v. *Quilligan,* CA No. 75-2057 (C.D. Cal., 1975).

51. *Maher* v. *Roe,* June 20, 1977.

52. Marshall, H.: Dorothea Dix, forgotten Samaritan, Chapel Hill, N.C., 1937, University of North Carolina Press.

53. Marshall, J. K.: Cited in The role of HEW's Bureau of Community Health Services, Women & Health Roundtable Report **2:** 1-6, May/June, 1978.

54. Marshall, T.: Dissenting opinion in *Maher* v. *Roe, Beal* v. *Doe* and *Poelker* v. *Doe,* June 20, 1977.

55. McGarraugh, R. E.: Sterilization without consent: teaching hospital violation of HEW regulations, Washington, D.C., Jan., 1975. Public Citizen's Health Research Group.

56. McIntosh, D., Supplemental Food Programs Division, Department of Agriculture, Washington, D.C.: Personal communication, May 4, 1979.

57. M.D.s lose suit on abortion privacy, American Medical News **21,** Dec. 8, 1978.

58. Medical Information System: Number of chronic renal disease beneficiaries ever en-

rolled since 7/1/73, Washington, D.C., June 30, 1979, Health Care Financing Administration.

59. Mintz, M.: The Medicare business, series of eight articles, The Washington Post, June 27, 1976 to July 4, 1976.

60. Mulhauser, K.: Report, NARAL Newsletter, **11:**2,3,7, July, 1979.

61. Mulligan, J. E.: Three federal interventions on behalf of childbearing women: the Sheppard-Towner Act, Emergency Maternity and Infant Care and the Maternal and Child Health and Mental Retardation Amendments of 1963, doctoral dissertation, University of Michigan, Ann Arbor, 1976.

62. Naierman, N., et al.: Sex discrimination in insurance, a guide for women, Washington, D.C., 1977, Women's Equity Action League (WEAL).

63. New York genetic risk case stirs controversy, The Nation's Health **9:**6, Feb., 1979.

64. New York State legislates pregnancy drug information, ACOG Newsletter, **22,** Oct., 1978.

65. New York State Task Force on Critical Problems: Insurance and women, Albany, N. Y., Oct., 1974.

66. OCs to be accompanied by brochures starting April 4, Family Practice News, March 15, 1978.

67. Oelsner, L.: Doctor held liable in abnormal births, New York Times, Dec. 28, 1978.

68. Oral contraceptive drug products: physician and patient labeling, Federal Register **41:**53633, 1976.

69. Pardee, R., Deputy Director, Office of Maternal and Child Health, Bureau of Community Health Services, U.S. Department of Health, Education and Welfare, Washington, D.C.: Personal communication, July, 1978.

70. Pardee, R., Deputy Director, Office of Maternal and Child Health, Bureau of Community Health Services, U.S. Department of Health, Education and Welfare, Washington, D.C.: Personal communication, April, 1979.

71. Patters, P., Office. of Professional Standards Review Organization, Division of Peer Review, U.S. Department of Health, Education and Welfare, Washington, D.C.: Personal communication, July 13, 1979.

72. Pearse, W. H.: ACOG Director: New York case may be precedent, The Nation's Health **9:**7, Feb., 1979.

73. Pilpel, H., et al.: Abortion: public issue, private decision, Public Affairs Pamphlet, no. 527, Sept., 1975.

74. *Poelker* v. *Doe,* June 20, 1977.

75. Public Law 95-623, signed Nov. 9, 1978.

76. *Relf* v. *Weinberger,* 372 Federal Supplement 1196, (D.D.C., 1974).

77. Requirements for patient labeling for progestational drug products, Federal Register **43:**47181, Oct. 13, 1978.

78. The Rideouts: case closed, issue open — questions on Oregon's landmark rape case, The Washington Post, p. B1, Dec. 12, 1978.

79: Rodriguez-Trias, H.: Guidelines on sterilization under attack, Women & Health **1:**30-31, Jan/Feb., 1976.

80. Rodriguez-Trias, H.: Sterilization abuse, The Women's Center, Reid Lectureship, Nov. 10-11, 1976, New York, 1978, Barnard College.

81. *Roe* v. *Wade,* no. 70-18, Jan. 22, 1973.

82. Rosen, G.: A history of public health, New York, 1958, M.D. Publications.

83. Rosen, G.: The first neighborhood health center movement — its rise and fall. Am. J. Public Health **61:**1620-1637, Aug., 1971.

84. Rosenfeld, M.: Foes of abortion sit in to "save lives," The Washington Post, Aug. 9, 1978.

85. Rothenberg, R.: Ophthalmia neonatorum due to Neisseria gonorrhea: prevention and treatment, Sex. Transm. Dis. **6**(suppl. A): 187-191, Sept., 1979.

86. Ryan, M. P.: Womanhood in America: from colonial times to the present, New York, 1975, New Viewpoints.

87. Schmidt, R. T. F.: ACOG president explains suit, ACOG Newsletter **21:**4, Sept., 1977.

88. Sinai, N., and Anderson, O. W.: EMIC (emergency maternity and infant care): a study of administrative experience, New York, 1974, Arno Press, Inc.

89. Slater, J.: Sterilization: newest threat to the poor, Ebony, p. 150, Oct., 1973.

90. Smillie, W.: Public health, its promise for the future, a chronicle of the development of public health in the United States, 1607-1914, New York, 1955, Macmillan Publishing Co., Inc.

91. Somers, H. M., and Somers, A. R.: Medicare and the hospitals: issues and prospects, Washington, D.C., 1967, The Brookings Institution.

92. State of New York, 13104, June 12, 1978. Signed, July 20, 1978.
93. Sterilization abuse of women: the facts, Health/Pac Bull., no. 62, Jan./Feb., 1975.
94. Sterilizations and abortions: federal financial participation, Federal Register **43:** 52146, Nov. 8, 1978.
95. Uri charges IHS with genocide policy, Hospital Tribune **11,** Aug., 1977.
96. U.S. Children's Bureau: Baby-saving campaigns: a preliminary report on what American cities are doing to prevent infant mortality, Infant Mortality Series no. 1, Washington, D.C., 1913, U.S. Government Printing Office.
97. U.S. Congress, House Subcommittee on Appropriations: Hearings on the First Supplemental National Defense Appropriation Bill, 1944, 78th Congress, 1st Session, Sept. 21, 1943.
98. U.S. General Accounting Office: Report to Hon. James C. Abourezk, B 164031(5), Nov., 1976.
99. U.S. Health Services Administration, Bureau of Community Health Services: Maternal and child health programs' legislative base, Washington, D.C., 1977, U.S. Government Printing Office. (Source: Rules and regulations for Title V of the Social Security Act, Subpart A of Part 51a as amended on Nov. 20, 1975, Federal Register **40.**)
100. U.S. Public Health Service: 200 years of child health in America. In Grotberg, E. H., ed: 200 years of children, no. (OHD) 77-30103, Washington, D.C., 1977. Office of Child Development, U.S. Department of Health, Education, and Welfare.
101. Vaughan, D., and Sparer, G.: Ethnic group and welfare status of women sterilized in federally funded family planning programs, Fam. Plann. Perspect. **6:**224-229, 1974.
102. Vazquez-Calzada, J.: La esterilización femenina en Puerto Rico, Revista de Ciencias Sociales **17:**281-308, Sept., 1973.
103. Venereal Disease Control Law Summary, July 1, 1972, Atlanta, Center for Disease Control.
104. Violence against the right to choose, Washington, D.C., Aug., 1979, National Abortion Rights Action League.
105. VonBargen, P., et al., editors: Health career opportunity grants for the disadvantaged. Health Resources Opportunity Programs, no. (HRA) 78-624, U.S. Department of Health, Education and Welfare, Washington, D.C., Feb., 1978, U.S. Government Printing Office.
106. Werner, C.: Pregnancy disability law: round two, NARAL Newsletter **11:**6, Aug., 1979.
107. Wolcott, I., editor: Regulations covering all federally funded sterilizations, Women & Health Roundtable Report **2:**3-4, Nov., 1978.
108. Woolston, H. B.: Prostitution in the U.S., Patterson Smith Reprint Series, New York, 1969.
109. Younger, M., and Hickman, P., Food and Nutrition Service, U.S. Department of Agriculture: Personal communications, May 11, 1979.

ADDITIONAL READINGS

Ad Hoc Women's Studies Committee Against Sterilization Abuse: Workbook on sterilization, Women's Studies, Sarah Lawrence College, 1978, Bronxville, N.Y.

Benson, H., et al.: Patient education and intrauterine contraception: a study of two package inserts, Am. J. Public Health **67:**446-449, May, 1977.

Blake, J.: The Supreme Court's abortion decisions and public opinion in the United States, Population and development Rev. **3:**45-62, March and June, 1977.

Bourque, D., et al., editors: Chartbook of federal health spending, 1969-1974, Washington, D.C., Aug., 1974, Center for Health Policy Studies, National Planning Association.

Burns, E. M.: The role of government in health services, Bull. N.Y. Acad. Med. **41:**753-794, 1965.

Cadena, M. A., and Trevino, M. C.: Utilization barriers to maternal-child health care programs of the urban low-income, Mexican-American family: implications for a national health policy, presented at the American Public Health Association Annual Meeting, Nov. 1, 1977, Washington, D.C.

Committee for Abortion Rights and Against Sterilization Abuse: CARASA News, CARASA, P.O. Box 124, Cathedral Station, New York, N.Y. 10025.

Caress, B.: Sterilization guidelines, Health/PAC Bull., no. 65, July/Aug., 1975.

Committee to End Sterilization Abuse (CESA): Sterilization abuse: the facts, CESA, Box A244, Cooper Station, New York, N.Y. 10003.

Chapman, C. B., and Talmadge, J. M.: The evolution of the right to health concept in the United States, the Pharos of Alpha Omega Alpha **34:**30-51, Jan., 1971.

Congressional Clearinghouse on Women's Rights, 722 HOB Annex No. 1, Washington, D.C. 20515, (202) 225-2947. (Readers may request to be added to mailing list through their local Congressperson.)

Cook, R. J., and Dickens, B. M.: A decade of international change in abortion law: 1967-1977, Am. J. Public Health **68:**637-644, 1978.

Cooper, W. K.: Maternity disability benefits: why not compromise? Personnel **54:**34-40, March/April, 1977.

Fleckenstein, L., et al.: Oral contraceptive patient information, J.A.M.A. **235:**1331-1336, 1976.

Fleshood, H. L., et al.: Is WIC reducing the prevalence of low birthweight and infant mortality? presented at the American Public Health Association Annual Meeting, Oct. 17, 1978, Los Angeles.

Food and Drug Administration Contractor's final report: survey of consumer's perceptions of patient package inserts for oral contraceptives, PB 248-739, Washington, D.C., 1975, NTIS.

Gray, A., editor: The Federal Monitor, Drawer Q, McLean, Va. 22101.

Gutwillig, J. G., chairperson: Interpretation of the Equal Rights Amendment in accordance with legislative history, Washington, D.C., Jan., 1974, Citizens' Advisory Council on the Status of Women.

Hertz, S. H.: The politics of the welfare mothers movement: a case study, Signs **2:**600-611, Spring, 1977.

House of Representatives, 94th Congress: Supplemental hearings before the Subcommittee on Health and the Environment of the Committee on Interstate and Foreign Commerce, Hearings on Bills H.R. 12937, 14309, and 14882 to establish a national system of maternal and child health care, and H.R. 14497 to establish a national health insurance system for maternal and child health care.

Hovey, M.: A doughty lady turns 50, Manpower **2,** March, 1970, reprinted Women's Bureau, Department of Labor, 1970.

Jaffe, F. S.: Public policy on fertility control, Sci. Am. **229:**17-23, July, 1973.

Johnson, A.: FDA: a slow starter and a slow runner, Trial **12:**22-25, Oct., 1976.

Johnson, A.: Letter to hearing clerk, Food and Drug Administration, regarding patient labeling for post-menopausal estrogens, Dec. 30, 1976.

Makarushka, J. L.: Workers' compensation: the long-term consequences of work-related injury for women, Sociology Department, Health Studies Program, Maxwell School, Syracuse University, 1977, Syracuse, N.Y.

Mechanic, D.: Considerations in the design of mental health benefits under national health insurance, Am. J. Public Health **68:**482-488, May, 1978.

Moore, K. A., and Caldwell, S. B.: The effect of government policies on out-of-wedlock sex and pregnancy, Fam. Plann. Perspect. **9:**164-169, 1977.

Muller, C. F.: Insurance coverage of abortion, contraception and sterilization, Fam. Plann. Perspect. **10:**71-77, March-April, 1978.

National Women's Health Network: An action index to your resources in Washington, Washington, D.C., June, 1977, National Women's Health Network.

North, F. A.: National health insurance for mothers and children, Am. J. Dis. Child. **13:** 17-20, Jan., 1977.

Reid, O. M., et al.: The American health-care system and the poor: a social organizational point of view, Welfare in Review **6:**1-12, Dec., 1968.

Report of the Second White House Conference on Standards of Child Welfare, Washington, D.C., 1920, United States Government Printing Office. (See particularly Appendix II: Minimum Standards for Public Protection of the Health of Mothers, 1919.)

Rettig, R. A.: The policy debate on patient care financing for victims of end stage renal disease, Law and Contemporary Problems **40:** 196-230, Autumn, 1976.

Roemer, M. I.: National health insurance as an agent for containing health-care costs, Bull. N.Y. Acad Med., second series, **54:**102-111, 1978.

Roemer, M. I., and Axelrod, S. J.: A national health service and Social Security, Am. J. Public Health **67:**462-465, May, 1977.

Rombauer, M. D.: Marital status and eligibility for federal statutory income benefits: a historical survey, Washington Law Review **52:**227-288, 1977.

Rosenfeld, B., et al.: A health research group's study on surgical sterilization: present abuses and proposed regulations, Washington, D.C., Oct., 1973, Health Research Group.

Ryan, K. J.: The FDA and the practice of medicine, N. Engl. J. Med. **297:**1287-1288, 1977.

Rye, J., and White, M.: Does objective based health education affect positive changes in the health status of WIC program clients? presented at the American Public Health Association Annual Meeting, Oct. 17, 1978, Los Angeles, Calif.

Schmidt, A. M.: Educating the public about health, J. Med. Educ. **50:**124-129, Feb., 1975.

Tenenbaum, S.: Women's Washington Report, 324 C Street, S.E., Washington, D.C. 20003, (202) 547-6606.

U.S. Public Health Service: Forward plan for health FY 1978-1982, no. 017-000-00172-8, Washington, D.C., Aug., 1976, United States Government Printing Office.

Wilner, D., et al.: Introduction to public health, New York, 1973, Macmillan Publishing Co., Inc. (See particularly Chapters 12 and 13.)

Wolcott, I., editor: Maternal and child health programs and policies, report on presentation by R. Hanft, Women & Health Roundtable Report **2,** Nov., 1978.

Wynn, K.: Second thoughts about sterilization, SISTER, 1977, 250 Howard Ave., New Haven, Conn. 06519.

Chapter 4

Women in the health care work force

HISTORICAL BACKGROUND

Women have always worked to provide health care. Although assisting in childbirth was a natural task for women, their role in health service delivery has not been limited to this function. Since the earliest priestess-physicians, women have been surgeons, internists, dentists, nurses, midwives, medical professors, public health workers, and hospital administrators as well as herb gatherers and lay healers.[43]

The exact number of women involved in any of these occupations is unknown. It is assumed, probably correctly, that in some fields, particulary surgery and dentistry, there were few females. The periods with waves of women's influence in medical care were probably a result of social and economic forces like those which are affecting women's participation today. For example, contemporary issues of access to university education, licensure, stratification of personnel and the attendant delegation of tasks and privileges, church influence on medical care, maldistribution of health personnel, shortage of males for the work force, and economic motivation all have their historical counterparts.

Since the establishment of universities, principally from the thirteenth century on, the admission of women to higher education and subsequently to licensure, has been blocked by Church, State, and social convention.[11] Surgical techniques and medical advances have been closely guarded secrets within a small male elite. The obstetrical forceps developed by the Chamberlen family in seventeenth-century England and kept secret by them for almost a century exemplify this, although Peter Chamberlen, III, offered to share his secret with the midwives on condition they agreed to work under his authority. After their refusal, the "secret" of the forceps was eventually disbursed among male obstetricians.[69]

Various types of women practitioners, for example empirics (apprentices to university-trained physicians), midwives, and nurses of the sixteenth and seventeenth centuries and registered nurses and licensed practical nurses of contemporary times, have been led to compete against each other in struggles for professional recognition and status.[59] Most dramatically, women healers have been the victims of open harassment and murder, especially during the fourteenth and fifteenth century witch-hunts in Europe when the "healing witch" was particularly vilified for her unauthorized (by the Church) practices, particularly her use of herbs and potions, believed by many to be the work of sorcery and the devil.[40]

Licensure

The issues of access to education, and therefore licensure, have probably had the greatest impact on women's role in the work force. Ostensibly, licensure functions to protect the public from quackery and unscrupulous practitioners, but it also functions to limit and control access to a profession. By establishing criteria, particularly educational criteria, certain groups of people may be excluded. In many instances this is of social benefit; in many other cases, however, licensure has served to benefit only a chosen few. The evolution of medical licensure is intricately interwoven with excluding women from medical practice.

From the twelfth century on, records exist of licensure laws and educational requirements for those who wanted to practice medicine. In 1224 Frederick II, Holy Roman Emperor, obliged a candidate for medicine to give evidence of elaborate classical studies. In 1225 he attempted to confer by authoritative Bull licenses to graduates of his new school at Naples. Gregory IX followed suit in 1229 in Toulouse, as did most of the other universities in the following years.

However, as early as 1220 the University of Paris had prohibited all from practicing medicine except their faculty, and since only bachelors could be admitted to this honor, an effective exclusion of women from the prestigious positions of medical practice began. The most famous test of this ruling came in 1322 when Jacoba Félicie de Almania was charged with practicing medicine without a license and was arraigned before the Court of Justice at Paris by the dean and masters of the faculty of Medicine.[56] She argued her case brilliantly on the grounds of the appropriateness of women being able to treat women. Despite much testimony about her skills and the lack of testimony, even in the charges against her, describing incompetence, she lost the case and was forced from practice. Since she had not been approved by them the faculty argued she must therefore be utterly ignorant in the art of medicine. Regarding her cures, they said they were "certain that a man approved in the aforesaid art could cure the sick better than such a woman."[47]

The ecclesiastical backing of licensure continued. In 1325 Pope John XXII urged Stephen, Bishop of Paris, to cooperate with the faculty to prevent all those ignorant of medicine from practicing in the city. In 1347 and 1350 the faculty again petitioned the Papacy for assistance.[11] Because of the educational barriers, women were still excluded.

By 1352 John Le Bon of France legalized the practice of medicine by specially qualified women and accorded equality between men and women surgeons,[9] although Guy de Chauliac (1300-1370), the influential surgeon, continued to favor exclusion of women because of their sex. Over the next 150 years in France, highly limited licensure was granted to women for specific tasks.

In England, where the universities were tightly closed to women, licensure based on education was particulary exclusionary. Although fourteenth-century records do mention some women being licensed, and although Queen Philippa (1314-1369), wife of Edward III, reputedly had a female surgeon in her services (Cecilia of Oxford), opposition to female licensing was organized and vocal. In 1421 a petition was submitted to Henry V (1387-1422) requesting that "no woman use the practice of fisyk (medicine) under payne of long imprisonment."

A subsequent draft of an act of Parliament in 1422 required all physicians, male and female, to be university graduates; women were thereby effectively excluded.[60]

In an act of 1511 Henry VIII established the College of Physicians and Surgeons and gave it, together with the Archbishop of Canterbury, the power of medical licensure throughout the realm. The act was directed at the "great multitude of ignorant persons," among whom were "common artificers, as smythes, weavers, and women" who took upon themselves "great cures and things of great difficulty in the whiche they partly use sorcerye and witchcrafte and noisome medicine."[41] This marks the beginning of effective regulation of medical practice in England.

The history of licensure in the United States has been well documented.[63] Although without doubt it has in many instances served the public good, one of the issues, the question of equitable access to the education that is a prerequisite for licensing, is still not resolved. Among other unresolved issues are those of vertical versus horizontal control (more skilled practitioners controlling the practice of those less skilled versus practitioners of equal skill regulating each other) and autonomous versus dependent practice (practitioners working independently versus working in a "team" concept with more skilled practitioners). There is also the overriding issue of consumer choice of provider, which licensing, by definition, limits. The controls exercised by licensure are particularly evident today with the resurgence of interest in midwifery. Many women want to use the services of midwives, and many others believe their practical experience acquired through attending several births has prepared them to sit the relevant state licensing examinations. Their lack of formal education and training is grounds for non-licensure in most states, although a few — for example, Maryland and Louisiana — in theory permit licensing by examination designed to prove competency.[81] Contemporary challenges to the law are still rare.[74] *Tait's Magazine* in June, 1841, made the following comment with surprisingly contemporary insight:

The accoucheur's is a profession nearly altogether wrested out of the hands of women, for which Nature has surely fitted them, if opinion permitted education to finish Nature's work. But women are held in the bonds of ignorance, and then pronounced of deficient capacity, or blamed for wanting the knowledge they are sternly prevented from acquiring.[44]

Midwives

In the United States, women's involvement in what would become modern medicine began with the arrival of the Mayflower and Mrs. Fuller, a midwife. She served until her death in 1664. Records are sketchy, but we do know that from 1620 until the growth of the Popular Health Movement in the 1830s and 1840s healing women worked chiefly as midwives, kitchen physics (visiting practitioners), and lay healers, both at home and in the community. A few were physicians.

Among the most notable of the midwives was Anne Hutchinson, who as a midwife, religious leader of the Antinomian dissidents, and a frequent organizer of women's meetings posed a threat to the stability of the Massachusetts Bay Colony by challenging the accepted definitions of God and divinity. Discredited when she attended the delivery of Mary Dyer, who gave birth to a deformed baby and when she herself expelled a hydatidiform mole, Hutchinson went to Rhode Island and then Pelham, New York, where she was killed in an Indian raid.[6]

Some of the other midwives recorded in the colonies were Widows Potter and Bradly, Goodwife Beecher, Elizabeth Phillips, the mother of William Lloyd Garrison, Margaret Jones, and Mrs. Wiat, for whom the town's epitaph written in 1705 read: "She assisted at ye births of one thousand, one hundred and odd children." However, the records do not show where these women trained, nor any details of their lives. Some undoubtedly acquired their skills in Europe and others by book and "clinical" experience. Some women were apprenticed to other midwives or physicians. Perhaps an argument for the importance of productive careers for women lies in the fact that many of these women had exceptionally long lives even by contemporary standards, living well into their eighties and nineties (this was also true of several women healers in Europe). Philadelphia records an "Elegy on the Death of the Ancient, Venerable, and Useful Matron and Midwife Mrs. Mary Broadwell, who rested from her labors, January 2, 1730, aged one hundred years and one day.[53]

Governmental regulation of the practice of both midwives and physicians in the United States seems to have first existed in the French colonies of Louisiana. A midwife named Marie Gissot successfully challenged the governor's regulations in refusing to nurse soldiers. Since many of them had scurvy, she argued that she might contaminate her midwifery cases. Between 1722 and 1723 three French midwives were examined by a committee of six physicians in Louisiana. Although they had diplomas from several European institutions, one woman was classed as a nurse or inferior midwife rather than as a skilled "obstetrician" and it was voted "she not be allowed to terminate labor before the arrival of a physician." The others were deemed fully competent for unsupervised practice.[43]

From 1760 on, licensure by examination existed in New York, and other states soon followed. Many experienced midwives who had previously been certified simply on the grounds of an oath "to be kind to the poor as well as the rich, and not to listen to lies as to the father of a baby, nor conceal the birth of bastards, nor produce miscarriages, nor operate needlessly on any women" still practiced, nonetheless.[36]

However, in 1753 James Lloyd had returned from Europe and introduced the fashion of male midwives. Despite protestations such as those of Dr. W. Beach, editor of the *American Practice of Medicine,* who charged that "prior to the sixteenth century not half the number of women died in childbirth as have died in a like period of time since the advent of the man-midwife,"[28] midwifery was doomed as an open avenue of employment for women in the health field.

In 1765 William Shippen, Jr., of Philadelphia proposed a course in midwifery for both men and women, and even as late as 1817 Dr. Thomas Ewell of Washington, D.C., proposed an elaborate scheme to establish a lying-in hospital where women might be instructed in midwifery. But opposition was vocal and strong from the developing medical establishment. Ewell's idea was finally rejected by the physicians, who, fearing competition, rationalized that midwives needed a total medical education and that licensure would merely legitimize second-class obstetrical care. Considering the prohibitions against women obtaining that medical education, such rationalizations accelerated the midwives' decline. Midwifery as an occupation was left with little prestige, although until the early twentieth century many midwives continued to work among the poor, immigrant working classes, blacks, and rural families.

At the beginning of the twentieth century it was estimated that midwives, both the "granny" and more formally trained, attended 50% of the nation's births. Although various studies and surveys in the early 1900s, including those of Williams and Baker, showed little difference in incidence of sepsis and fetal outcome between physician- and midwife-attended deliveries, the opposition to midwives and the stereotype of the dirty, drunk midwife were overwhelming.[21] Despite the lack of definitive data, Williams concluded in 1912 that "reform (in obstetrics) is urgently needed and can be accomplished more speedily by radical improvement in medical education than by attempting the almost impossible task of improving midwives."[78]

Two schools kept the midwife concept alive in the United States – the New York Maternity Center Association's school founded in 1931 and the Kentucky Frontier Nursing Service's school founded in 1939. Both have done much toward fostering today's growth of nurse-midwives as valued health team members.

Physicians

Records of women physicians of the early colonies are even more sketchy than those of midwives. Some of the names available, although with few details, include Jane Hawkins, Doctress Joanna Smith (cousin to Anne Hutchinson), Mrs. Ann Eliot of Roxbury, Massachusetts, Sarah Sands – the doctor of Block Island, Rhode Island – and Mrs. Allyn, who received 20 pounds for her services as an army surgeon.[43]

In spite of early attempts at licensure of physicians, the concept was not firmly established until the 1880s. Although several states had licensure laws by 1830, these were soon repealed during the 1840s and 1850s under the influence of the Popular Health Movement and its eclectics.[62]

The Popular Health Movement, formed by a coalition of feminists and working-class radicals, sought a total redefinition of health care. It drew support from all elements of a society that was becoming increasingly liberal, hostile to all professionalism, and generally disenchanted with physicians' arrogance and their noticeable lack of curative success. Members viewed the body and mind not as separate entities but as important factors in a person's well-being. Balance of these factors had to be achieved for health.[45]

Various sects within the Popular Health Movement had individual theories, such as hydropathy, herbalism, animal magnetism, and homeopathy on how to achieve this balance. This lack of unity undoubtedly contributed to the movement's decline, but several significant changes occurred nonetheless. One was the formation of Ladies' Physiological Reform Societies. In an effort to combat growing female invalidism – the fashion of middle- and upper-class women to be weak, helpless, and sickly – lectures on elementary anatomy, sex, general hygiene, diet, sensible dress (no corsets), and contraception were given to interested groups of women. Teachers often were graduates of the female sectarian medical colleges established by sects in the Popular Health Movement.

These numerous schools opened up medical education for women and blacks. One teacher was Lydia Folger Fowler (1822-1879). After graduation in 1850 from the Central Medical College of New York, which taught eclecticism and homeopathy, Fowler was appointed professor of midwifery at one of the college's splinter schools, the Rochester Eclectic Medical College. She thus became the first woman professor in a legally authorized medical school in the United States.[47]

The Popular Health Movement and its efforts to open the health profession to women faced strong opposition from the American Medical Association (AMA). Formed in 1847 as the professional organization of one sect, the allopaths, the AMA was all male, white, and well organized. Its opposition was served by the Flexner Report of 1910,[7] which, in establishing standards for medical education, effectively produced the decline of all marginal and proprietary medical schools; women had been disproportionately concentrated in these schools. Only one school, the Woman's Medical College of Pennsylvania founded in 1850, remained open for women; now the Medical College of Pennsylvania, it admitted its first male students in 1970.

Although the Popular Health Movement as a whole became in time more institutionalized into neo-Thomsonianism and eclecticism and was ultimately submerged by the regular schools, it did substantially alter the numbers of women physicians and foster demands among them for admission to regular medical schools.

Following Elizabeth Blackwell's historic achievement in 1849 of being the first woman graduate from a regular medical college, other notable women quickly joined the ranks of practitioners: Hannah Myers Longshore (1851), Nancy Talbot Clarke (1852), Harriet K. Hunt (1853), Emily Blackwell (1854), and Marie Zakrzewska (1856), who founded the New England Hospital for women and children in 1862.[58] By 1877 there were five hospitals managed by and for women, and between 1850 and 1895 19 medical schools for women had been established, including the Blackwells' Women's Medical College, part of their New York infirmary (see Fig. 4-1). The New England Female Medical College, chartered in 1856, granted the first medical degree to a black woman, Rebecca Lee, in 1864.[44]

By 1881, 470 women were known to have taken medical degrees (excluding graduates of eclectic and homeopathic schools). To a questionnaire sent out, 300 full replies were received, and partial information was obtained on 130 more. Dr. Sophia Jex-Blake, herself a graduate of the Blackwells' school, described the findings:

Of these 430 women, 390 are found to be engaged in active practice, 11 have never practiced at all, while 29 have practiced for a time and then retired. Of the latter, 12 have ceased practice on account of marriage, 7 from ill-health, 5 have engaged in other work, while the remainder give no reasons. These women are scattered over twenty-six States of the Union, New York, Pennsylvania and Massachusetts having the largest number. There are, so far as we know, no women physicians in the Southern States, with the exception of Maryland, Virginia, West Virginia, and Texas; also none in Arkansas, Kentucky, and

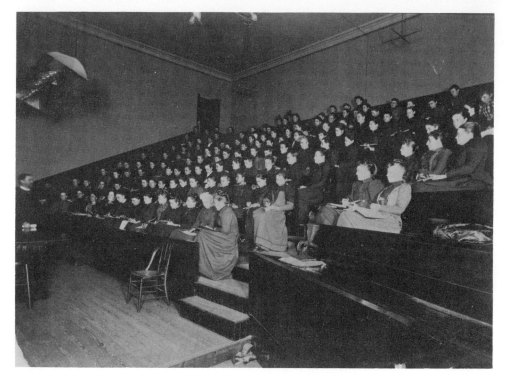

Fig. 4-1. Classroom scene, 1890. (Courtesy Archives and Special Collections on Women in Medicine of the Medical College of Pennsylvania, Philadelphia.)

Nevada. While Boston, New York, Philadelphia, and Chicago have each quite a large number, many of the answers have come from small villages and towns. Seventy-five percent were single on beginning the study of medicine, 19 percent were married, and 6 percent were widows. Their average age was twenty-seven years, and the average time of study before engaging in practice was four and a half years.

From 362 replies to enquiries respecting the financial results of practice, it appeared that 226 were satisfied with their position, and that most of the remainder had been in practice too short a time to give a definite answer. Only 11 out of the 362 seem to have practiced over two years and to have failed to become self-supporting.

Beside their work in private practice, thirty-four percent of this list of physicians are or have been employed as attending or resident physicians in various institutions. The most distinctive work of women in this direction has been the founding and management of hospitals and dispensaries for women and children in several of the large cities.[44]

Many of these women had been educated either at the Woman's Medical College of Pennsylvania or the Blackwells' school (see Fig. 4-2). Others were educated at the Department of Medicine and Surgery of the University of Michigan at Ann Arbor, which had been open to women since 1879. Syracuse University was incorporated on March 25, 1870, and, unlike the University of Michigan, did not hold separate classes for women. Their first female medical graduates

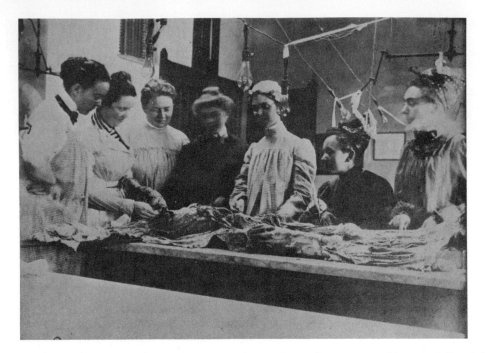

Fig. 4-2. Students in anatomy laboratory, about 1903. (Courtesy Archives and Special Collections on Women in Medicine of the Medical College of Pennsylvania, Philadelphia.)

were in 1875. The University of California at Berkeley was organized in 1868 and admitted women "on equality with men," although they comprised only about one-fifth of any class. Attendance at three full courses of 5 months was required before graduation in medicine. The Universities of Iowa, Minnesota, Colorado, Oregon, and Buffalo soon followed; Columbian College in Washington, D.C. (later George Washington University) admitted women in 1882 but 10 years later refused them. Johns Hopkins University also admitted women, but initially, writes Richard Shryock, "women students were allowed to examine men only above the neck—here male modesty entered the picture—with resulting embarrassment when women were later assigned to men's wards."[62] However, male modesty soon dissolved with the economic incentive of an endowment of almost a half-million dollars from Elizabeth Garrett Anderson, an English physician who served as Dean of the London School of Medicine for Women from 1883 to 1903, on condition that the university remove all restrictions by sex. Abraham Flexner noted that her act made it the first American medical school "of a genuine university type," implying a more comprehensive approach to medical education.[29]

As the regular institutions reluctantly began to admit women, many of the women graduates, including the Blackwell sisters, urged attendance at these well-established schools. Women's schools closed. In retrospect, it is debatable whether women's understandable push for respectability has paid off.

The opportunity for coeducation at the established schools did not mean

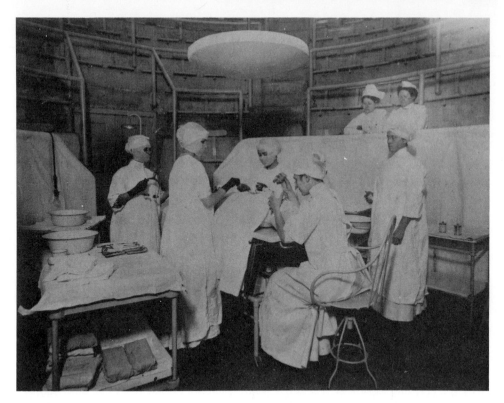

Fig. 4-3. Operating room scene, 1911. (Courtesy Archives and Special Collections on Women in Medicine of the Medical College of Pennsylvania, Philadelphia.)

equal opportunity for women, nor did it mean acceptance as providers of health care to the rich or elite. The closure of the women's colleges dramatically diminished the medical school slots available. As the increase in the number of women physicians leveled off, the opportunities for women technicians, nurses, and other health workers increased. (See Fig. 4-3.) Even when opportunities for women began to increase, the percentage of women physicians was for many years still smaller than it had been in the early 1900s. From 1900 until 1973, for example, the percentage of female medical students only rose from 4% to 13%. By 1975 and with the use of affirmative action, an estimated 22.2% of first-year medical students were women (18% of total medical school enrollment), and approximately 11% of the graduates were women. Although some institutions are reporting that 50% of their entering classes are made up of women, most medical schools seem to have leveled off in 1978 and 1979 with about 25% to 30% of students being women.[8]

Nurses

Nursing care was historically provided through religious or charitable institutions or by unpaid female relatives in the home. Prior to the development of hospitals, this was also essentially true in the United States. One of the earliest attempts at formalizing nursing came during the Civil War, when Dorothea Dix established the Sanitary Commission of the Union Army. Despite tremendous opposition from the Army Medical Corps, she organized nursing care on the battlefield. Many of the women so trained returned to their neighborhoods and utilized their skills, particularly in public health nursing. They were especially interested in hygiene, nutrition, and preventive health habits for mothers and children.

However, most members of earliest nursing staffs of hospitals were drawn from society's rejects: drunks, prostitutes, immigrants, and the poor.[59] Middle-class women who saw in nursing a chance to move out of the home and/or to perform a valuable social service were frequently made the supervisors; class differences shaped the nursing hierarchy. In either case, until the establishment of hospital training schools, nursing education consisted of on-the-job training, sometimes from physicians but more often from the experienced nurse to the newcomers.[14]

Although some types of nursing training programs were already in existence, the first formal nursing school was organized in 1871 at the New England Hospital for Women and Children founded in Boston in 1862 by Marie Elizabeth Zakrzewska.[58] Although "training nurses for the care of the sick" was one of the stated founding objectives of the hospital, this goal had run into problems during the first 10 years of the hospital's existence. Zakrzewska insisted on a 6-month committment for a training period, and few women had therefore applied. In 1871 the training period was set at 1 year; applicants had to be between 21 and 31 years old, "well and strong," of good character and disposition, and with a "good knowledge of general housework desirable."[58] The New England Hospital also admitted the first black woman into nursing training, Mary Eliza Mahoney, who graduated in 1879.

As hospitals grew in size, number, and importance, nurses were defined as physician helpers. In their student status, nurses represented an accessible, cheap (unpaid) source of labor. Between 1880 and 1900, for example, nursing schools grew in number from 15 to 432, with the number of students increasing from 323 to 11,000.[14]

Even though by 1920, untrained nurses outnumbered trained nurses three to two, nursing schools were firmly established. Those which had functioned independently of hospitals had by and large disappeared; the student nurse was welcomed into the hospital structure. Noted Lavinia Dock, nursing historian: "Discipline and strict subordination of the school makes it possible for the hospital to exact from (the student nurse) an amount of work it would be quite impossible to exact from women over whom it had no special hold. . . ."[24]

Graduates of nursing schools frequently worked as private duty nurses for the wealthy, in their homes or in hospitals. There they were accused of spreading discontent because they were exempt from performing the extensive and frequently menial work of the student nurse — cooking, cleaning, and laundering.

But nursing leaders (educators) began by the 1920s to voice their concerns. Nursing training was frequently in second place to service. The content of nursing education was under the control of the directors of the hospital, and the quality of "trained" nurses varied widely. In her landmark report of 1923, Josephine Goldmark outlined these concerns and suggested a classification of nurses according to their training; the nursing hierarchy was becoming a reality.

More significantly, the Depression forced the two national nursing organizations, the National League of Nursing Education (originally established in 1894 as the Society of Superintendents of Training Schools for Nurses, changed to the NLN in 1912) and the American Nurses' Association (organized in 1896 as the Nurses Association Alumnae of the United States and Canada, changed to ANA in 1911), to establish policies that altered the pattern of nursing. The ANA agreed to an 8-hour day to share the available work and ease unemployment, and the NLN, in a probable effort to limit the supply of nurses, pushed for the minimum nursing education standards set out in the Goldmark Report.[17,59]

The Depression also reduced the demand for private duty nurses, and graduates returned to work in the hospitals to which increasingly large numbers of the sick and not so sick (e.g., parturient women) were being confined.

By the 1930s, hospitals were staffed by practical ("untrained") nurses and trained nurses (registered nurses, RNs). To avoid friction between these two groups, the incipient hierarchy was solidified. Aided by the ANA, whose RNs controlled licensing boards and set forth educational criteria, the states required licensure of practical nurses. Clear demarcations were made also between these groups and nursing aides; by 1945, for example, 212,000 women had been certified as nursing aides through American Red Cross programs and by 1950, 216,000 aides, attendants, and orderlies were employed in the United States.[14] This hierarchical structure continues as a major characteristic of the United States nursing profession.

GENERAL CHARACTERISTICS OF HEALTH CARE DELIVERY TODAY

Today health work can still be characterized as women's work. From the historical development just outlined has come a legacy of underrepresentation of women in the higher echelons of health service delivery and of overrepresentation in the lowest. Even where women are predominant, for example, in nursing and dental hygiene, they are still subservient to male-dominated professions.

Today approximately 3 million women work in the health sector (Tables 4-1 and 4-2). Over 80% of all health service and hospital workers are women, and the percentage is rising. As the overwhelmingly female lower ranks expand (e.g., the number of practical nurses grew by 80% between 1960 and 1970),[10] the pyramid of power is increasingly concentrated at the top among the approximately half million (usually male) physicians, administrators, health corporation managers, medical school educators, and insurance company executives.[10]

Some typical generalizations can be made about women's participation in the health service industry, which also apply to their participation throughout the work force (see Chapter 5). They receive less pay than their male counterparts (64% of male income in the professional and technical worker category, 58% for service workers),[80] are in less prestigious specialties, have fewer opportunities

Table 4-1. Employed persons in selected health professions, United States, 1978*

Professions	Total number (000)	Percent distribution	
		Female	Black or other minority
Total employed, all occupations	94,373	41.2	11.2
Physicians, dentists, related practitioners	756	10.4	7.3
Medical and osteopathic physicians	424	11.3	9.7
Dentists	117	1.7	4.3
Pharmacists	136	16.9	6.6
Nurses, dieticians, and therapists	1351	92.9	11.7
Registered nurses	1112	96.7	11.7
Therapists	189	70.4	9.0
Health technologists and technicians	498	70.9	12.9
Clinical laboratory	208	73.6	14.4
Radiological	97	67.0	9.3
Social and recreation workers	505	61.0	19.2
Social workers	385	62.3	19.0
Recreation workers	121	57.0	20.7
Health administrators	184	46.2	7.6
Secretaries, medical	83	98.8	7.2
Health service workers	1846	89.9	23.6
Dental assistants	130	98.5	3.8
Aides and trainees (excluding nursing)	276	86.2	19.6
Nursing aides, orderlies, attendants	1037	87.0	27.6
Practical nurses	402	97.0	22.4

*Based on data from U.S. Department of Labor Bureau of Labor Statistics: Employment and earnings **26:**172, 173, 179, 180, Jan., 1979.

Table 4-2. Persons employed in the health industry, United States, 1978*

Place of employment	Total number (000)	Percent distribution	
		Female	Black or other minority
Offices of physicians	753	67.2	4.8
Offices of dentists	360	67.2	3.3
Hospitals	3781	75.8	19.4
Convalescent institutions	1009	88.1	19.2
Offices of health practitioners†	83	57.8	‡
Welfare services	788	70.9	23.5
Residential welfare facilities	119	60.5	20.2
Drug and medicine companies	185	38.4	10.4
Optical and health services supply companies	231	51.5	6.9

*Based on data from U.S. Department of Labor Bureau of Labor Statistics: Employment and earnings **26:**172, 173, 179, 180, Jan., 1979.
†Not elsewhere classified.
‡Unavailable.

for upward mobility, have a higher turnover because of their related spouse/parent roles, and yet are among the most highly skilled workers of all industries. Health service work also conforms to the many helping and nurturing roles that women are traditionally socialized to fill. Although women obviously could "nurture" as physicians, there are relatively few opportunities and encouragements to do so.

For most women, and minority women in particular, employment in the health sector is one sure avenue of employment outside the home. In a society where relatively few occupations are open in any degree to women (according to the 1970 census, seven occupations, one of which was nursing, contained 43% of all women workers), the subordinate positions, low pay, and confining and dead-end nature of many women's jobs must be weighed against no employment opportunities whatsoever. Dr. Carol Brown also points out that the relatively low pay women receive in the health sector must be compared with their pay elsewhere: "Median full-time earnings in hospital employment are above the median for workers in all industries for the categories of white women, black men and black women. Median earnings in hospital employment are well below the median only for white men."[10]

Issues

Women health workers in all occupations face many common issues. The most frequently discussed are issues of unequal pay, unequal advancement opportunities, hours not conducive to combining spouse/parent/employment roles, stratification within the health care industry, sexism, and a prevailing belief that women cannot fill the relevant top jobs as chiefs-of-staff, administrators, or supervisors. General criticisms of women in the top professions reflect beliefs that women are less competent, are best employed as health care providers to children, and are generally less productive. Of the less than 2% of dentists who are women, the majority of specialists are pedodontists. In 1976, although there was some change, the specialties of pediatrics (19.4% of women residents) and psychiatry, especially child psychiatry (10.9% of women residents), continued to be popular residencies for women. Internal medicine ranked highest, with 22.5% of women residents.

But other issues such as establishing professional identity, control of licensure, and unionization are specific to certain categories of health workers, and although crucial in the struggle for women's more equitable participation in health care delivery, frequently function to divide the ranks of women health workers and obscure the more fundamental economic, class, and social questions. In recognizing needs and goals of specific groups we must not lose sight of the forces that have produced the issues.

Upper level health occupations

Physicians. Women have been constantly challenged with the argument that they have neither the intellect nor the temperament to be physicians. An 1848 text on obstetrics says: "She (woman) has a head almost too small for intellect but just big enough for love."[62, p. 184] In 1905 F. W. Van Dyke, president of the Oregon State Medical Society, noted that: "hard study killed sexual desire in women, took away their beauty, brought on hysteria, neurasthenia, dyspepsia, astigmatism, and dysmenorrhea."[12, p. 75] Educated women, he added, could not bear children with ease because study arrested the development of the pelvis at the same time it increased the size of the child's brain, and therefore its head. This caused extensive suffering in childbirth.[12] Even in 1970, Hubert Humphrey's physician, Edgar Berman, stated that "women could not fill leadership roles because of the influences of their periodicity, that is, their menstrual cycles and menopause."[47, p. 75]

By 1975 after a depression, two world wars, and the advent of the women's movement and affirmative action, "scientific" findings and attitudes had changed. For minority women, however, the change was miniscule (Table 4-3).

In 1976, 8.3% (28,966 of 348,443) of the active physicians with known

Table 4-3. Total enrollment and graduates of selected schools for the health professions, United States, selected years*†

Profession	Academic year	Total number enrolled	Female (%)	Minority (%)	White (%)
Total enrollment					
Medicine	1976-1977	57,765	22.4	11.0	89.0
Osteopathic medicine	1978-1979	4,220	16.5	4.4‡	95.6‡
Dentistry	1976-1977	21,013	11.2	10.1	89.9
Optometry	1976-1977	4,033	13.4	7.4	92.6
Pharmacy	1976-1977	24,082	36.8	8.9	91.1
Podiatry	1976-1977	2,204	7.1	6.1	93.9
Veterinary medicine	1976-1977	6,571	28.2	3.0	97.0
Nursing§	1974-1975	196,389	94.0	13.6	86.4
Total graduates					
Medicine	1976-1977	13,607	19.2	6.8	93.2
Osteopathic medicine‖	1978-1979	1,012	16.1	NA¶	NA
Dentistry	1975-1976	5,336	4.6	9.3	90.7
Optometry	1974-1975	752	4.4	NA	NA
Pharmacy	1974-1975	5,414	26.1	NA	NA
Podiatry	1974-1975	353	1.1	NA	NA
Veterinary medicine	1974-1975	1,165	14.2	NA	NA
Nursing§	1974-1975	52,207	92.7	#	#

*Based on data from U.S. Department of Health, Education and Welfare: Minorities and women in health fields, Pub. No. (HRA) 76-22, Bureau of Health Manpower, Sept., 1975, and No. (HRA) 79-22, Oct., 1978, Washington, D.C., U.S. Government Printing Office.
†For various exceptions, inclusions, and limitations of data, see sources.
‡Data from 1976-1977 academic year.
§All programs.
‖Data from American Osteopathic Association: Staff study #4: Role of women in osteopathic medicine, an appreciation and projection, Chicago, 1979, DRAFT Document.
¶NA = Not available.
#In those programs answering questions on racial/ethnic category, 9.2% of graduates were black, 5.5% were of Spanish background, and 3.3% were American Indian or Oriental.

addresses were women. In medical schools about 22% of the 1979 graduating class and 25% of the 1979 entering class were women. Although the numbers of women are increasing, many barriers are still to be faced. When women medical or dental students drop out of school, they do so primarily for role conflict and social reasons, whereas for men the primary reason is academic failure. Even when admitted to health profession schools, women still face sexist attitudes and discriminatory treatment, well documented to date within medical and dental schools.[13,18] Unfortunately, these attitudes can be so pervasive that women students may adopt the mentality of the oppressor and in turn transmit the stereotypical and sexist thinking to their practices. Support for women students is rare and where it is available, such as at the Medical College of Pennsylvania, it is highly valued.[30]

It is frequently argued, too, that women health professionals (e.g., physicians, dentists) are not acceptable to the public. In a 1974 study by Dr. Edgar B. Engleman of 500 New York City Clinic patients, 80% said they would prefer a male to a female doctor, although more than half had never been treated by a woman physician. Patients cited reasons that women were less competent and less experienced, but at the same considered them to be cleaner, more emotional, more trustworthy, and more concerned about poor patients. One third of young black women expressed a preference for a woman physician and 80% of those who had actually been treated by a woman viewed the experience positively.[48]

Another study published in 1975 found that 34% of a sample of 409 patients preferred a woman gynecologist, 19.3% did not, and 36% had no preference. The researchers believed that patients who preferred female gynecologists were most likely to find gynecological examinations difficult and be critical of gynecologists' understanding of women's psychological and sexual problems.[35]

Another study in 1976 of three different types of clinic populations measured women's experience with female physicians and their preference between paraprofessionals and physicians to perform specific gynecologically related procedures. The study demonstrated that when women had experienced care from a female physician, they preferred her. They also preferred treatment mostly from physicians, although no mistrust of paraprofessional performance was implied.[46]

However, it appears that experience with women physicians, on which acceptance or preference is built, will be severely limited for many years. According to the American College of Obstetricians and Gynecologists, as of July 25, 1978, of the 20,348 fellows of the college, only 1423, or 6.9%, were women.[4] Of the approximately 28,966 active women physicians on AMA records for 1976, only 3205 were in surgical specialties.[32] Although the number of women fellows of ACOG has approximately doubled since 1974, the increasing entry of women into obstetrical-gynecological residencies may reflect not women's interest in the specialty or hospitals' and schools' acceptance of women as much as the fact that there are more available slots in that field. In 1974, for example, 15% of residency positions were unfilled, and about 50% of residents on duty were foreign medical graduates.[72] By 1976, according to the AMA's *Directory of Accredited Residences* only 214 (5.2%) of the 4113 available residencies in

Table 4-4. Distribution within specialization of active physicians, United States, 1976*

Activity	Total physicians†	Total female physicians‡	Percentage female physicians
All physicians	348,443	28,966	8.3
Total patient care	318,412	25,896	8.1
General practice	54,332	3,064	5.6
Medical specialties	89,213	9,664	10.8
Surgical specialties	95,102	3,205	3.4
Other specialties	79,765	9,963	12.5
Medical teaching	6,935	844	12.2
Administration	11,689	1,077	9.2
Research	8,514	816	9.6
Other	2,893	333	11.5

*From Goodman, L. J.: Physician distribution and medical licensure in the U.S., 1976, Chicago, 1977, The American Medical Association. Reprinted with permission from the American Medical Association.
†Excludes 22,117 inactive, 30,129 not classified, and 8757 address unknown.
‡Excludes 3535 inactive, 5078 not classified, and 1182 address unknown.

Table 4-5. Distribution of men and women within selected medical specialties, United States, 1976

Specialty	Men (%)	Women (%)
Anesthesiology	86.1	13.9
General (family) practice	94.2	5.7
Internal medicine	92.3	7.7
Obstetrics and gynecology	91.5	8.5
Pediatrics (includes pediatric allergy and cardiology)	76.7	23.3
Psychiatry (includes child psychiatry)	85.1	14.9
Radiology	90.7	9.3
Surgery	97.7	2.3
All other	93.8	6.2

*Based on data from Goodman, L. J.: Physician distribution and medical licensure in the U.S., 1976, Chicago, 1977, American Medical Association; and Minorities and women in the health fields, Bureau of Health Manpower, (HRA) 79-22, Washington, D.C., 1979, U.S. Government Printing Office.

obstetrics and gynecology were unfilled and about 26% of the residents on duty in obstetrics and gynecology were foreign medical graduates.[22]

In medicine, women traditionally have been counseled or channeled into or have selected the specialties of pediatrics, pathology, psychiatry (especially child psychiatry) anesthesiology (with detrimental effects on their fertility—see Chapter 5), general medicine, and public health (18% of public health physicians are women), although, as noted, increasing numbers of women are selecting internal medicine. In general terms, the specialty classifications of active women physicians in 1976 were as follows: medical, 32%, general practice, 11%, surgical, 11%, and all others, 45%[32] (see Table 4-4).

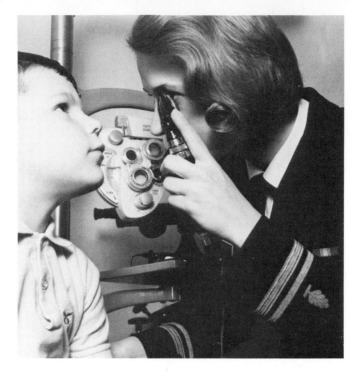

Fig. 4-4. Naval optometrist. (Courtesy Women's Bureau, U.S. Department of Labor.)

Although changes in the age distribution, country of medical education, and geographical location of women physicians are likely to bring changes in specialty choice, traditional male specialities such as surgery and internal medicine are exceedingly popular and correspondingly slow to accept women. Similarly, coveted medical school appointments are predominately filled by men. Table 4-5 shows the percentage of women in various specialties in 1976. In 1978, only 15.0% of medical school faculties were women and those were overwhelmingly in library positions. When only physician faculty were considered, women comprised less than 10%. Only 5% of professors were women, no deans were women, and 1976 data show that 31% of instructors and 28% of lecturers were female.[26] In 1978 about 38% of all female physicians were under age 35 as compared to 26% of all male physicians. About 15% of the foreign-trained physicians in the United States were women and between 6% and 7% of the United States and Canadian graduates in the United States were female. (See Figs. 4-4 and 4-5.) The majority of women physicians are in the Northeast, followed by the North Central, South, and West. The most recent data (1972) indicate that about 40% of women physicians who are specialists are board certified as are 50% to 60% of male physician specialists[79] (see Table 4-6). All these characteristics affect hours worked and income, displayed in Table 4-7. On the average, women physicians' income is about 57% that of men's.

Productivity of female physicians has recently been documented and an

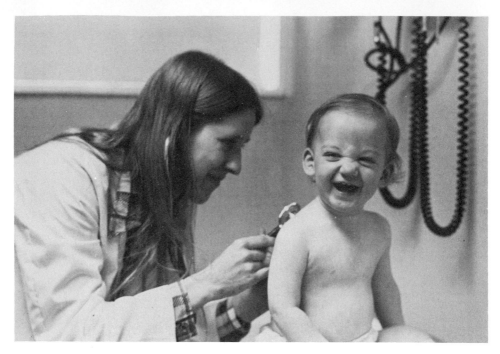

Fig. 4-5. Pediatrician. (Courtesy Health Sciences Information Services, University of Washington, Seattle.)

Table 4-6. Percent of specialists board certified, United States, 1972*†

Specialty	Males certified (%)	Females certified (%)
All specialties	53.9	39.6
Anesthesiology	60.9	51.5
General (family) practice	13.4	7.9
Internal medicine	49.9	22.6
Obstetrics and gynecology	74.3	39.7
Pediatrics (includes pediatric allergy and cardiology)	80.6	54.9
Psychiatry (includes child psychiatry)	53.4	33.3
Radiology	85.7	78.9
Surgery	74.4	60.6
All other	56.0	54.3

*From Kehrer, B. H.: Professional and practice characteristics of men and women physicians. In Profiles of Medical Practice, 1974, Chicago, 1974, American Medical Association. Based on a sample survey of about 1400 women and 7100 men physicians. Reprinted with permission from the American Medical Association.
†This is the most recent data available. The American Board of Medical Specialties estimates that these total percentages are still adequately representative. Attempts are being made to update data.

Table 4-7. Selected practice characteristics of physicians by specialty and sex*

Specialty	Specialists, 1972		Average net income from medical practice, 1972		Average hours of direct patient care per week, 1973		Source of 1972† net income (average %)‡					
							Direct fee-for-service		Shared practice		Salary or retainer	
	Male (%)	Female (%)	Male	Female	Male	Female	Male	Female	Male	Female	Male	Female
All specialties	100.0	100.0	$47,945	$27,558	46.5	37.4	56.9	50.2	41.7	31.4	19.2	38.1
Anesthesiology	4.8	10.6	50,898	35,543	48.3	43.5	38.7	53.9	32.0	12.8	29.8	33.5
General (family) practice	22.9	15.8	41,634	22,339	47.9	39.2	72.7	62.4	17.6	11.4	9.5	27.5
Internal medicine	16.3	9.7	45,043	23,267	47.5	40.7	58.4	44.3	21.8	12.2	20.2	45.0
Obstetrics and gynecology	7.3	9.0	53,940	32,864	49.2	37.4	46.8	57.8	31.2	17.8	21.7	24.1
Pediatrics	5.8	17.6	40,529	23,549	45.8	37.0	52.6	40.4	30.7	11.0	17.5	48.4
Psychiatry	5.8	18.3	40,433	24,797	40.8	32.1	68.9	61.9	4.1	1.2	27.5	36.2
Radiology	4.2	3.0	58,891	33,308	41.9	34.9	13.2	10.5	58.5	31.6	27.4	52.6
Surgery	24.5	5.1	56,377	40,000	48.0	37.8	57.8	60.2	25.4	15.6	16.8	24.2
All other	8.4	10.9	44,910	27,711	39.7	35.8	44.6	30.9	21.8	19.0	33.8	51.5

*From Kehrer, B. H.: Professional and practice characteristics of men and women physicians. In Profiles of medical practice, 1974, Chicago, 1974, American Medical Association. Based on a sample survey of about 1400 women and 7100 men physicians. Reprinted with permission from the American Medical Association. (See also Kehrer, B. H.: Factors affecting the incomes of men and women physicians: an exploratory analysis, Human Resources **11**:526-545, 1976.)

†Most recent data available.

‡The sum of the three percentages added horizontally for either male or female physicians will not be 100% because each column is based on a different number of observations.

effort made to correct previous studies. In one glaring error, the Carnegie Commission Report of 1970[39] states that only 45% of women physicians worked, either full or part-time, when the correct figure was 91.1%. Such a mistake probably passed three readers because it reflects widely held beliefs.

In their sample the 1975 researchers found that women physicians work nearly nine-tenths as much as do men physicians. The difference in the work ratios between men and women is due to time taken out by women for mothering obligations. This finding is consistent with those of many previous studies and forms the basis for flexible residency schedule demands of both men and women.[37,75] The researchers observe: "In addition to noting the heavy work load of women (the majority are married and have responsibilities for households with children), we found that women take little time out from the work force compared to men who do not have these added responsibilities."[37] They found that physicians of both sexes worked too hard and that the high suicide, substance abuse, and early death rates among physicians supported this view. The effects on patient care of physician work overload can be only speculated on.

Relatively little research has been done on the interactive effects of income, practice patterns, and specialty of top women health professionals. A 1974 study of Michigan health professionals in dentistry, optometry, medicine, veterinary medicine, pharmacy, and osteopathy found that, in general, women preferred to work in group situations and to be employees rather than employers. Such arrangements gave greater flexibility for combining motherhood and working roles. Relatively few women were found in optometry and dentistry, where the mode of practice is self-employment.[15]

The acceptance of women in other top level health professions has not been well documented. Many of the 45.1% of female health administrators in 1977 were in church-owned institutions, where there has been wider acceptance of female officials. There is also a disproportionate representation of women administrators by type of hospital. Women predominately administer small, rural, proprietary facilities, and throughout administrative ranks they are in lower-paying positions.[70] A 1973 survey in California found that women made up only 24% of the middle- and upper-administrative cadre and that they were "located in such traditional 'women's' departments as housekeeping, dietetics, and nursing. Only a small fraction were found in institution-wide policy-making positions."[5]

Women wanting to be veterinarians have had an additional hurdle, since they have been judged not strong enough to handle large animals. Even if this were found to be true, given the enormous small pet population in the United States and the amount spent for pet veterinary services, such an argument is invalid for keeping large numbers of women out of the profession. A recent report on the New York State College of Veterinary Medicine at Cornell University indicates that the class of 1981 is over 50% female and that this increase is partly because it is recognized that "with the introduction of tranquilizers, women are now capable of handling large animals."[8]

Dentists. Of the 134,415 dentists in the United States in 1979, 2391, or 1.9%, were women (Table 4-8). The majority (as is true for all dentists) are in the Middle

Table 4-8. Practice characteristics of professionally active women dentists, United States (including possessions), 1979*

Occupation or specialty	Number
Primary occupation	
Practicing dentist (more than 30 hours per week)	1034
Practicing dentist (less than 30 hours per week)	373
Dental school faculty/staff member	147
Armed forces dentist	46
Other federal services (e.g., VA, PHS dentist)	42
State and local government employee	97
Hospital staff dentist	22
Intern/resident/student	141
No longer practicing dentistry/retired	404
Health/dental organization staff member	12
Unknown occupation	73
TOTAL	2391
Specialty	
General practice	1701
Oral surgery	6
Endodontics	4
Orthodontics	49
Pedodontics	61
Periodontics	24
Prosthodontics	4
Oral pathology	1
Public health	2
Full-time faculty of dental school	96
Full-time in state public health program	18
Retired/no longer practicing dentistry	425
TOTAL	2391
TOTAL INCLUDING UNLOCATED DENTISTS	2644

*From Distribution of dentists in the United States by state, region and county, Chicago, 1979, American Dental Association. Copyright by the American Dental Association. Reprinted by permission.

Atlantic and East North Central regions of the United States. Because of the nature of dentistry, about 80% are self-employed, compared with 94% of male dentists. By the 1978-1979 academic year women comprised about 15.9% of first-year dental students, and 14% of total enrollment.[23]

The American Dental Association states that dentistry is an ideal profession for women because of the many fringe benefits, the fact that practitioners can set their own hours, and the high earnings. They note that women have "inherent gentleness, patience and sympathy with patients,"[1] yet the profession, recognized as one of the most conservative in the United States, has done little to encourage women to join its ranks.

On the other hand, the profession has encouraged women to participate in its dental auxiliary programs. In 1975, 99.4% of dental hygienist enrollees were women; of enrollees in dental laboratory technology, 29.5% were women; and 99.8% of those enrolled in dental assistance courses were women (see Fig. 4-6).[79]

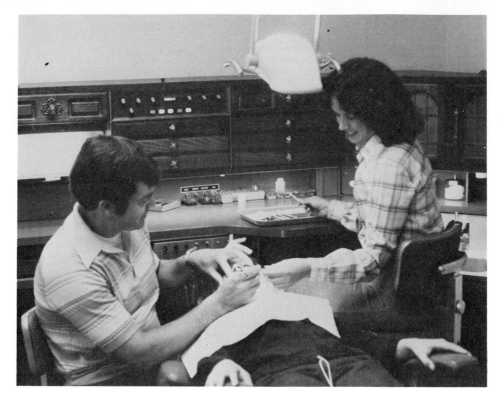

Fig. 4-6. Dental assistant and dentist.

Table 4-9. Employed registered nurses, United States, 1972*

Position	Total	Male	Female	Percent female
All types of positions	778,470†	10,989	766,416	98.5
Administrator or assistant	29,752	897	28,855	97.0
Consultant	6,681	125	6,556	98.1
Supervisor or assistant	80,648	1,733	78,915	97.8
Instructor	32,657	480	32,177	98.5
Head nurse or assistant	119,905	1,657	118,248	98.6
General duty or staff	432,976	3,461	429,515	99.2
Other specified type	54,841	2,135	52,706	96.1
Not reported	21,010	501	20,509	97.6

*From American Nurse's Association: Facts about nursing, 72-73, Kansas City, 1974, The Association. Reprinted by permission of ANA. (Most recent data available.)
†Includes 1065 employed RNs whose sex was not reported.

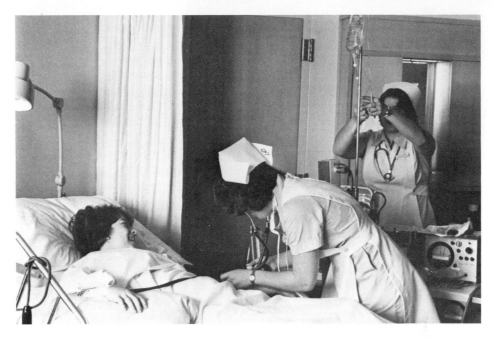

Fig. 4-7. Nursing students. (Courtesy Seattle University, Seattle.)

Midlevel health occupations

Nurses. Since the 1920s the nursing profession has struggled to be recognized as an independent profession. Yet for an occupation that has about 1.5 million members (1.1 million RNs, 400,000 LPNs), including related nursing services, has two national organizations, and is vital to health service delivery, it wields singularly little power. Brown observes that "although some of the middle-ranking (nursing) occupations assert some controls over lower-ranking occupations following the physicians' model, they cannot assert power because they have little or none to assert."[10]

Many of the characterizations that pertained to the top-level health professions pertain to nursing. Although men comprise only about 3% of the total RN population, they are 16% of the supervisors and 14% of head or assistant head nurses and are disproportionately represented as general duty nurses. Men are also paid more in all nursing categories.[25] (See Table 4-9.)

Today's nursing work force is clearly stratified along the lines suggested in the 1880s. Today there are baccalaureate registered nurses (RNs), diploma school RNs, associate program RNs, licensed practical nurses (LPNs) or licensed vocational nurses (LVNs in California and Texas), and nurses' aides, who are usually trained on the job. Nurse-practitioners are generally baccalaureate or master's degree RNs with additional specialty training in, for example, pediatrics or obstetrics. They have more status than baccalaureate RNs, who in turn have more status than RNs from 2-year programs. At the top of the hierarchy are the nursing leaders-educators in the field. (See Fig. 4-7.)

The quest for a professional identity has led nursing to push for 4-year programs for all RNs. The wisdom of this policy is highly debatable as RNs move to fill administrative and paperwork positions, drifting away from patient care. The patient care tasks are increasingly done at lower cost by LPNs and aides. RNs may eventually price themselves out of the market. Furthermore, this quest for professionalism in the name of improved patient care succeeds in limiting access to nursing careers; the medical profession's elitism and exlusivity are emulated by nurses. The very object—good patient care—suffers in the struggle for respectability.

The concept of institutional licensure[38] is opposed by nursing leaders.[3] Although it would clearly provide job mobility and flexibility of task delegation and do much to relieve the dead-end nature of many midlevel and lower level jobs, such licensure (though not explicitly stated by nurses) would remove control of nursing occupations from the nursing leaders themselves. There is also concern that individual hospitals would have discretion regarding professional licensing at the expense of the nursing boards' current authority.

Another major issue confronting nursing is the problem of turnover. Nurses cite "impoverished work environment," meaning inadequate staff, low pay, subordination to physicians, degrading behavioral expectations (maintaining traditional feminine roles), and few opportunities to utilize nurses' considerable skills as reasons for the turnover. According to one study, relocation of husbands or of nurses themselves contributed substantially to the turnover rate.[34] Yet another study suggested that nurses viewed themselves as secondary earners—as their husbands' incomes reached a certain level, nurses quit.[34] The work environment was not sufficiently appealing to sustain commitment.

Public health, medical records, and physical and occupational therapy personnel. With the exception of nursing, public health educational programs have a higher percentage of women than those of any other health profession. The bulk of women graduates from schools of public health in 1972 went into public health nursing, nutrition, education, and maternal and child health (see Table 4-10). By 1976 a high percentage of women went into health administration. Of the 1975 and 1976 graduates of public health programs who were United States citizens, women comprised 76.3% of those with bachelor's degrees, 48.1% of master's degree graduates, and 35.6% of those with doctorate degrees.[33]

Medical record administration and medical technology programs are still overwhelmingly occupied by females even though the number of bachelor's degree level graduates has declined in the last few years (see Table 4-11). In the 1977-1978 academic year about 97% of students in medical records programs were women and about 85% of students in medical technology programs were women. The percentages decline as more advanced degrees are sought.[49]

Similar patterns of declining numbers of women seeking higher degrees exist in the physical and occupational therapy fields, with only about half the master's graduates in physical therapy being women (total graduates in these fields are small). These professions have also experienced stratification similar to that of the nursing profession. For example, physical therapy aides are the vocational auxiliaries to physical therapists, and recreational therapists are an outgrowth of

Table 4-10. Specialization of United States students in schools of public health, 1975 and 1976*

Specialty	Total students	Female			Male		
		Number	Percent in specialty	Percent of all female specialists	Number	Percent in specialty	Percent of all male specialists
All specialties	5394	2635	48.9	100.0	2759	51.1	100.0
Health administration	1576	767	48.7	29.1	809	51.3	29.3
Hospital administration	177	53	29.9	2.0	124	70.1	4.5
Public health education	295	193	65.4	7.3	102	34.6	3.7
Environmental health	703	170	24.2	6.5	533	75.8	19.3
Public health nursing	235	225	95.7	8.5	10	4.3	0.4
Epidemiology	760	329	43.3	12.5	431	56.7	15.6
Nutrition	226	184	81.4	7.0	42	18.6	1.5
Maternal and child health	157	107	68.2	4.0	50	31.8	1.8
Biostatistics	383	157	41.0	6.0	226	59.0	8.2
Occupational health	146	40	27.4	1.5	106	72.6	3.8
Dental public health	30	12	40.0	0.5	18	60.0	0.7
Mental health	68	39	57.4	1.5	29	42.6	1.1
Population studies	164	107	65.2	4.0	57	34.8	2.1
Behavioral and social services	75	39	52.0	1.5	36	48.0	1.3
Other and unknown	399	213	53.4	8.1	186	46.6	6.7

*Data provided by William B. Parsons, Project Director, Data Collection Center, Association of Schools of Public Health, Washington, D.C.

Table 4-11. All graduates of medical record librarianship, medical technology, occupational therapy, and physical therapy programs, United States, 1975 and 1976*

Degree	Medical record administration		Medical technology		Occupational therapy		Physical therapy	
	Total graduates	Female graduates (%)	Total graduates	Female graduates (%)	Total graduates	Female graduates (%)	Total graduates	Female graduates (%)
Bachelor's	521	93.4	5445	80.0	1478	94.4	2091	77.4
Master's	9	88.8	266	51.5	166	82.5	167	67.6
Doctorate	—	—	—	—	—	—	1	0

*Based on data from Earned degrees conferred 1975-1976 summary data, no. 017-080-01868-3, Washington, D.C., 1978, National Center for Education Statistics.

the occupational therapy profession. Each group tries to define its tasks as separate and tends to categorize tasks as professional versus practical or vocational.

New health professionals (NHPs). NHPs make up a broad category of mid-level workers that includes some professionals who are not new but who are enjoying a renaissance, or a formal status, in the United States scene. Midwives, physicians' assistants, nurse-practitioners, women's health care specialists, therapists (e.g., inhalation, occupational, mental health) nurse-anesthetists, radiology technicians, and others all fall in this group.* For some categories the percentages of females are shown in Table 4-1. In many instances the new health professions have also provided opportunities for upward mobility of minorities, particularly for those who were formerly armed forces corpsmen. Initially believed to be a major influence in medical cost containment, the growth of NHPs is largely determined by their acceptability to the older, established professions.

NHPs, male and female, face many issues in common. Their substitutability for physicians depends on their cost, their relative productivity, the degree to which the physician's tasks can be safely delegated, and their legitimization by professional bodies and the public. Depending on state licensure and/or certification, NHPs may function as independent free-standing practitioners. Over the last decade, NHPs, and particularly nurse-practitioners, have been setting up independent practice. Few third party payors will reimburse them, and they frequently have to use covering clinics or empathetic physicians to arrange reimbursement. At present this is the biggest obstacle to their growth.

Public Law 95-210 (the Rostenkowski-Clark bill) would, under specified circumstances, provide reimbursement to various free-standing personnel, including physicians' assistants, nurse-midwives, and nurse-practitioners, in certified rural clinics not affiliated with hospitals. Although the law does not change state practice laws and is only effective in states where these personnel are recognized, passage of the law should encourage the growth of NHPs.[57]

Licenses to prescribe drugs are another issue for NHPs. In Washington State in July, 1977, the Nurse Practice Act was passed, under which certain types of NHPs, including certified nurse-midwives who registered as certified registered nurses (CRNs), are able to prescribe. In August, 1979, the Board of Nursing adopted rules and regulations on CRN prescriptive authority.

NHPs are also seeking admitting privileges to hospitals. This is particularly appropriate for nurse-midwives, several of whom are participating in birth centers or home births simply because admitting privileges, and therefore the chance to practice to the full scope of their abilities, are denied them. Another key issue is access to diagnostic laboratories, which is crucial for independent practice. Again, cover arrangements are generally made.

In 1979, salaries for NHPs ranged between $15,000 and $25,000. As a general rule, male NHPs outearn their female counterparts. This has been particularly irritating to nurse-practitioners, who have usually undergone more

---

*References 2, 16, 19, 52, 66-68, 71.

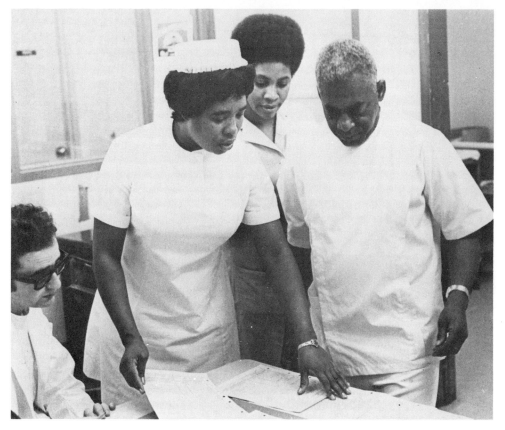

Fig. 4-8. Health care team. (Courtesy National Union of Hospital and Health Care Employees, Local 1199.)

extensive formal training than have their male counterparts, the physician's assistant or Medex. However, considering the breadth of on-the-job experience of, for example, former military corpsmen, the relevance of the formal training is sometimes questionable.

Hierarchical conflicts are particularly significant for NHPs, many of whom have more direct experience in their particular field than does the physician who is their superior. Social workers in institutions constantly face this problem (of the 325,000 social workers, about 60% are women) when they must take third place in the hierarchy of psychiatrist or psychiatric resident, psychologist, and social worker, even though they may have more knowledge of the case. Conflicts may also be horizontal, notes Brown, as, for example, "whether physician assistants, standing in loco medicus, can give orders to nurses or whether nurses as independent professionals can give orders to physician assistants."[76] A suit filed in this regard in Washington State (1978) was settled in 1980 and affirmed that RNs must take orders from physician assistants.[76]

Nurse-midwives. After almost disappearing at the turn of the century, there are now about 2000 nurse-midwives in the United States. Although they are still responsible for only about 1% of the nation's births (as compared with 80% in parts of Europe, the United Kingdom, and Scandinavia) their numbers are growing. Nurse-midwifery services are available through clinics, voluntary and public hospitals, physician-midwife teams in private practice, and in some cases nurse-midwives in independent practice with physician backup.

The American College of Nurse-Midwives (ACNM) stresses that nurse-midwives are interdependent members of the health team always working in conjunction with physicians. The college defines the nurse-midwife as

a registered professional nurse who by virtue of her added knowledge and skill gained through an organized program of study and clinical experience recognized by the ACNM, has extended the limits (legal limits where they obtain) of her practice into the area of management of care of mothers and babies throughout the maternity cycle so long as progress meets criteria accepted as normal.[77]

On graduation from one of 18 ACNM-recognized basic programs, a nurse-midwife is eligible to take the ACNM national examination for certification. Successful candidates may then use the initials "CNM" (Certified Nurse-Midwife) after their name. In many states possession of a nurse-midwifery degree is a prerequisite for licensure as a midwife, although a few states permit licensure by examination if the candidate has graduated from an "approved school of midwifery" with an appropriately rigorous training. Such laws permit the licensure of the estimated several hundred foreign-trained midwives currently in the United States. These women frequently were trained in schools of midwifery common outside the United States. Although nursing is incorporated into midwifery in such programs, a nursing qualification is not a prerequisite for entry. Many of these women are highly skilled individuals, and it is a mistake to categorize them, as is the practice in the United States, together with lay midwives, who may or may not be skilled, but who have no formal training.

Interest in and demand for nurse-midwifery services are increasing in the United States for reasons of economy, physician shortage and/or maldistribution, appreciation of the midwife's style of obstetrical care, recognition of the superior maternal and infant morbidity and mortality statistics in countries where midwives are widely utilized, and recognition of the important contribution nurse-midwives can make to strengthening contraceptive, maternal, and health education services.

Although the nurse-midwife is capable of utilizing surgical and technological procedures such as episiotomy and fetal monitoring, she is encouraged in her training to use these only when necessary, with a resultant reduction of both financial and physical costs. She has been trained to do external version in the event of a breech position and to do a vaginal delivery of a breech presentation, although current obstetrical practice discourages such techniques. She stays with the mother throughout labor and delivery; hence the name "midwife," Middle English for "with woman." Nurse-midwives can be male; as of 1977 three nurse-midwives were men.

Lower level health occupations

Lower level health workers are overwhelmingly female: 93.5% of clerical workers and 82.5% of service workers. Minority women (minority men also work in this group) comprise about 30%.[51]

Clerical workers include secretaries, medical record clerks, billing and collection clerks, ward clerks, and bookkeepers. Service workers include aides, orderlies, janitorial and housekeeping staff, porters, and others. Together these groups comprise about 54% of all health workers. Their pay is low—an average of about $9000 annually, which includes fringe benefits.

Fundamental issues that confront this group are no different from those with which women in the higher levels must deal. They include problems of low and lesser pay, parent/spouse/work role conflict (child care is particularly crucial for those with low incomes because domestic help is too expensive), lack of job mobility, and lack of decision-making opportunities. Occupational hazards may also be a problem.

Unions, which can be of benefit to all health workers, are particularly impor-

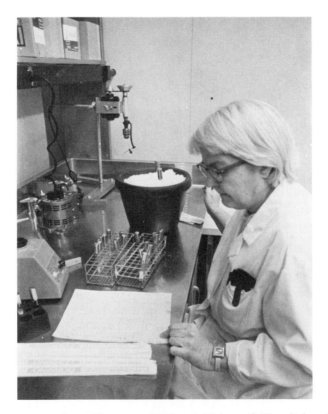

Fig. 4-9. Laboratory worker. (Courtesy National Union of Hospital and Health Care Employees, Local 1199.)

tant for lower level health workers. In the National Union of Hospital and Health Care Employees (NUHHCE), Local 1199, at least 80% of the members are women and comprise an estimated 90% of its Hospital Division membership. Union leadership has been mostly older white men, but this is a result of Local 1199's origin as a predominately male drug workers' union. Women officers are being trained by the leadership, and in 1978 two of four executive vice-presidents were women, as were five of the 21-member national executive board.[50]

Union organizing is concerned mostly with the basic bread-and-butter issues of hours and wages. Of special significance to women has been the abolition of job classifications by sex, equal pay for equal work, and requiring management contributions to training programs that enable women to upgrade their job status. Unions nationally have done little to provide child care services, although Local 1199's experience, for example, shows that child care services at place of employment are wanted in rural areas but not by metropolitan workers. Recently Local 1199 has begun to make efforts also to organize nurses, who are becoming less resistant to unionization. Increasingly, union membership is seen to be compatible with perceived professional status, including the right to strike. Unionization by professionals has perhaps been helped by the 1974 amendments to the National Labor Relations Act, which provided in part that professionals could not be compelled to be members of bargaining units with nonprofessionals.

Nonconventional health care occupations

Nonconventional health workers are those who work outside the organized system. Perhaps the largest category in this group is indeed conventional: the female family member who provides unpaid care in the home. With over a million persons estimated to be receiving care within the home for chronic conditions and many persons receiving care for acute illnesses, particularly childhood diseases, the health care industry needs this worker. Some research into the issues faced by the unpaid female worker is now being done,[55] but her health care services have long been presumed to be readily available, freely, even lovingly, given, her moral responsibility, and her primary responsibility, taking precedence over other demands, including her regular employment.

The suggested solution of paying women to provide care in the home is a possibility but one that invites abuse. Yet the economic realities that families confront when one member must cease paid employment to care for another demand a solution from a rational health care delivery system. Adequate recognition is long overdue of the need for home health care workers and the important health care job performed by family members.

Volunteer workers also play an important role in the health care system. Predominantly women, they are indispensable in the daily caring aspects of hospital services. They function in varied community organizations such as Meals-on-Wheels and senior citizen services, filling tasks as diverse as fund-raising or writing letters for the incapacitated.

Other nonconventional health workers are lay midwives (as distinguished from nurse- or foreign-trained midwives), herbalists, folk healers, curanderas, naturopaths, spiritual and psychic healers, moxibustionists (practitioners who burn a herb on the skin according to the principles of acupuncture), root doctors, and, where they are outside the formal system, acupuncturists.

Women are represented in all these groups, although their exact number is unknown. In a recent study the median estimate of some use of these healers by Californians was as high as 30%.[61] In 1973 there were an estimated 3000 lay midwives in the United States. These are men and women who by clinical experience and/or tradition have established themselves as midwifery practitioners. In some states (e.g., Texas) they may practice if legally registered.

INTERNATIONAL PERSPECTIVES

The United States has a lower percentage of female physicians than any other industrialized country except Spain. In 1972, when 11% of medical students in the United States were women, Ecuador had 18%; Paraguay, 31%; and the Dominican Republic, 48%.[20] The United States also compares unfavorably in dentistry. In Europe, for example, between 20% and 80% of dentists are women. In Poland 80% of the dentists and 46% of the physicians are women. In France 13.5% of the physicians and 26.6% of the dentists are women.[79] In Lebanon 6.7% of the physicians, 5.5% of the dentists, and 24.2% of the pharmacists are women.[65] In Israel, 31% of the physicians and 80% of the nurses are women[65] (see Table 4-12).

Where international comparative data are available, the specialties that have the most women are similar to those in the United States. In Finland, about 28% of physicians are women, as are 70% of dentists; among the specialists, 24% are women.[79] They are heavily represented (either near or over 50% of the total specialists) in child psychiatry, venereal diseases, dermatology, pediatrics, ophthalmology, and pulmonary diseases. In Sweden, where about 18% of the physicians are women, 13.2% of specialists are female. They are 30% of the psychiatrists, 25% of the anesthesiologists, and 23% of the pediatricians. In both Sweden and Finland, women comprise 19% of the obstetrician-gynecologists.[79]

Some analyses of comparative status suggest that these top health professions have lower status in countries other than the United States. Whether the professions had lower status and women were therefore permitted to enter or whether women's relatively higher participation lowered the status of the profession is undetermined. Nonetheless, women's greater participation in these professions, which, regardless of their relative status, are still highly valued and among the most highly paid in all countries,[31] may also be a reflection of women's superior social integration in these countries compared with that in the United States.

However, although the participation of women in the health care work forces of many countries is more equitable than in the United States, similar discrimination still exists in many other countries in hiring, mobility, pay, and educational opportunities based on gender and superimposed on class biases. In many countries the majority of women have relatively no access to education. In Arab countries, for example, 62.4% of girls who are of school age never enter school.

Table 4-12. Distribution of student enrollees and graduates in the medical sciences, selected countries, selected years*†

Country and status of student	Year	Total	Male	Female	Percent female
Australia					
Enrollees	1970	12,844	8372	4472	34.8
Graduates	1970	2179	1311	868	39.8
Cameroon					
Enrollees	1971	132	116	16	12.1
Graduates	1969	NA‡	NA	NA	NA
Colombia					
Enrollees	1970	7749	NA	NA	NA
Graduates	1969	939	NA	NA	NA
Finland					
Enrollees	1971	3638	2071	1567	43.1
Graduates	1971	728	414	314	43.1
France					
Enrollees	1971	142,720	NA	NA	NA
Graduates	1966	5528	3397	2131	38.6
Philippines					
Enrollees	1969	24,947	4743	20,204	81.0
Graduates	1968	4251	807	3444	81.0
Poland					
Enrollees	1971	36,766	8758	28,008	76.2
Graduates	1970	10,564	1876	8688	82.2
Sweden					
Enrollees	1971	11,642	6867	4775	41.0
Graduates	1971	4790	1763	3027	63.2
United Kingdom					
Enrollees	1969	20,015	13,758	6257	31.3
Graduates	1970	6589	4976	1613	24.5
USSR§					
Enrollees	1970	321,023	141,748	179,275	55.8
Graduates	1970	7800	NA	NA	NA

*United Nations Educational, Scientific, and Cultural Organization: Statistical yearbook, 1973, Louvain, Belgium 1974, UNESCO Press.
†Includes anatomy, dentistry, medicine, midwifery, nursing, optometry, osteopathy, pharmacy, physiotherapy, public health, and similar subjects.
‡*NA* = Not available.
§Includes public health, physical culture, and sports.

Lack of money leads to placing priorities favoring men on educational opportunities and therefore access to income-producing employment; places go to men and members of the upper classes.[65]

Union of Soviet Socialist Republics (USSR)

In the USSR in 1970, the majority of physicians were women—73.7%. Women comprised 77.4% of the dentists, 82.9% of the feldshers (paramedics), 94.9% of the pharmacists, and 99.1% of the nurses. More than 50% of all USSR physicians work in the Russian federation, the largest republic. A study of that region showed that over 60% of women physicians specialized in therapies (defined as hematology, physiotherapy, cardiorheumatology, endocrinology, gastroenterology), pediatrics, obstetrics and gynecology, and stomatology (study of diseases of the mouth).[54] Nearly 6% of Soviet women physicians specialize in surgery, compared with 3% in Sweden, 2.3% in Finland, and 1.4% in the United States.

Women are also better represented in administration in the Soviet Union; in 1975 "twelve women [were] vice-ministers at Ministries of Health of the USSR and union republics; three women [held] posts as Ministers of Health in autonomous republics, and 48 [were heads of] main departments and departments of ministries."[54]

In addition to midwives, the USSR has another midlevel women's health worker known as an *akusherka*. Similar to the obstetrical nurses being developed in the United States, the *akusherka* is widely used to implement the preventive care philosophy of Soviet medicine. In cancer screening clinics, for example, all women age 25 years and over are brought in for cytology tests for cervical carcinoma. These tests are conducted by an *akusherka*, or obstetrical assistant (the name is a diminutive of *akusher*—obstetrician).

In women's advisory clinics, which appear to be dispensaries forming part of the polyclinic-hospital combination in urban centers, *akusherkas* deliver basic gynecological care, but here they are under closer physician supervision. They treat minor pelvic disorders and vaginitis and do complete pelvic examinations, referring complications to the physician.[82] Young girls also receive gynecological care from *akusherkas*.

The other important function of this midlevel practitioner (and also of the feldsher) is to provide health education. It is an integral part of the prophylaxis offered in a polyclinic or rural health center.

In rural areas of the USSR, midwives and feldsher-midwife auxiliaries (a personnel category that is disappearing) handle basic gynecological care as part of their practice. Dr. Daniel Flauhault, chief medical officer, training of auxiliary personnel, World Health Organization, indicates that special training programs have been implemented for midwives to do routine laboratory work related to minor gynecological conditions. For example, gonorrhea is managed in rural areas by a midwife and in urban areas by an obstetrical assistant.[73] Contraception is provided by midwives, abortions are referred to the *uchastok* (district) physician, and sexuality problems, which might be a logical inclusion in this scope of practice, are not mentioned in the literature.

People's Republic of China

Much has been written on the rural barefoot doctors in China—half of whom are women.[64] In addition to their basic primary health care responsibilities, the barefoot doctors may practice obstetrics and do family planning, in which they may be assisted by a midwife.

In urban China auxiliary health workers who have particular significance for women are utilized. Urban auxiliary health workers are known as Red medical workers and function on "Lane Committees," smaller health unit subdivisions of the neighborhoods. These Lane Committee health station workers are always women, frequently local housewives. They usually receive about a month's basic training at their district hospital and are subsequently visited by a physician from that facility about three times a week. Red medical workers screen for cervical cancer, provide contraceptive education, and make routine house calls to encourage contraceptive compliance. (As a mark of their success, the Sidels report that in one Lane Committee health station, the birth rate was as low as 8 per 1000, whereas in rural areas the crude birth rate is slightly under 24 per 1000.)[64]

Both Red medical workers and barefoot doctors receive training in traumatology and treatment of the newborn. They may insert intrauterine devices, and in the absence of more highly trained personnel, a very experienced worker may perform abortions and vasectomies.[27] Auxiliary personnel may also be used within industrial centers to promote health education, contraceptive utilization and routine screening.

OTHER GENERAL CHARACTERISTICS OF WOMEN'S WORK FORCE PARTICIPATION

In addition to licensure discussed at the beginning of this chapter, several factors have interacted and continue to interact to inhibit women's equitable participation in health care delivery.

By and large, women have not cared for groups exerting power within society. With the exception of a few royal midwives, women health care workers throughout history have generally treated, as they do today, the powerless: children, other women, those seeking public health services, and the mentally ill. They have not had the benefits that wealthy clients and patronage can bring.

Women have also lacked the economic independence to seek out health careers that required long periods of training. For the most part, the women who became physicians in the early United States came from comfortable family circumstances and had strong psychological support from their families. Since, in general, women have little financial independence and are not encouraged to participate productively in society, they remain isolated from one another and from life itself. This isolation serves to control women's development. That such control has been considered desirable is emphasized by the fact that one of the charges brought against witches in Europe, Anne Hutchinson in America, and feminists of all times is that they organized women and met in groups.

The growth of technology curtailed women's participation in healing but only because a specific education from which women were excluded was deemed necessary to use the technology. The development of the forceps in the seventeenth century, the use of which was reserved to physicians, and the advances in surgical technique today are examples of this. Such distinctions made in task delegation have led to an ever-narrowing definition of the skills that women health workers possess, a definition which can then be used to block women's participation.

Hierarchies within health care delivery have been particularly harmful to women. Intergroup competition became readily apparent among women healers after the rise of the universities, and male-controlled opposition to them increased. Physicians and empirics were differentially treated from midwives, who in turn were rated above nurses and old wives. This latter group were clearly in many cases persecuted by the midwives themselves, who were attacking as a defense to being attacked.

• • •

Intergroup competition contains an important lesson for women health workers today. It is apparent as physicians consider themselves to be separate from the rest of the health care team, as nurses stratify themselves into six ranks, and as both view themselves as being several rungs above clerical and service workers, or as physical therapists and social workers develop their own aides and divide themselves into "professionals" and "workers." Not only does patient care suffer in this process, but the mutual support that might encourage women's more equitable participation in health care delivery is dissipated. As Kate Campbell Hurd-Mead, a historian and physician of the early twentieth century, stated:

It is not a substitution of women for men that will bring about a new impetus to medical efficiency, but a closer union of women themselves, together with truer comradeship between men and women doctors, and a wider and deeper education in cultural subjects as well as in medical sciences which will result in an ever increasing service to humanity.[42]

SUGGESTED TOPICS FOR DISCUSSION, FURTHER RESEARCH, AND FIELD PROJECTS

1. What happens to men who enter professions traditionally occupied by women? What degree of status and social acceptance do they experience in comparison with women? How do their salaries compare with women's? Some suggested fields are social work, nursing and occupational and rehabilitative therapy. To what degree do men in these professions compare in status and social acceptance with men in traditionally male professions?

2. Should health workers be unionized? What are some factors that explain why only some health workers have unionized? Should health workers have the right to strike? If so, should this right be universal or limited to only certain health workers?

3. What are the licensing laws for midwives and new health professionals, for example, the Medex, nurse-practitioner, and paramedics in your state? Can they receive third party reimbursement? Can they prescribe drugs? Are women evenly distributed in the various categories of new health professionals?

4. Study the nurses' "1985 proposal." What are the pro and con arguments? Who will benefit and lose if the proposal is passed? How will the "1985 proposal" affect nursing as we know it today? How does the "1985 proposal" fit in with nursing's historical development in the United States? (A suggested initial reference: Dolan, A. K.: The New York State Nurses Association 1985 Proposal: who needs it? J. Health Politics and Law, **2:**508-531, Winter, 1978.)

5. Research the numbers and ranks of academic personnel at the nearest medical school. What percentage and which ranks are comprised of women? Is there a salary differential between men and women in the same rank? NOTE: in most state-supported medical schools, salaries are in the public record, which is usually available in libraries.

6. Contact local health workers' unions. What are their chief organizing issues? SUGGES-
   TION: Contact NUHHCE 1199, 310 W. 43rd St., New York, N.Y. 10036.
7. Contact local professional societies, for example, medical, veterinary, and dental.
   What percentage of their members are women? In what specialties do they practice?
   What hours do they work and in what type of practice settings?
8. Research the status of nontraditional health care workers in your area, for example,
   naturopaths, curanderas, lay midwives, and root doctors. What groups do they serve?
   How are they reimbursed? How do their fees compare with traditional practitioners?
   What is their legal status? What is the distribution of men and women?
9. Many women's groups (including the Women's Bureau of the Department of Labor)
   support the philosophy of "equal pay for work of equal value" rather than "equal pay
   for equal work." What are the implications of the two approaches? What effects would
   each philosophy have on health care workers?
10. What have been/are the effects, both historically and at the present, of seeking "pro-
    fessionalism" for women health workers? Who has gained and who has lost by "profes-
    sionalization?" What has been won or lost?

REFERENCES

1. ADA News, Report on women in dentistry, Aug. 2, 1971.
2. Adamson, E. T.: Critical issues in the use of
   physician associates and assistants, Am. J.
   Public Health **61:**1765-1779, 1971.
3. Agree, B.: The threat of institutional licensure, Am. J. Nurs. **73:**1758-1763, 1973.
4. American College of Obstetricians and Gynecologists: Personal communication, Oct. 5,
   1978.
5. Appelbaum, A.: Women in health care administration, Hospitals **49:**52-59, 1975.
6. Barker-Benfield, G. J.: Anne Hutchinson
   and the Puritan attitude toward women,
   Feminist Studies 1:65-96, Fall, 1972.
7. Berliner, H.: A larger perspective on the
   Flexner Report, Int. J. Health Serv. **5:**573-
   592, 1975.
8. Bluestone, N.: The future impact of women
   physicians on American medicine, Am. J.
   Public Health **68:**760-763, 1978. (Also,
   Medical education in the U.S. 1977-1978,
   Appendix II, Table 2, J.A.M.A. **240:**2892-
   2894, 1978.)
9. Bolton, C.: Early practice of medicine by
   women, J. Sci. pp. 1-15, Jan., 1881.
10. Brown, C.: Women workers in the health
    service industry, Int. J. Health Serv. **5:**173-
    183, 1975.
11. Bullough, V. L.: The development of medi-
    cine as a profession, New York, 1966,
    Hafner Press.
12. Bullough, V., and Voght, M.: Women,
    menstruation and nineteenth century medi-
    cine, Bull. Hist. Med. **47:**66-82, 1973, p. 75.
13. Campbell, M.: Why would a girl go into
    medicine? Old Westbury, N.Y. 1973, The
    Feminist Press.
14. Cannings, K., and Lazonick, W.: The de-
    velopment of the nursing workforce in the
    United States: a basic analysis, Int. J. Health
    Serv. **5:**185-216, 1975.
15. Carpenter, E.: Women in male dominated
    health professions, Int. J. Health Serv. **7:**
    191-208, 1977.
16. Cohen, E., editor: The new health profes-
    sionals, Rockville, Md., 1977, Aspen Sys-
    tems Corp.
17. Committee for the Study of Nursing Edu-
    cation: Nursing and nursing education in
    the United States, New York, 1923, Mac-
    millan Inc.
18. Coombs, J., and Drolette, M.: Discrimina-
    tion—the case of the female dental student,
    Women & Health, **2:**12-21, July/Aug., 1977.
19. Day, L. R., et al.: Acceptance of pediatric
    nurse practitioners, Am. J. Dis. Child **119:**
    204-208, 1970.
20. DeFigueroa, T. O.: Young, woman and Latin
    American, Gazette 7 (no. 1), pp. 8-11. (Pub-
    lication of the Pan American Health Organi-
    zation [no date].)
21. Devitt, N.: The statistical case for the elimi-
    nation of the midwife. Fact versus prejudice:
    1890-1935, Women & Health **4:**81-96,
    Spring, 1979.
22. Directory of accredited residencies 1977-78,
    Chicago, 1978, American Medical Associa-
    tion.
23. Distribution of dentists in the United States
    by state, region, district & county, Chicago,

1979, Bureau of Economic Research & Statistics, American Dental Association.

24. Dock, L.: The relation of training schools to hospitals. In Hampton, I., editor: Nursing of the Sick, 1893, New York, 1949, McGraw-Hill Book Co.

25. Facts about nursing 1976-77: Kansas City, Mo., 1977, American Nurses Association.

26. Farrell, K., et al.: Women physicians in medical academia: a national statistical survey, J.A.M.A. **241:**2808-2812, 1979. (Additional data obtained from Braslow, J., Association of American Medical College Faculty Roster, Association of American Medical Colleges, Washington, D.C.: Personal communication, Aug., 1979.)

27. Faundes, A., and Luukkainen, T.: Health and family planning services in the Chinese Peoples' Republic, Stud. Fam. Plann. **3:**165-176, July, 1972.

28. Findley, P.: Priests of Lucina: the story of obstetrics, Boston, 1939, Little, Brown & Co., p. 346.

29. Flexner, A.: Medical education in the United States and Canada, New York, 1910, Carnegie Foundation.

30. Gantz, P.: Medical schools embrace older women. Med. Dimensions **5:**30-33: April, 1976.

31. Glaser, W. A.: Paying the doctor: systems of remuneration and their effects, Baltimore, Md., 1970, the Johns Hopkins, University Press.

32. Goodman, L. J.: Physician distribution and medical licensure in the U.S., 1976, Chicago, 1977, American Medical Association.

33. Graduates U.S. schools of public health 1975-1976, June 30, 1976, Association of Schools of Public Health.

34. Grissum, M., and Spengler, C.: Womanpower & health care, Boston, 1976, Little, Brown & Co.

35. Haar, E., et al.: Factors related to the preference for a female gynecologist, Med. Care **13:**782-790, 1975.

36. Haggard, H. W.: Devils, drugs and doctors, New York, 1929, Harper & Row, Publishers.

37. Heins, M., et al.: A comparison of the productivity of women & men physicians, Office of The Assistant Secretary for Planning & Evaluation, U.S. Department of Health, Education and Welfare, Washington, D.C., 1976, U.S. Government Printing Office.

38. Hershey, N.: An alternative to mandatory licensure of health professionals, Hosp. Prog. **50:**71-74, March, 1969.

39. Higher education and the nations's health: policies for medical and dental education, Carnegie Commission of Higher Education, New York, 1970, McGraw-Hill Book Co. (For commentary on the report, see reference 37.)

40. Hole, C.: A mirror of witchcraft, London, 1957, Chatto & Windus, Ltd.

41. Hughes, M. J.: Women healers in mediaeval life and literature, New York, 1943, King's Crown Press.

42. Hurd-Mead, K. C.: The seven important periods in the evolution of women in medicine, address to the Woman's Medical College of Pennsylvania, June 11, 1930, Bull. Woman's Med. College of Pennsylvania, **81:** 1-15, 1930.

43. Hurd-Mead, K. C.: A history of women in medicine from the earliest times to the beginning of the nineteenth century, Conn., 1938, The Haddam Press.

44. Jex-Blake, S.: Medical women, Edinburgh, Oliphant, Anderson and Ferrier, 1886, Source Book Press. p. 23.

45. Kett, J. F.: The formation of the American medical profession, New Haven, Conn., 1968, Yale University Press.

46. Marieskind, H. I.: Gynaecological services: their historical relationship to the womens' movement with recent experience of self-help clinics and other delivery modes, doctoral dissertation, #762-5222-01500, Ann Arbor, Mich., 1976, Xerox University Microfilms.

47. Marks, G., and Beatty, W. K.: Women in white, New York, 1972, Charles Scribner's Sons.

48. Medical Tribune Report: Patients found mistrustful of women M.Ds., Med. Tribune **15:**13, May 1, 1974.

49. National Center for Educational Statistics: Earned degrees conferred 1975-76, Stock no. 017-080-01868-3, Washington, D.C., 1975, U.S. Government Printing Office.

50. National Union of Hospital and Health Care Employees, Local 1199: Personal communication, Oct. 13, 1978.

51. Navarro, V.: Women in health care, N. Engl. J. Med. **292:**398-402, 1975.

52. Ostergard, D. R., et al.: A training program for allied health personnel in family planning and cancer screening, J. Reprod. Med. **7:**40, 1971.

53. Packard, F. R.: History of medicine in the United States, vol. 1, New York, 1931, Hafner Press, p. 49.

54. Piradova, M.: USSR—women in the health professions, Women & Health **1**:24-29, May/June, 1976.

55. Polansky, E.: The social and economic impact on the family members who care for the chronically ill at home, doctoral dissertation, New York, 1980, Columbia University School of Social Work.

56. Power, E.: Some women practitioners of medicine in the middle ages. In Proceedings of the Royal Society of Medicine: History of Medicine, section XV, no. 6, London, 1922.

57. Public Law 95-210. Regulations finalized during 1978.

58. Punnett, L.: Women-controlled medicine—theory and practice in 19th century Boston, Women & Health **1**:3-10, July/Aug., 1976.

59. Reverby, S.: The emergence of hospital nursing, Health/PAC Bull., no. 66, pp. 7-15, Sept./Oct., 1975.

60. Riley, H. J., editor: Memorials of London. Cited in Jones, I. B.: Popular medical knowledge in fourteenth century English literature, part I, Bull. Inst. History Med. **5**:519-520, May, 1937.

61. Schwartz, P. J., and Gibbens, S. F.: Boundary medicine. A preliminary estimate of health care outside of the conventional medical system, Report to Health Planning and Intergovernmental Relations, Sacramento, 1975, California State Department of Health.

62. Shryock, R. H.: Medicine in America: historical essays, Baltimore, 1966, The Johns Hopkins University Press.

63. Shryock, R. H.: Medical licensing in America, 1650-1965, Baltimore, 1967, The Johns Hopkins University Press.

64. Sidel, R., and Sidel, V.: The delivery of medical care in China, Sci. Am. **230**:19-27, April, 1974.

65. Silver, G.: International innovations in health policy regarding women. The geography may change a lot: the situation very little, paper presented at Conference on Women in Health, region III, Philadelphia, June, 1976.

66. Smith, K. R.: Manpower substitution in ambulatory care. In Rafferty, J., editor: Health, manpower, and productivity, Lexington, Mass., 1974, Lexington Books.

67. Smith, M. R., et al.: The R.N. obstetric assistant: a clinical trial, Obstet. Gynecol. **38**:308-312, Aug., 1971.

68. Smith, R. A., et al.: A strategy for health manpower: reflections on an experience called Medex, J.A.M.A. **217**:1362-1367, 1971.

69. Spencer, H. R.: The history of British midwifery from 1650-1800, London, 1927, John Bale, Sons & Danielsson, Ltd.,

70. Spillane, E. J.: Top management compensation in Catholic-sponsored hospitals, Hosp. Prog. **53**: 41, Nov. 1972.

71. Steinwachs, D. H., et al.: The role of new health practitioners in a prepaid group practice, Med. Care **14**:95-120, 1976.

72. Stevens, R.: Critical questions for medicine's future, Prism, **3**:10, Feb, 1975.

73. U.S.S.R. Ministry of Public Health: Detection of gonorrhea in the population. The role of womens' consultation stations in the Ukranian S.S.R., INT/VDT/183, Geneva, Nov. 16, 1962, World Health Organization.

74. Ventre, F.: The making of a legalized lay midwife, Birth & the Family Journal **3**: 109-115, Fall, 1976.

75. Wallace, J.: Part-time internships and residencies: programs to be encouraged, J. Am. Med. Wom. Assoc. **24**:566-570, 1969.

76. *Washington State Nurses' Association* vs. *Board of Medical Examiners For The State of Washington and Doctor Robert F. Wilkins, Its Chairman, and the State of Washington:* No. 6850-I, 1978.

77. What is a nurse-midwife? Washington, D.C., 1974, The American College of Nurse-Midwives. (Also see Nurse-midwifery in the United States, 1976-1977, Washington, D.C., 1978, The American College of Nurse-Midwives.)

78. Williams, J. W.: Medical education and the midwife problem in the United States, J.A.M.A. **58**:1-7, 1912.

79. Women in health careers, chart book for International Conference on Women in Health, Bureau of Health Manpower, stock no. 017-041-00104-1, Washington, D.C., 1975, U.S. Government Printing Office.

80. Womens' Bureau: The earnings gap between women and men, Employment Standards Administration, U.S. Department of Labor, Washington, D.C., 1976, U.S. Government Printing Office.

81. Womens' Rights Project of the Center for Law & Social Policy, Washington, D.C.

82. World Health Organization. MCH in the

U.S.S.R., Public Health Pap. **11:** entire issue, 1962.

ADDITIONAL READINGS

Association of American Medical Colleges (AAMC): Participation of women and minorities on U.S. medical school faculties, (HRA) 76-91, contract no. NOI-MI-24401, Washington, D.C., March, 1976, U.S. Government Printing Office.

Barringer, E. D.: Bowery to Bellevue, the story of New York's first woman ambulance surgeon, New York, 1950, W. W. Norton & Co.

Blake, J. B.: Women and medicine in ante-bellum America, Bull. Hist. Med. **39:**99-123, March/April, 1965.

Boquist, C., and Haase, J.: An historical review of women in dentistry. An annotated bibliography, (HRA), 77-643, June, 1977, U.S. Department of Health, Education and Welfare.

Bullough, B.: Barriers to the nurse practitioner movement: a problem of women in a woman's field, Int. J. Health Serv. **5:**225-233, 1975.

Campbell, R.: Minorities in nursing, January, 1973, California Nurses' Association, 185 Post St., San Francisco, Calif.

Cleland, V.: Sex discrimination: nursing's most pervasive problem, Am. J. Nurs. **71:**1542-1547, 1971.

Cooper, V.: Women as health workers—the lady's not for burning, Health/PAC Bull., no. 15, pp. 2-7, March, 1970.

Dillon, T. F., et al.: Midwifery, 1977, Am. J. Obstet. Gynecol. **130:**917-926, 1978.

Fried, F. E.: Women in medicine—the training years, J. Operational Psychiatry **5:**101-102, 1974.

Funkenstein, D. H.: Medical students, medical schools and society during five eras: factors affecting the career choices of physicians 1958-1976, Cambridge, Mass. 1978, Ballinger Publishing Co.

Gordon, T. L., and Johnson, D. G.: Study of U.S. medical school applicants, 1976-1977, J. Med. Educ. **53:**873-897, 1978.

Hasselbart, S.: Women doctors win and male nurses lose—a study of sex role and occupational stereotypes, Sociology of Work and Occupations, **4:**49-62, Feb. 19, 1977.

Heins, M., et al.: Comparison of the productivity of women and men physicians, J.A.M.A. **237:**2514-2517, 1977.

Hooyman, N. R., and Kaplan, J. S.: New roles for professional women: skills for change, Public Administration Review **36:**374-378, July/Aug., 1976.

Hurd-Mead, K. C.: Medical women of America, New York, 1933, Froben.

Institute of Personality Assessment and Research, University of California, Berkeley: Bibliography of longitudinal study of physicians in training and in practice, Harrison G. Gough, Ph.D., director, May, 1978.

Jenkins, G.: 1985: closing the door on nurses New York style, Health/PAC Bull., no. 78, Sept./Oct., 1977.

Jussim, J., and Muller, C.: Medical education for women: how good an investment? J. Med. Educ. **50:**571-580, June, 1975.

Kobrin, F. E.: The American midwife controversy: a crisis of professionalization, Bull. Hist. Med. **40:**350-363, July/Aug., 1966.

Levy, B., et al.: Reducing neonatal mortality rate with nurse-midwives, Am. J. Obstet. Gynecol. **189:**50-58, 1971.

Linn, E. L.: Professional activities of women dentists, J. Am. Dent. Assoc. **81:**1383-1387, 1970.

Lopate, C.: Women in medicine, Baltimore, 1968, Johns Hopkins University Press.

Nerlinger, J.: Things looking up—but not too far for women M.H.A.S., Modern Hospital **120:**47, Jan. 1973.

Nutting, A., and Dock, L. L.: History of nursing, 4 vols., New York, 1907-1912, G. P. Putnam's Sons.

Pollitt, A.: Social and Psychological Characteristics in Medical Specialty and Geographic Decisions, Graduate Medical Education National Advisory Committee, Department of Health, Education and Welfare, Health Resources Administration, (HRA) 78-13, Washington, D.C., 1978, U.S. Government Printing Office.

Proceedings of the International Conference on Women in Health: June 16-18, 1975, U.S. Department of Health, Education and Welfare, (HRA) 76-51, Washington, D.C., 1975, U.S. Government Printing Office.

Radcliffe Program in Health Care, Haase, J. V., project director: A study of the participation of women in the health care industry labor force, U.S. Department of Health, Education and Welfare, 1976 (HRA), 77-644, Washington, D.C., 1976, U.S. Government Printing Office.

Reverby, S.: Health: women's work, Health/PAC Bull., no. 40, pp. 15-20, April, 1972.

Roeske, N. A.: Women in psychiatry: a review, Am. J. Psychiatry **133:**365-372, April, 1976.

Scher, M.: Women psychiatrists in the U.S., Am. J. Psychiatry **130:**118-122, Oct., 1973.

Shamban, N.: R.N's strike, Health/PAC Bull., no. 60, Sept./Oct., 1974.

Slome, C., et al.: Effectiveness of certified nurse-midwives. A prospective evaluation study, Am. J. Obstet. Gynecol. **124:**177-182, 1976.

Spieler, E.: Division of laborers, Health/PAC Bull., no. 46, pp. 3-9, Nov., 1972.

Student National Medical Association Inc.: Minority medical students, U.S. Department of Health, Education and Welfare, Health Resources Administration, (HRA) 78-635, Washington, D.C., 1977, U.S. Government Printing Office.

Urban and Rural Systems: Exploratory study of women in the health professions schools, Women's Action Program, U.S. Department of Health, Education and Welfare, contract HEW-05-74-291, Washington, D.C., 1976, U.S. Government Printing Office.

U.S. Department of Health, Education and Welfare: Minorities and women in the health fields: applicants, students, and workers, (HRA) 76-22, Washington, D.C., 1975, U.S. Government Printing Office.

Walsh, M. R.: Doctors wanted: no women need apply, New Haven and London, 1977, Yale University Press.

Werther, W., and Lockhart, C.: Labor relations in the health professions, Boston, 1976, Little, Brown & Co.

Williams, P. A.: Women in medicine: some themes and variations, J. Med. Educ. **46:**584-591, July, 1971.

Wiseman, J. P.: Social forces and the politics of research approaches: studying the wives of alcoholics. In Olson, V., editor: Women and their health: research implications for a new era, (HRA) 77-3138, National Center for Health Services Research, Washington, D.C., 1975, U.S. Government Printing Office.

Women in the workplace: a special section, Monthly Labor Review **97:**3-84, May, 1974.

Women health workers, a slide show, Philadelphia, 1976, Women's Health Collective, 5027 Newhall St., Philadelphia, Pa. 19144.

Women's Work Project of the Union for Radical Political Economics: U.S.A.—women health workers, Women & Health **1:**14-23, May/June, 1976.

Yerxa, E. J.: On being a member of a "feminine" profession, Am. J. Occupational Therapy **29:**597-598, 1975.

Chapter 5

Women and occupational health

Much of women's greater longevity (see Chapter 1) has been attributed to their lack of exposure to the work environment and the assumption, in contradiction to mental health statistics, that there is less stress in their lives. Conversely, the fact that United States males' longevity is eighteenth in the world while United States females' is ninth[94] has been attributed to the more predominant exposure of men to the factory environment, with its less stringent health and safety standards than in many other industrialized countries.

Today, women are rapidly entering traditional male jobs and are reaffirming in massive numbers what has been known for centuries — that the average work place is safe for neither men nor women.

HISTORICAL BACKGROUND

In the United States, women's first major participation outside the home in the productive work force was as slaves; their appalling work conditions on one plantation have been documented by Kemble.[50] Womens' first major participation in the paid industrial work force was in the mid-nineteenth century as textile workers in the mills of New England, where women and children* comprised 90% of the work force. Women's work of that era was characterized (as it still generally is today) by lower pay, exposure to occupational hazards[96] (see Table 5-1), inadequate union representation, and increased opportunities when men were occupied elsewhere, as, for example, during war.[29]

Early efforts by women to improve their lot through unionization were opposed, and in the 1870s, only the cigarmaker's union and the typographical union admitted women. By the 1880s the Knights of Labor were organizing women workers and, together with women's own organizing efforts, this led in 1903 to the establishment of the Women's Trade Union League;[28, pp. 410-413] this essentially died in 1941, although a skeletal staff continued until 1950 and a New York branch continued until the early 1950s.

---

*Child labor was finally regulated by the Fair Labor Standards Act of June 4, 1938. The act provided a basic wage and a maximum work day in interstate industries, established enforcement methods, and provided the opportunity for subsequent establishment of a national minimum standard of child labor. See Bradbury, D. E.: Five decades of action for children: a history of the children's bureau, Washington, D.C., 1962, U.S. Department of Health, Education and Welfare.

Table 5-1. Mortality by age per 1000 textile mill workers and nonworkers in Fall River, Massachusetts, 1912*

Ages	Men workers	Men nonworkers	Women workers	Women nonworkers
15 to 19 years	2.48	4.64	4.91	2.85
20 to 24 years	4.41	5.22	5.68	3.07
25 to 29 years	4.47	4.13	7.66	5.04
30 to 34 years	8.46	8.70	11.30	7.09
35 to 39 years	11.69	5.67	11.57	5.90
40 to 44 years	7.20	9.99	14.57	7.61

*Data collected by the Federal Bureau of Labor and published as part of their "Report on the Condition of Women and Child Wage Earners in the United States," vol. XIV, Washington, D.C., 1912. Adapted from Hamilton, A.: Do women in industry need special health legislation? In The health of women and children, New York, 1977, Arno Press, Inc.

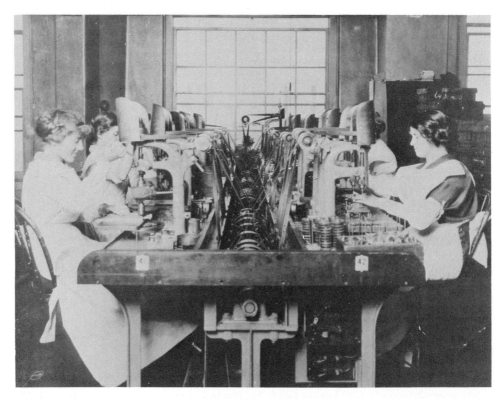

Fig. 5-1. Working the drill presses, early 1900s. (Courtesy Women's Bureau, U.S. Department of Labor.)

Early occupational studies

Various reports on occupational hazards, particularly in the tobacco industry, had been issued throughout the nineteenth century and served to highlight the need for worker protection.[63] Demands by work force leaders[76] with support from feminists, volunteer charity workers, and other middle-class women eventually led to a congressional inquiry from 1908 to 1911 on the status and conditions of women and children's work.[96] Over the subsequent decades, reported hazards and tragedies, some of which are described here, aroused public attention. This has culminated today in formally organized study of women's occupational health.

In 1908 an investigation was conducted of the phosphorous match factories, where about half the work force was women and children. It was found that 5.9% (151) of the industry's 2540 workers had been poisoned by phosphorus, resulting in bone degeneration, and in particular a deformity of the jaw known as "phossy jaw."[101] In 1937 the Factories Act finally prohibited the use of poisonous white phosphorus in the manufacture of matches.

The Triangle Shirtwaist Factory fire of March 25, 1911, lasted for only 20 minutes, but during this time about 150 women and young girls burned or jumped to their deaths. The building lacked fire escapes or alarms, the fire was several stories up in the building, and the company owners had bribed fire marshals to report fire-safe working conditions. The factory owners were tried and acquitted, although one was subsequently fined $20.00.[13]

From its establishment in 1912, the Children's Bureau, originally in the Department of Labor and now in the Department of Health, Education and Welfare, together with the Women's Bureau established in 1920 in the Department of Labor, published data and supported epidemiological studies of women's health, particularly as they related to fetal and infant outcome. One report demonstrated that in two New England mill-town communities, high infant mortality rates were occurring. The 1913 data from New Bedford, Massachusetts, showed an infant mortality rate for children of women "gainfully employed" prior to giving birth of 154.5 per 1000 as compared with 108.8 for infants of unemployed mothers.[17] Similarly, in 1914 in Manchester, New Hampshire, the rates for the infants of the employed and unemployed groups were 199.2 and 133.9, respectively. Further analysis of women working away from home and unemployed women showed infant mortality rates of 227.5 and 149.8 per 1000 live births.[98] These rates were consistent with 1897 findings from England on perinatal and infant mortality among lead workers. The 212 pregnancies among women lead workers in 1897 resulted in only 61 living children. The number of miscarriages and stillbirths among women who worked in lead after marriage was triple that of women working at housework only.[35] Explanations for these differences noted the poverty and early return to work of all the employed groups, in addition to exposure to the work environment.

In 1929, 42 cases of degenerative bone tissue and severe anemia were found among watch dial painters and were attributed to the ingestion of the radioactive paint used for marking the luminous numbers. Of the victims, 80% were women;

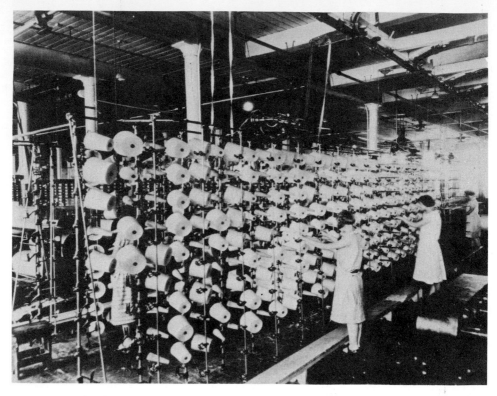

Fig. 5-2. Textile factory, 1930s. (Courtesy Women's Bureau, U.S. Department of Labor.)

as the women twisted the brushes in their mouths to make a fine tip, the paint was being absorbed. Subsequent studies of these workers showed an abnormally high cancer incidence.[74]

One of the most thorough studies of women's occupational health was sponsored by the U.S. Army and was authored by Dr. Anna Baetjer[6] of Johns Hopkins University. Published in 1946, *Women in Industry* delineated the many areas in which research was needed and reported on the potential effects on the fetus of benzene, turpentine, carbon monoxide, carbon disulfide, hydrocarbon, lead, mercury, and radiation, as well as discussing typical sweatshop conditions. Baetjer concluded that particular protective measures should be taken for pregnant women workers, but she reviewed all available data and stated that, contrary to widespread opinion, nonpregnant women did not appear to be any more susceptible than men to poisoning from toxic substances such as lead.[6]

A more recent report on yet another occupational health hazard was published in 1974 by the American Society of Anesthesiologists (ASA), supported by the National Institute for Occupational Safety and Health (NIOSH). By retrospective review the study showed that female operating room personnel had higher rates of spontaneous abortion, cancer, and hepatic and renal disease, and that their children had higher rates of congenital abnormalities than was true for comparable professional groups who were not exposed to operating rooms. The study noted that "this increased risk of congenital abnormalities was also present among the unexposed wives of male operating room personnel." Because of the suggested relationship between exposure to anesthetic gases and the cited medical conditions, the report strongly recommended adequate venting of gases from operating rooms.[3]

Alice Hamilton

Throughout the nineteenth and twentieth centuries, of all the various reports filed, the work of Alice Hamilton (1869-1970) particularly stands out in developing national concern for women's occupational health problems. Strongly in favor of special protective legislation for women (discussed later), Hamilton focused several of her studies on the effects of the workplace on pregnant women.[35]

Alice Hamilton grew up in Fort Wayne, Indiana, and attended one of the small eclectic medical colleges of the Midwest. After transferring to the University of Michigan and graduating in 1893, Hamilton became interested in pathology. She pursued further study in this field in Leipzig, Germany, and returned to the United States in 1896. Hamilton found little interest in her skills and after some additional study at Johns Hopkins, moved to Chicago where she joined Jane Addams at Hull House. Her enthusiasm for social medicine grew, and she soon opened a well-baby clinic.

Alice Hamilton's interest in occupational health began in 1902 with her investigation into a typhoid epidemic among Chicago's poor. This, combined with her contacts with working class peoples through her activities at Hull House, provided Hamilton with evidence of the effects and extent of poisoning from toxic chemicals in the workplace.

In 1910 Hamilton was appointed to a commission in the State of Illinois to study occupational illness and began a full-time commitment to this emerging specialty. Hamilton was assigned to investigate lead poisoning and proceeded to visit factories, workers' clubs, homes, and unions. She was spurred on by her embarrassment at the paucity of U.S. data compared with those of European countries. These countries' efforts to ensure industrial safety were demonstrated to her when she was the U.S. representative to the International Congress on Occupational Accidents and Diseases in Brussels in 1910.

Over the next decades, in addition to her pacifist, socialist, and femininst activities, Alice Hamilton reported on the paint, explosives, and munitions industries, the hazards in stone-cutting and copper-mining work, and the dangers of lead, carbon monoxide, mercury, viscose rayon, and a variety of solvents, including benzol.[36] She identified silicosis, industrial anemia, "caisson disease," paralysis, and insanity as a result of workplace conditions.[37]

In 1918 Hamilton was appointed to a professorship at the Harvard Medical School, overcoming accusations of being pro-German because of her pacifist beliefs (reluctantly abandoned after visits to pre–World War II Nazi Germany). As the first woman professor it was made clear to her she was hired because no male who could teach industrial medicine could be found; "she must not use the

Harvard Club available to all other faculty members, she must not demand her quota of football tickets, and she must not embarrass the faculty by marching in the graduation procession or by sitting on the commencement platform."[31]

Hamilton retired from Harvard in 1935 as professor emeritus of industrial medicine, and at that time was convinced that with the strength of the labor movement and interest from professionals, occupational hazards would be minimized. She died in Connecticut at age 101.[19] Much of Alice Hamilton's work is only now being recognized, and her interests are gradually becoming a focus for contemporary health activists.[26]

WOMEN AT WORK
Female work force

During the first four decades of the twentieth century the rate of women's (over 14 years) participation in the labor force rose steadily from 20% to 29% (see Table 5-2). Although the rapid influx of women workers during World War II subsided after the war, many women continued in the work force. The postwar female labor force was increasingly married and middle class, with the most rapid growth occurring among women aged 35 and older. More recently, despite the less than 1 million licensed day-care slots, the most rapid increase in participation has come among wives aged 20 to 24 years with children under 6 years of age. In 1960, 19% of women in this group worked; by 1974 this had almost doubled to 37% (see Table 5-3).[103]

In 1979 the labor force was about 42%[79] female with 50.1% of women 16 years and over employed. Women are still predominantly employed, however, as

Table 5-2. Women in the labor force, selected years, 1890 to 1979*†‡

Date	Number	Percent of all workers	Percent of female population
1890 (June)	3,704,000	17.0	18.2
1900 (June)	4,999,000	18.1	20.0
1920 (January)	8,229,000	20.4	22.7
1930 (April)†	10,396,000	21.9	23.6
1940 (March)	13,783,000	25.4	28.9
1945 (April)	19,290,000	36.1	38.1
1950 (April)	17,882,000	29.1	33.0
1960 (April)	22,985,000	33.3	37.4
1965 (April)	25,831,000	35.0	38.8
1970 (April)	31,293,000	38.1	43.2
1974 (April)	35,165,000	39.3	45.0
1979 (January)	42,362,000	42.0	50.1

*Based on data from Women's Bureau, U.S. Department of Labor: 1975 Handbook on women workers, 1975, U.S. Government Printing Office; and current data from the Bureau of Labor Statistics.
†The number of working women is underestimated because, at least until 1930, farm women were generally not counted as employed.
‡Prior to 1968 females aged 14 and over were counted as women; after 1968 females aged 16 and over were counted as women.

clerical, service, and professional or technical workers (see Table 5-4). More detailed and recent breakdowns of women's employment by occupation (see Table 5-5), and industry (see Table 5-6) show that within these major occupational and industrial groupings, women work in the lower-paying positions with less upward mobility and in "traditional" female slots.

The shift of women to nontraditional jobs is occurring, however, most notably in the skilled trades. In 1960, 277,000 women worked in skilled occupations (craft and kindred worker group) as compared with 495,000 in 1970. The rate of increase was twice that for women in all occupations and eight times the rate for men in skilled trades. Specifically, the proportion of female carpenters changed from 0.4% in 1960 to 1.3% in 1970; of electricians, from 0.7% to 1.8%; of plumbers, from 0.3% to 1.1%; of auto mechanics, from 0.4% to 1.4%; of painters, from 1.9% to 4.1%; of tool and die makers, from 0.6% to 2.1%; and of machinists, from 1.3% to 3.1%.[103]

Text continued on p. 172.

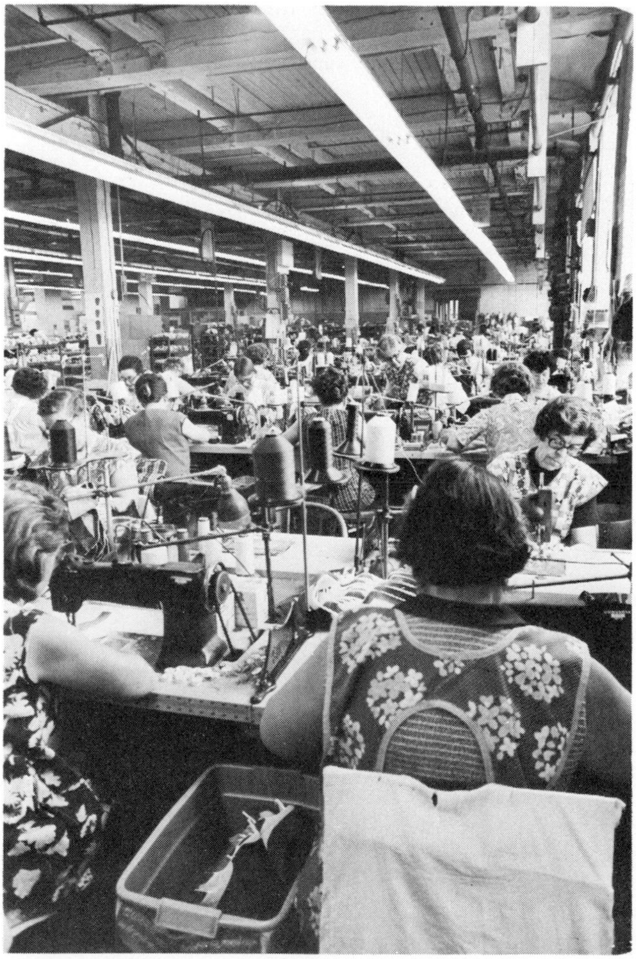

Fig. 5-3. Shoe factory, 1970s. (Courtesy Betty Medsger © Copyright 1975.)

Table 5-3. Labor force participation of mothers and of all women, selected years, 1940 to 1974*†

Year	Percent of female population employed‡	Percent of all mothers in labor force		
		With children under 18	With children under 6§	With children 6 to 17 years of age only‖
1940	28.2	8.6	NA#	NA
1946¶	31.2	18.2	NA	NA
1948	31.9	20.2	13.0	31.0
1952	33.8	23.8	16.0	35.0
1956	35.9	27.5	18.0	40.0
1960	36.7	30.4	19.0	43.0
1964	37.4	34.5	25.0	46.0
1968	41.6	39.4	29.0	50.0
1972	43.9	42.9	32.0	53.0
1974	45.2	45.7	37.0	54.0

*Based on data from Women's Bureau, U.S. Department of Labor: 1975 Handbook on women workers, 1975, U.S. Government Printing Office.
†Prior to 1968 females aged 14 and over were counted as women; after 1968 females aged 16 and over were counted as women.
‡Annual averages.
§May also have older children. Numbers rounded to the nearest percent.
‖Numbers rounded to the nearest percent.
¶Compare with Table 5-1 data for 1945 (38.1%) and note the rapid drop of female participation at the end of World War II.
#*NA* = Not available.

Table 5-4. Major occupational groups of employed women, selected years, 1959 to 1974*†

Major occupational group	Percent distribution				Women as a percent of total persons employed, April, 1974
	1959	1964	1969	April, 1974	
Professional, technical workers	12.1	13.0	13.8	15.6	41.6
Managers, administrators	5.1	4.6	4.3	5.0	18.6
Sales workers	7.8	7.3	6.9	6.8	41.7
Clerical workers	29.9	31.2	34.3	34.5	77.2
Craft and kindred workers	1.0	1.0	1.2	1.4	4.2
Operatives	15.4	15.3	15.4	13.1	31.6
Nonfarm laborers	.5	.4	.5	1.0	8.3
Service workers	23.5	23.9	21.6	21.3	62.5
Private household	9.0	8.4	5.5	3.9	98.5
Other	14.4	15.5	16.1	17.4	57.8
Farm workers	4.8	3.3	2.0	1.4	15.0
TOTAL	100.0	100.0	100.0	100.0	39.0

*Based on data from Manpower report of the President, April, 1974; and U.S. Department of Labor, Bureau of Labor Statistics: Employment and earnings, May, 1974; adapted from Women's Bureau, U.S. Department of Labor: 1975 Handbook on women workers, Washington, D.C., 1975, U.S. Government Printing Office.
†Women aged 16 and over.

Table 5-5. Occupations in which over 40% of employed persons are women (age 16 and over), 1978*

Occupations	Total number employed, both sexes (000)	Percent of total employed	
		Female	Black or other minority
White collar workers	47,205	52.1	8.1
Professional and technical	14,245	42.7	8.7
Librarians, archivists, and curators	202	80.7	6.9
Librarians	187	84.5	7.0
Personnel and labor relations workers	405	43.7	12.3
Nurses, dieticians, and therapists	1,351	92.9	11.7
Registered Nurses	1,112	96.7	11.7
Therapists	189	70.4	9.0
Health Technologists and technicians	498	70.9	12.9
Clinical laboratory technologists and technicians	208	73.6	14.4
Radiologic technologists and technicians	97	67.0	9.3
Psychologists	106	48.1	8.5
Social and recreation workers	505	61.0	19.2
Social workers	385	62.3	19.0
Recreation workers	121	57.0	20.7
Teachers, except college and university	2,992	71.0	9.8
Adult education	81	49.4	11.1
Elementary school	1,304	84.0	10.6
Prekindergarten and kindergarten	299	96.5	15.7
Secondary school	1,154	51.6	8.8
Others†	224	75.9	4.5
Radio operators	53	47.2	9.4
Vocational and educational counselors	171	52.6	14.6
Athletes and kindred workers	101	40.6	4.0
Editors and reporters	184	42.4	4.9
Painters and sculptors	186	44.6	2.2
Public relations specialists and publicity writers	131	40.5	4.6

*Based on data from U.S. Department of Labor, Bureau of Labor Statistics: Employment and earnings, vol. 26, no. 1, Jan. 1979.

†Not elsewhere classified.

Continued.

Table 5-5. Occupations in which over 40% of employed persons are women (age 16 and over), 1978—cont'd

Occupations	Total number employed, both sexes (000)	Percent of total employed	
		Female	Black or other minority
White collar workers—cont'd			
Buyers, wholesale and retail trade	170	40.0	5.3
Health administrators	184	46.2	7.6
Managers and superintendents, building	157	50.3	6.4
Office managers†	370	65.1	2.4
Sales workers	5,951	44.8	5.0
Demonstrators	96	94.8	4.2
Hucksters and peddlers	203	80.8	5.4
Real estate agents and brokers	555	45.0	2.7
Sales workers and sales clerks†	4,247	46.4	5.2
Sales clerks, retail trade	2,338	71.5	6.4
Sales workers, services and construction	169	43.2	7.7
Clerical workers	16,904	79.6	10.5
Bank tellers	449	91.5	8.0
Billing clerks	168	88.1	7.7
Bookkeepers	1,830	90.7	5.0
Cashiers	1,403	87.1	10.6
Clerical supervisors†	204	63.2	11.5
Collectors, bill and account	78	57.7	11.5
Counter clerks, except food	377	77.2	10.1
Enumerators and interviewers	53	75.5	15.9
Estimators and investigators†	451	53.4	10.6
File clerks	273	85.7	23.4
Insurance adjustors, examiners and investigators	169	51.5	11.2
Library attendants and assistants	172	80.8	11.0
Mail handlers, except Post Office	162	49.4	19.1
Office machine operators	827	74.2	15.4
Bookkeeping and billing machine	45	86.7	13.3
Computers and peripheral equipment	393	58.3	13.2
Key punch	273	95.6	18.3
Payroll and timekeeping clerks	241	75.5	7.1
Receptionists	588	96.9	9.5

Secretaries	3,590	99.2	6.2
Legal	162	99.4	3.1
Medical	83	98.8	7.2
Other†	3,345	99.2	6.3
Statistical clerks	377	76.1	11.7
Stenographers	94	90.4	10.6
Teachers aides, except school monitors	342	92.1	18.1
Telephone operators	311	94.2	12.5
Ticket, station, and express agents	128	40.6	11.7
Typists	1,044	96.6	16.2
All other clerical workers	1,674	41.9	14.3
Blue collar workers	31,531	18.3	12.4
Bakers	128	48.4	10.2
Decorators and window dressers	125	70.4	6.4
Assemblers	1,164	52.1	16.4
Bottling and canning operators	56	44.6	17.9
Checkers, examiners, and inspectors; manufacturing	736	48.8	11.8
Clothing ironers and pressers	126	80.2	42.9
Cutting operatives†	263	31.9	14.4
Dressmakers, except factory	116	97.4	12.1
Laundry and drycleaning operatives†	174	67.8	26.4
Packers and wrappers, excluding meat and produce	675	62.5	17.6
Photographic process workers	96	50.0	12.5
Sewers and stitchers	814	94.8	17.4
Shoemaking machine operatives	78	76.9	7.7
Textile operatives	374	59.9	25.7
Spinners, twisters, and winders	151	66.2	29.1
Winding operatives†	68	54.4	13.2
Bus drivers	337	45.1	21.1
Animal caretakers	83	51.8	9.6
Service workers	12,839	62.6	19.8
Private households	1,162	97.7	33.0
Child care workers	486	98.1	7.6
Cleaners and servants	530	97.0	52.5
Housekeepers	118	99.2	44.1

Continued.

Table 5-5. Occupations in which over 40% of employed persons are women (age 16 and over), 1978—cont'd

Occupations	Total number employed, both sexes (000)	Percent of total employed	
		Female	Black or other minority
Blue collar workers—cont'd			
Service workers, except private household	11,677	59.1	18.5
Cleaning workers	2,430	35.3	28.1
Lodging quarters cleaners	179	97.2	40.8
Building interior cleaners†	862	53.6	32.3
Food service workers	4,283	68.9	13.7
Cooks	1,186	57.2	20.2
Food counter and fountain workers	463	85.7	11.4
Waiters	1,383	90.5	7.2
Food service workers†	514	74.7	20.6
Health service workers	1,846	89.9	23.6
Dental assistants	130	98.5	3.8
Health aides, excluding nursing	276	86.2	19.6
Nursing aides, orderlies, and attendants	1,037	87.0	27.6
Practical nurses	402	97.0	22.4
Personal service workers	1,760	74.0	15.3
Attendants	306	57.2	13.1
Child care workers	425	94.8	15.3
Hairdressers and cosmetologists	542	89.1	9.2
Housekeepers	135	68.1	19.3
Welfare service aides	96	87.5	34.4
Farm laborers, unpaid family workers	299	69.6	2.7
TOTAL	94,373	41.2	11.2

Table 5-6. Industries in which over 40% of employed persons are women, 1978*

Industries	Total number employed, both sexes (000)	Percent of total employed	
		Female	Black or other minority
Agricultural services, except horticultural	245	40.8	8.2
Electrical machinery, equipment, and supplies	2,144	41.5	9.9
Electrical machinery†	1,409	42.9	9.7
Professional and photographic equipment and watches	560	42.5	7.1
Scientific and controlling instruments	160	40.6	5.6
Optical and health services supplies	231	51.5	6.9
Miscellaneous manufacturing industries	591	48.4	10.7
Canning and preserving (fruits, vegetables, seafood)	271	46.9	14.0
Confectionery and related products	94	55.3	20.2
Textile mill products	871	47.0	17.8
Knitting mills	196	64.3	10.2
Yarn, thread, and fabric mills	514	44.6	21.2
Apparel and other fabricated textile products	1,285	77.4	16.4
Apparel and accessories	1,128	79.6	16.7
Miscellaneous fabricated textile products	157	61.8	14.6
Soaps and cosmetics	143	42.0	11.2
Miscellaneous plastic products	379	45.1	8.4
Leather and leather products	283	62.5	9.2
Footwear, except rubber	189	69.8	7.4
Leather products, except footwear	68	58.8	5.9
Services incidental to transportation	177	58.8	5.1
Communications	1,311	44.8	11.2
Telephone (wire and radio)	1,065	48.3	11.5
Wholesale and retail trade	19,253	45.5	8.1
Dry goods and apparel	91	40.7	8.8

*Based on data from U.S. Department of Labor, Bureau of Labor Statistics: Employment and earnings, vol. 26, no. 1, Jan., 1979. *Continued.*

†Not elsewhere classified.

‡*NA* = Not available.

Table 5-6. Industries in which over 40% of employed persons are women, 1978—cont'd

Industries	Total number employed, both sexes (000)	Percent of total employed	
		Female	Black or other minority
Retail trade	15,636	50.3	8.4
Department and mail-order establishments	2,030	68.4	9.8
Limited-price variety stores	160	76.9	8.1
Direct-selling establishments	350	78.3	5.1
Miscellaneous general merchandise stores	218	71.1	6.9
Grocery stores	2,055	42.8	8.7
Dairy products stores	62	62.9	9.7
Retail bakeries	140	65.7	5.0
Food stores†	168	48.2	9.5
Apparel and accessory stores, except shoe stores	674	76.6	8.8
Shoe stores	132	45.5	5.3
Eating and drinking places	4,015	60.7	11.2
Drugstores	473	59.8	7.4
Jewelry stores	133	57.9	6.0
Retail florists	148	66.2	4.1
Miscellaneous retail stores	883	57.4	6.9
Finance, insurance, and real estate	5,406	55.6	9.0
Banking	1,442	70.9	10.3
Credit agencies	441	65.1	7.0
Insurance	1,776	53.8	9.1
Real estate, including real estate—insurance—law offices	1,478	43.3	8.6
Service industries	31,682	56.6	14.1

Employment and temporary help agencies	188	70.7	16.0
Business management and consulting services	268	51.5	6.0
Computer programming services	156	40.4	7.7
Business services†	623	50.7	7.1
Personal services	3,826	74.4	21.5
Private households	1,396	87.2	31.1
Hotels and motels	693	61.2	22.1
Laundering, cleaning, and other garment services	363	63.6	26.4
Beauty shops	553	89.0	9.2
Dressmaking shops	41	97.6	7.3
Miscellaneous	252	45.2	9.9
Bowling alleys, billiard and pool parlors	82	40.2	6.1
Professional and related services	18,327	65.1	13.3
Offices of physicians	753	67.2	4.8
Offices of dentists	360	67.2	3.3
Hospitals	3,781	75.8	19.4
Convalescent institutions	1,009	88.1	19.2
Offices of health practitioners†	83	57.8	NA‡
Health services†	687	68.9	15.1
Legal services	650	48.5	2.6
Elementary and secondary schools	5,180	70.6	13.2
Colleges and universities	1,996	49.1	11.4
Libraries	167	81.4	11.4
Educational services†	277	67.1	10.1
Museums, art galleries, and zoos	67	47.8	9.0
Religious organizations	618	42.4	8.4
Welfare services	788	70.9	23.5
Residential welfare facilities	119	60.5	20.2
Nonprofit membership organizations	464	53.0	11.6
Accounting, auditing, and bookkeeping services	445	44.9	3.6
Miscellaneous professional and related services	370	42.4	5.4
TOTAL	94,373	41.2	11.2

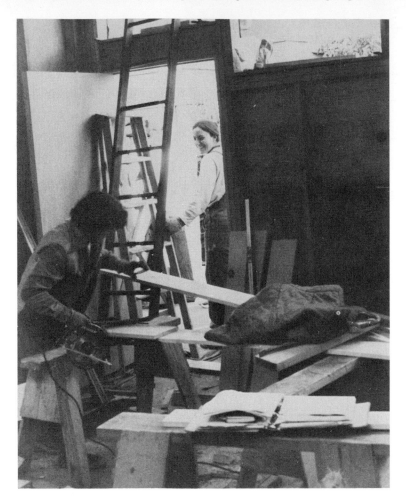

Fig. 5-4. Carpenters.

Salaries for women lag behind men's, and the differential has increased. Full-time women workers (age 14 and over) earned a median of about $3000 in 1957, about 64% of the men's median of $4700. In 1973, women workers (age 14 and over) had a median income of $6335 which was about 57% of the men's median of $11,186.[105] By 1977, women (age 16 and over) earned a median of $8618, 58.9% of the $14,626 earned by men.[105]

Differences between employment patterns of minority and white women are narrowing as opportunities for minority women increase and larger proportions of young minority women enter clerical and professional/technical work rather than service occupations (see Table 5-7).

Table 5-7. Major occupational groups of employed women, March, 1973*

Major occupational group	White		Minority races	
	16 to 34 years	35 years and over	16 to 34 years	35 years and over
Total number of women employed (000)	12,810	15,137	1,840	2,138
Percent distribution				
Professional, technical workers	16.7	14.5	13.5	11.6
Managers, administrators (except farm)	2.8	7.5	2.6	2.9
Sales workers	6.5	8.1	2.9	2.0
Clerical workers	39.0	32.5	35.5	15.0
Craft and kindred workers	1.0	1.7	0.8	1.2
Operatives (except transport)	11.1	14.5	16.8	14.1
Transport equipment operatives	0.4	0.6	0.1	0.4
Laborers (except farm)	0.9	0.7	0.9	1.1
Private household workers	3.4	2.5	6.0	20.9
Service workers (except private household)	17.1	15.7	20.3	29.8
Farmers and farm managers	0.2	0.4	†	†
Farm laborers and supervisors	0.8	1.3	0.6	1.0

*Based on data from U.S. Department of Labor, Bureau of Labor Statistics: Special Labor Force Report No. 164; adapted from Women's Bureau, U.S. Department of Labor: 1975 Handbook on women workers, Washington, D.C., 1975, U.S. Government Printing Office.
†Not available.

PROTECTIVE LEGISLATION
Historical background

Because of the massive numbers of female workers who have entered the work force, there has been a refocus on the question of special protective legislation for women. The concept was originally suggested by Hamilton, Baetjer, and other early occupational health researchers in an effort to protect the pregnant woman worker, or more correctly, her fetus. Hamilton also believed that women were more susceptible to poisoning from toxic substances than were men, and therefore advocated special legislation for women themselves.[36] This belief explained her opposition to the Equal Rights Amendment (discussed below), a position from which she withdrew in 1952.[19] When protective legislation was first proposed, it was in response to the appalling working conditions of women — sweatshop conditions for minimal pay. Protective legislation was seen then by its supporters as the only way to improve women's conditions in the work force, and it was believed that its benefits would outweigh its costs.

Other support for protective legislation derived from mixed motives. Protective legislation effectively served to keep women out of the job market or confined to specified tasks. Considering the economic hardships faced by many male workers, this was to their advantage. It reinforced myths of women as frail, inferior, and unreliable workers because of possible illness. It was also hoped that protective legislation would improve the workplace for men; it was believed that limits on weights to be lifted and established working hours for women might be a means of gaining benefits for men from "behind women's petticoats."[10] Still other support came with the idea that if women were singled out for special protection, the workplace would not have to be cleaned up and therefore made safe for all workers as a whole; universal protection could be avoided.[87, Chap. 1]

On the whole, protective legislation has fostered the improvement of working conditions for all workers. The first example came in 1908 in *Muller* v. *Oregon* in which the U.S. Supreme Court held that a 10-hour work day limit could be imposed for women. The importance of this ruling lay in the fact that it overturned a 1905 Supreme Court decision which held that the State of New York could not restrict the hours of work in a place of private employment (*Lochner* v. *New York*). Having established the possibility of collective contracts concerning working conditions, male workers soon sought a limit to their working day. Granted in 1917 in *Bunting* v. *Oregon*, the gain was made "on the basis of sexist generalities about the special weaknesses and biological roles of women."[87]

Various state laws soon followed pertaining to night work, weight loads, hours, and types of employment. Frequently contradictory, most ignored the weights lifted and the hours (including nights) women worked in traditional occupations such as nursing. The Women's Bureau sponsored several studies attempting to document incidences of occupational hazards and hence the need for protective legislation. Finally, on June 4, 1938, the Fair Labor Standards Act was passed, as much for children as for men and women, providing a floor for wages and a ceiling for hours; this was amended in 1974 to cover children who worked in agriculture and subsequently again amended in 1978 to permit child labor in agriculture (discussed later).

The work of Dr. Anna Baetjer in 1946 had begun to shift the focus for protective legislation to the pregnant woman worker rather than all women. When the war ended and the assumption generally prevailed that women would leave the work force, little attention was paid to her recommendations. Today myths still abound as to women's susceptibility; consequently, discrimination based on "protection" still exists. Still existing, too, in many cases is the question of the degree of risk from toxic substances faced by offspring of working women, by offspring of previously employed women currently not working, and by offspring of women never employed outside the home.

It has therefore become relatively easy for employers to move women of childbearing years out of jobs, in theory for their protection, and to demand pregnancy tests, sterilization, and compulsory maternity leaves during pregnancy, usually without appropriate compensation for pay or seniority lost. The obvious and employee-desired alternative of converting the workplace to a hazard-free environment safe for fetus and female and male workers has been deemed impracticable. The need for such action, however, is becoming increasingly evident to factory owners and male-dominated unions as more is learned about the effects of toxic exposure on male reproductive capacity.

Current federal laws

In attempts to remedy discriminatory practices, four major federal laws have been passed: the Equal Pay Act of 1963, effective June 11, 1964; Title VII of the Civil Rights Act of 1964, effective July 2, 1965; Executive Order 11246 which was amended to cover sex, effective October 14, 1968, by Executive Order 11375; and the Age Discrimination in Employment Act of 1967, effective June 12, 1968.

The Equal Pay Act establishes "equal pay for equal work," but because standards for work and job responsibilities rely on individual employers' judgment, many loopholes can be found.

Title VII prohibits discrimination on the basis of sex, race, color, religion, and national origin in all terms, conditions, or privileges of employment. The act as amended in 1972 now covers public and private employers of 15 or more persons, public and private employment agencies, public and private educational institutions, labor unions with 15 or more members, and state and local governments. A separate section covers the Civil Service Commission; excluded are Indian tribes and private clubs.

Defense of Title VII suits frequently focuses on the statutory exemption of sex as a "bona fide occupational qualification" (e.g., in the case of an actor or wet-nurse) or when the sex of the employee is related to a "business necessity." Employer practices of "protecting" fertile women from hazardous exposure, thus causing them to lose their jobs, seniority, and/or pay levels, has led to several suits under Title VII. Increasing evidence of equal hazards to the reproductive capacity of male workers is providing the basis for Title VII action by demonstrating that both men and women are at risk and women alone cannot therefore be "protected" out of their jobs. Similarly, if working conditions are maintained that are inherently unsafe for the fertility and reproductive capacity of only one sex and from which only one sex is excluded, Title VII is considered to be violated on the grounds of discriminatory treatment and a discriminatory impact. Notes one commentator on Title VII:

Exclusion of only fertile women from a toxic workplace may evidence both discriminatory treatment and discriminatory effect which are presumptively unlawful. The narrow bona fide occupational qualification exception will not be applicable because femaleness does not prevent these fertile women from doing their jobs, which they must be given a free choice to keep or give up. Nor will the "business necessity" defense save employers, as cleaning up the workplace will always be a less discriminatory alternative available to excluding the fertile woman. In short, exclusion of fertile women should violate Title VII.[93]

Executive Order 11246 as amended by Executive Order 11375 basically prohibits discrimination in federal employment or by federal government contractors; it also requires the development of affirmative action plans.

The Age Discrimination in Employment Act applies to employers of 20 or more persons and prohibits discrimination in hiring, firing, promotion, and other employment practices of persons 40 to 65 years old. It is particularly pertinent to women, many of whom return to the labor force at an older age.

Other federal legislation concerns safety and health. The Occupational Safety and Health Act of 1970, effective April 28, 1971, states its purpose as "to assure so far as possible every working man and woman in the nation safe and healthful working conditions and to preserve our human resources."* The act provides for the establishment of the Occupational Safety and Health Administration (OSHA) in the Department of Labor, with the power to establish and enforce standards, inspect the workplace, and conduct appeals.

Also established by the act, is the National Institute of Occupational Safety and Health (NIOSH) in the Department of Health, Education and Welfare. This agency is responsible for writing criteria documents containing recommendations for federal standards, and for conducting occupational health research. To date, the work of both OSHA and NIOSH has been hampered by inadequate staff and funds and characterized by slowness in carrying out the purposes of the law.

The Nuclear Regulatory Commission (NRC), formerly the Atomic Energy Commission, also has responsibility for establishing safe standards pertaining specifically to radiation. On considering the fetus and radiation, however, the NRC suggested pregnant women could delay having children, ask to be moved, or leave their jobs.[40]

Equal Rights Amendment

When the Equal Rights Amendment was first proposed, Alice Hamilton, the Women's Trade Union League, and a number of other women's organizations were opposed; they believed that what protective legislation did exist would be nullified and the meager protection women then had would vanish. Changing her mind in 1952, Hamilton stated:

My long opposition to the Equal Rights Amendment has lost much of its force during the 30 years since the movement for it started. The health of women in industry is now a matter of concern to health authorities, both state and federal, to employers' associations, insurance companies, and trade unions. I do not believe that this situation would be changed by the passage of the amendment now.[19]

Hamilton's optimism seems somewhat unfounded, and ratification of the Equal Rights Amendment would do much for women's health in employment by guaranteeing that "equality of rights under the law shall not be denied or abridged by the United States or any State on account of sex." This would include ensuring equal job opportunities, providing more basis for enforcing that the workplace be equally safe for men and women thereby guaranteeing equal rights to employment and rendering unconstitutional discriminatory "protective" labor practices.

SPECIFIC EXAMPLES OF OCCUPATIONAL HEALTH HAZARDS TO WOMEN

In this section the health hazards faced by all women workers will be discussed, as well as those which have a particular bearing on the pregnant woman. Hazards that affect large numbers of women in specific occupations will then be described.

---

*OSHA: Section 2(b); 29 USC Section 652(b).

Women workers: a separate issue

Hricko[40] has classified the hazards that women workers face in four categories: (1) those common to both men and women who are employed in about equal numbers in a job category (e.g., assembly line work); (2) those related to jobs that typically have been "men's work" but into which women are moving (e.g., skilled trades, police work); (3) those related to jobs that are stereotypically "women's work" where the work force is primarily female (e.g., secretarial, domestic service, and hospital work); (4) those which affect fertility or sexual and reproductive functions where both men and women may be affected, but where women with developing fetuses may have special risks (e.g., exposure to radiation, lead, and anesthetic gases).

In this latter category two types of agents are of particular concern: mutagens and teratogens. Unlike carcinogens, which are substances that can cause cancer in those who are exposed, mutagens and teratogens can harm unborn generations. Mutagens are substances or agents that can cause mutations or changes in the genetic material of living cells. Of particular concern are mutagens that cause changes (mutations) in germ cells (sperm or egg), which are passed on to the offspring when conception occurs. Teratogens are substances or agents that can cause birth or other abnormalities in offspring by interfering with the development of the fetus after conception. The agents (e.g., the drug thalidomide) are transferred through the mother's placenta and may result in miscarriage or the birth of a deformed baby.

Despite the fact that the health of all workers has not been a top concern of industry or government, and that many if not all health hazards also affect men, women's health needs are of special concern. This is because occupations that are predominantly female, especially nonindustrial jobs such as clerical work and housework, have been particularly neglected. Where women are entering nontraditional occupations, studies of health hazards, when studies exist, have generally not considered the possibilities of women workers. As noted earlier, employers, not knowing the risks for fertility and pregnancy, have frequently sought to exclude women, thereby denying them equal access to usually more lucrative employment. It is therefore critical that research be done to provide a more rational approach to current arguments.

Certain hazards are common to male and female workers in many jobs. Exposure to chemicals and physical agents may result for both men and women in lowered fertility, skin irritation, skin and various organ diseases, vision disturbances, dizziness, nausea, and poisoning in the children of those exposed,[7,16,24] and, specifically for women, in menstrual problems and damage to the fetus.[5,40,58,78] Exposure to carcinogenic agents, for example, vinyl chloride or estrogens, may cause cancer in the worker and in the offspring of the worker, and may also cause potentially cancerous conditions in members of the worker's household.[33,45,89]

Physical requirements of various jobs may produce disability in both men and women. For example, continuous standing can contribute to varicose veins, and lifting heavy weights may induce back strains.[65,74a] Fatigue, lack of ventilation, high noise levels, and constant monotony may also contribute to disabling conditions, to stress, or more directly to less attention to safety, with subsequent increases in industrial accidents.*

Considerations of fatigue and stress are particularly pertinent to women who, in addition to the demands of their employment, in the vast majority of instances, must still work "another shift" at home. Women may also be subject to sexual harrassment at work, a matter recently investigated and in some instances settled in favor of the women by the courts. Poorly represented in unions, women are beginning to seek amelioration of these conditions.

Pregnancy and work

On the basis of their own experience, it was presumed for many decades by those who owned the companies and made the laws that pregnant women did not work. When men returned after World War II, women were expected to go home or move to less risky jobs. Occupational hazards to the fetus therefore were of little concern. However, current interest in the well-being of pregnant women workers, although long overdue and to be encouraged, has also raised some fears. Many women recognize the value of the research for their own and their babies' well-being but fear that, as hazards are documented, job opportunities will be narrowed for them and, on the grounds that they might be or become pregnant, they will once more be subject to illegal discrimination. Hricko and Marrett[41] note, however, that the Occupational Safety and Health Act mandates that OSHA set standards which "most adequately assure(s) that no employee (i.e., male or female) will suffer material impairment of health or functional capacity." Hricko and Marrett also say, "Without question that mandate must include consideration of any adverse effects of chemical exposures on the genes, the genital organs, sexual functions, fertility, and reproductive functions, and on any transplacental effects of exposure that might harm the fetus."[41]

For other workers the new focus and a few studies to date are demonstrating that reproductive hazards are not women's alone. For example, as noted earlier, the study on operating room personnel also found an increased risk of birth defects among the unexposed wives of male operating room workers.[3] In addition, other data indicate links between exposure to carbon disulfide,[57] diethylstilbestrol,[46] pesticides,[90, p. A18] and impotence in males, while studies of radiation exposure and lead poisoning show that these can affect spermatogenesis and lead to chromosomal aberrations in male workers.[44] These new findings, tragic though they are, may provide the impetus needed to get the workplace made safe, and pregnant women and their babies will benefit. The goal should be, then, a workplace equally safe for all.

The Department of Labor estimates that annually about 1.5 million babies will be born to working mothers. Exposure to the following substances (not an all-inclusive list) is of particular concern to pregnant women because of their impact on fertility and fetal development, on the chance of a live birth, and on behavioral adaptation[85]: lead, vinyl chloride, organic solvents such as aromatics (e.g., benzene), chlorinated hydrocarbons, anesthetic gases, estrogens, ionizing radiation, pesticides, mercury, carbon monoxide, carbon disulfide, polychlorinated

---

*References 12 and 87 (Chapters 2 and 3).

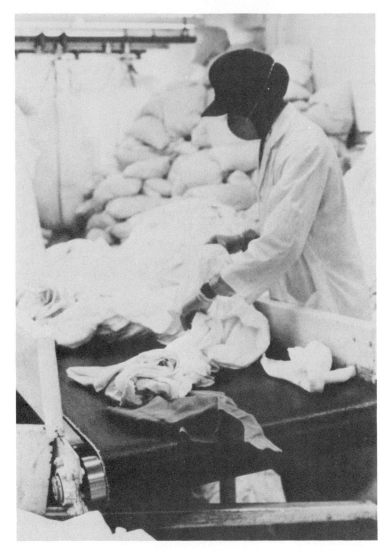

Fig. 5-5. Hospital laundry worker. (Courtesy Health Sciences Information Service, University of Washington, Seattle.)

biphenyls (PCBs), radiant energy (e.g., x rays, lasers, ultraviolet light, microwaves), biological agents, cadmium, beryllium, polybrominated biphenyls (PBBs), and certain pharmaceuticals. Also of concern are the effects of dust, exhaustion, diseases, infections, vibration, noise, heat and thermal stress, and psychological stress exacerbated by the simultaneous role demand of pregnancy.[1,40,42,87] Finally, after the baby is born, absence of opportunities to maintain breastfeeding while the mother is working may impair her sense of well-being and deprive the infant of optimal nourishment.[47]

Acknowledgment that pregnant women work (there has also been recognition that productive employment may be one of the most effective agents for regulating fertility)[9] has led to a variety of tactics on the part of industry, ostensibly to protect women and their children. However, Olga Madar, president of the Coalition of Labor Union Women (CLUW), notes:

Industry's worry about harm to a fetus stems not from humanitarianism, but from fear that the fetus may be born deformed and live to sue them successfully for its injuries. As remote a possibility as that is, it weighs heavier on their minds than taking the steps necessary to prevent such harm to any of the offspring of either male or female workers by cleaning up the workplace.[87]

Whatever industry's motives, in the name of protection, women workers of childbearing years have been subjected to required pregnancy testing to demonstrate their nongravid condition,[60] (ironic and somewhat ridiculous, since almost all tests take at least 42 days after the last menstrual period to be positive and most fetal damage occurs in the first few weeks following conception); sterilization (led to a suit in which OSHA has joined);[86] and transferral to other jobs (some of which paid less).[70, p. 379] Furthermore, childbearing women become particularly vulnerable to lay-offs during periods of high unemployment.[55]

To facilitate safe working conditions for all workers, including pregnant women, several guidelines have been developed, including those of the Women's Bureau and the American College of Obstetricians and Gynecologists. All stress the right of workers, including pregnant women, to work in a hazard-free environment and stress that the choice between maintaining fertility or keeping a job is untenable. Topics included in some or all of the guidelines are maternity leaves, the option of working until onset of labor, maternity benefits and health insurance, maternal and fetal health during pregnancy, and unemployment and disability compensation,[1,43,104] where much reform of the 50 different state programs is needed.[51] Most critically, effective April 29, 1979, Public Law 95-555 of October 31, 1978, mandates that employers will not be allowed to refuse sick leave or disability benefits to women who are unable to work because of pregnancy. Furthermore, employers with 15 or more employees and a company health plan may not refuse coverage of normal pregnancy and delivery costs in their company health plan or reimburse less for this than for other medical conditions. Opposition to this law centers on costs, but it is an equitable and long overdue recognition of the fact that pregnant women work.[107]

Cosmetologists, hairdressers, and beauticians

In 1978 approximately 542,000 persons were employed as beauty operatives, of whom 89.1% were women and 9.2% were minorities (see Table 5-5). Mortality data for this occupational group are scarce. Further research is needed, particularly on the relationship between carcinogenic properties of chemicals used in the industry, for example, hair dyes (see later),[81] and outcome. Morbidity data that have been collected reveal several potential hazards, including varicose veins from excessively long periods of standing in a fixed position, eye damage from shampoos containing cationics as germicides and nonionics as cleansing agents,[39] exposure to carcinogens from aerosol hair sprays and hair dyes, abnormal lung cell pathology, chronic respiratory disease, pulmonary thesaurosis

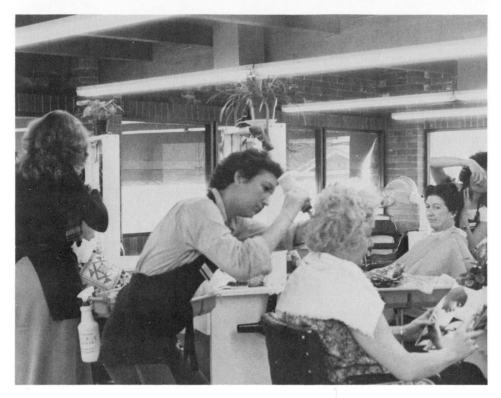

Fig. 5-6. Cosmetologists. (Courtesy M. A. Maurer.)

(a lung storage disease), and sarcoidosis (a granuloma-forming disease that can occur in the lung and also throughout the body) from the hair spray resins and lacquer, which stiffen the lung fiber. Other hazards include skin irritations from dyes and permanent wave solutions, the development of allergies, which may lead to asthma, exposure to mutagens from hair dyes, exposure to asbestos from hair dryers, and, not unexpectedly, stress. Many of these hazards are exacerbated by the small, inadequately ventilated, and humid work locations typical in this field.[40, Chap. 22] Workers involved in the manufacturing of these products may also experience similar hazards.

Although some beauticians are returning to the hand pump for hair spray, aerosol hair sprays are still in widespread use. Containing resins, plasticizers, solvents, additives, and a propellant, usually Freon or other fluorocarbons, aerosol hair sprays have been implicated through several studies of lung function and sputum cytology as causing pulmonary dysfunction and possibly cancer.[31,32,71,72,107]

Hair dyes, mostly "permanent" hair colorings, are used by an estimated two of every five American women. The industry states that of every dollar spent on hair dyes, 75 cents is for the "permanent" type.[95] Hair dyes were extensively studied in the early 1970s, and 89% of the "permanent" type were found to cause mutations in bacterial laboratory cultures; carcinogenic properties were also suspected.[4] Because hair dyes can be absorbed through the scalp, researchers have recommended studies of birth defects and cancer among both users and those who work with dyes. Links between breast cancer and hair dye exposure have also been suggested,[80] but have been disputed by the industry, which cites several studies[14] showing no link between the two. Additionally, chromosomal damage and hair dyes have been associated.[52]

Clerical workers

In 1978 there were approximately 16.9 million persons employed as clerical workers; of these, 79.6% were women and 10.5% minorities (see Table 5-5). Office work has been generally regarded as safe work, but on the basis of one California study in 1959, an annual disability total of 40,000 injuries and more than 200 deaths have been projected.[8,67] Most injuries are sustained through falls incurred when moving equipment or file cabinets, when opening file cabinets, or when walking on slippery surfaces.

In general, health hazards in the office involve back and muscle strain and/or fatigue from improperly designed furniture or long hours of typing or sitting in one position (may also cause varicose veins and hemorrhoids); eyestrain from intense focusing in poorly lit work areas; hearing impairment from excessive noise levels; exposure to toxic chemicals (e.g., those contained in duplicating and stencil machines); and stress from monotony or job dissatisfaction.* Constant repetitive tasks such as typing have also produced the condition known as tenosynovitis — a painful, swollen wrist condition.[54,102]

The study of ergonomics — the relationship between biology and technology — is pertinent to clerical workers, since many of the hazards, particularly those related to muscle and back strain, could be alleviated by having furniture and equipment designed to conform to the physical needs of those who use them. For example, office chairs that support the lower back, typing tables at an appropriate height, and desks that are well lit, appropriately sized, and avoid the need for constant stretching to reach necessary items would all reduce health hazards. Similarly, more comfortable conditions could alleviate tension, stress, and boredom, which may contribute to accidents.

Office machines require chemicals, such as typewriter cleaner, stencil fluid, and copy machine toners, that contain potentially hazardous chemicals. For example, the trichloroethylene in a type cleaner can cause visual disturbances, mental confusion, fatigue, and sometimes nausea and vomiting.[61] In this regard, ventilation is extremely important to diffuse the concentrations of the chemicals, particularly where ammonia or methanol is used in duplicating machines.[2]

Although it provides some ventilation, the widespread use of air conditioning also creates other hazards. Asbestos fibers, which were used to fireproof many office buildings prior to 1970, are coming loose and are now being circulated through air conditioners. A 1975 study by the Environmental Science Laboratory of Mt. Sinai School of Medicine documented dangerously high levels of asbestos

---

*References 40 (Chapter 20), 61, 87.

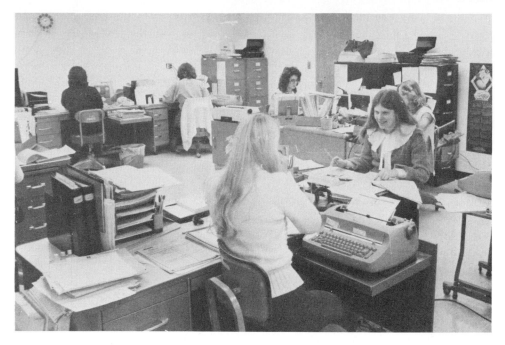

Fig. 5-7. Secretaries. (Courtesy Bill Ransdell.)

in some New York buildings. These have been known to cause mesothelioma, cancer of the lining of the lung.[91,99]

Textile workers

In 1978 approximately 2.2 million persons were employed as apparel and textile workers. Among apparel workers, 77.4% were women and 16.4% were minorities; among textile workers, 47% were women and 17.8% were minorities (see Table 5-6). As with other occupations, there is scant documentation of morbidity and mortality, but one British study of 900 females who worked with asbestos and textiles (the asbestos was used as a fire retardant in the fabrics) showed by 1968 significant increases in deaths from lung and pleura (lung lining) cancer, other cancers, and respiratory diseases.[40,68]

Health hazards in the textile industry include dangerous machinery; workplaces with inadequate lighting and high heat, humidity, and noise levels; and exposure to toxic chemicals used in bleaching, in synthetic fabric manufacture, and in making fabrics flame retardant, waterproof, shrink resistant, and permanent press. These hazards may cause skin irritation, deafness, loss of vision, eye irritation, cancer, fatigue, headaches, back strain, menstrual difficulties, psychological disturbances, and respiratory problems.

Most important, large numbers of textile workers (close to 1 million) are constantly exposed to cotton dust, which frequently causes byssinosis, or brown lung disease. Beginning as an allergic-type reaction to the cotton dust, the condition may progress to asthma, chronic bronchitis, emphysema, or byssinosis. In 1977, 2030 workers died from dust diseases of the lung; in 1971 it was estimated that 25% to 30% of all United States workers in cotton factories had byssinosis.[40]

A mid-1970s study of the approximately 400,000 workers in the men's apparel industry (85% of whom are women) documented the hazards to which these workers are exposed. The researcher, Dr. Peter Nord, in a study for NIOSH, noted that "before a garment is completed, as many as 10 different chemicals may be put on the fabric to make it permanent press or flame retardant."[59] Despite the unionization of many workers in the garment industry in the early 1900s (International Ladies Garment Workers, Amalgamated Clothing Workers), Nord found conditions that paralleled the turn of the century sweatshops.[59]

Dental assistants

In 1978 approximately 130,000 persons were employed as dental assistants; of these, 98.5% were women and 3.8% were minorities (see Table 5-5). Of particular concern from an occupational health perspective is the exposure of these workers, especially the women because of pregnancy, to mercury. Mercury contained in the mercury-silver amalgam material used to restore decayed teeth readily vaporizes and may be inhaled.[78] Early symptoms of mercury poisoning include inflammation of the mouth and gums, metallic taste, emotional instability, chest pains, and headache. Higher exposure levels can produce kidney damage, unconsciousness, respiratory complications, blindness, loss of memory, brain damage, and death.[40,77] Organic (methyl) mercury, which is more toxic to the nervous system than inorganic mercury, was the cause of the disastrous teratogenic effects in the Minimata victims;[83,84] teratogenic effects of inorganic mercury are as yet undocumented.

A 1976 study[34] in California verified earlier reports of mercury exposure. Every dental office surveyed was contaminated in various degrees with elemental mercury, and the extent of contamination depended on the "number of amalgam restorations prepared per day, the method of mixing the amalgam, the type of floor covering and chair covering, housekeeping procedures, and the type of ventilation."[77]

Flight attendants

In 1977 approximately 39,000 persons were employed as flight attendants; of these, 94.8% were women and 1000 were minorities, all of whom were women.[106] Research into the health hazards faced by these workers is only beginning, but preliminary reports suggest that the hazards include exposure to radiation from both cosmic and natural sources and from leakage of radioactive materials carried in the cargo holds of commercial airliners; unlevel work surfaces; deafening noise levels; vibration; and poorly fastened equipment. These hazards may be responsible for the health problems common to flight attendants: kidney ailments, menstrual disorders, alcoholism, fatigue, muscle pain (from constantly walking on an incline during flights on larger planes), burns, and a nerve condition that resembles multiple sclerosis.[59]

Craft workers

In 1975 the Associated Council on the Arts determined that of people over 16 years of age in the United States, about 56.7 million (39% of the population) were working as either a career or a hobby, in weaving, pottery, ceramic, wood, or other crafts, and that 21.8 million (16%) were working in painting, drawing, or sculpture. It is estimated from several surveys that of these 50% to 72% are women.[64]

Although the hazards and their effects vary in degree of extremity, some toxic materials associated with crafts include silica in glazes, which may cause silicosis (nodular fibrotic changes in the lung); heavy metals such as lead, which may cause poisoning; and solvents such as benzene, which may cause headaches, dizziness, or even leukemia or aplastic anemia. Poor ventilation may cause dizziness and headaches and will exacerbate the effects of the other hazards.[64] Some craft tools are potentially hazardous, particularly those used in woodworking, metal casting, welding, and glassblowing. Woodworkers have also been found to have 500 times more nasopharyngeal cancer than the general population.[88]

Children of craft workers may also be affected because of their greater susceptibility and because much craft work is done in the home. Lead poisoning in an 18-month-old child of stained glass artists has been documented.[64] When the mother works at home, breast-feeding may be more convenient but may contribute to toxicity in children. Children are likely to be affected also because many women, because of their traditional child care function, may bring their young infants to work with them in studios. For craft workers, hazards to the fetus can be expected to be similar to those recorded for factory workers[42] but are as yet undocumented.

Housewives

In 1978 an estimated 25.1 million women, married with husband present, were not in the labor force; presumably a large percentage of these worked as unpaid houseworkers.[21] (The value of housewives' labor is generally estimated at about $4.00 per hour.) Accidents are a leading cause of mortality among housewives (and among all persons) and several studies have demonstrated that many accidents, fatal and nonfatal, happen in the home. Of all victims of non-transport-related accidents, housewives comprise one of the largest occupational groups. These accidents involve fires, falls, fractures, and use of consumer products (in 1977 women sustained 3,594,677 injuries from this latter category), including chemicals, drugs, medical equipment, and flammable clothing.[20,25,92,100]

Another recently published study has found a significant excess of cancer mortality among housewives in an Oregon metropolitan area, "whether calculated by separate estimation of housewife population at risk or by assumption that housewives included all women unemployed or not in the labor force."[66] The researchers also discovered a higher incidence of cancers (typically breast, ovary, colon, lung, uterine corpus, stomach, and lymphomas) among housewives than among paid household workers. Data suggest that the housewife (and the working woman who keeps house) may be exposed to carcinogens in the home in the form of household products; some cited are surfactants, quarternary ammonium compounds, benzene, chlorinated hydrocarbons, naphthas, a variety of petroleum distillates, phenolic substances, chromic acid, acrylate polishes, aromatic nitrates, and halides. In addition, few homes, if any, have the protective clothing or equipment used by exposed workers in industrial settings. The need for further investigation is stressed.[66]

ENVIRONMENTAL HAZARDS

Hazards to women's health do not come from occupational employment alone. Nor do they come only from externally imposed exposure; some, such as smoking (linked also with low-birth-weight babies and spontaneous abortion)[27,53] and diet, are to a large extent, self-imposed. Other hazards, which essentially are from self-imposed exposure, are nonetheless derived from external exposure to promotional publicity and advertising. This is particularly true of exposure to cosmetics and household, personal hygiene, and baby care products, the advertising for which appeals to women because of their socialization, which teaches them to want to be the prettiest and the best smelling possible and to have the cleanest home and the healthiest child. Many environmental hazards, unlike occupational hazards, are totally out of individual control, short of relocation after knowledge and/or exposure.

Hexachlorophene

The introduction of hexachlorophene as an antiseptic in 1941 is an example of externally imposed exposure; in the United States in the 1960s it was added to many products, including soaps, face lotion, hair tonics, antiperspirants, toothpaste, and hand creams. In 1972 following a University of Washington study demonstrating that brain damage occurred among newborn infants who were routinely washed with hexachlorophene solutions, the Food and Drug Administration (FDA) restricted the pharmaceutical marketing of the substance to physician prescription and hospital use. A recent Swedish study has now implicated hexachlorophene in an excess of congenital malformation in infants born to nurses who have been heavily exposed to the antiseptic.[38] It is now suspected that hexachlorophene use may also be a confounding variable in the high rates of congenital anomalies and miscarriages among operating room personnel, which were discussed earlier.[11] Until further study, the National Institute of Child Health and Human Development is advising pregnant women not to use it.

Chemical dumping

The Love Canal situation, publicized in 1978, is an example of a hazard, exposure to which is beyond the control of the individual. An area near Niagara Falls in New York had been used several decades earlier as a dumping ground for chemicals. These began to leach out, were probably responsible for an excess of congenital anomalies and stillbirths, and resulted in the evacuation of the residents.[69] The Environmental Protection Agency estimates that there are 32,254 similar sites in the nation.

Plutonium contamination

Plutonium contamination, exemplified by the as yet unresolved 1974 case of Karen Silkwood and Kerr-McGee, has also been studied in Jefferson County, Colorado. Preliminary data suggest that there is a measurable effect on the rate of congenital malformations in the contaminated area.[48] The development of nuclear power and the potential of contamination from plutonium and radioactive wastes raises similarly the possibility of the presence of teratogens and carcinogens, but on an even larger scale because of the planned widespread use of nuclear power.[15]

Crop spraying

The use of pesticides and herbicides for spraying crops, clearing bush, and maintaining roads presents an environmental hazard of as yet unknown duration; evidence has already established immediate effects of some of the chemicals. On the basis of an excess number of miscarriages among women in Alsea, Oregon, an area subject to spraying over the past 5 years with 2,4,5-T, which contains dioxin, the Environmental Protection Agency prohibited its use nationwide on February 28, 1979.[18] Pesticides and herbicides may also contaminate infants through their mothers' milk.[56]

Concerns about the effects of pesticides on children have led to recommendations from OSHA and NIOSH to the Department of Labor to prohibit the employment of 10- and 11-year-olds (prepubescents) to pick crops, particularly strawberries and potatoes, for which child labor is especially welcomed. The Department of Labor ignored the recommendations and on August 18, 1978, issued a regulation implementing an amendment to the Fair Labor Standards Act allowing a waiver of the child labor laws specifically to permit the employment of these young children in harvesting. More recently, for the 1979 harvest, the Department of Labor forbade employment of these young children except under special circumstances for which a waiver had to be granted. Although the laws pertain only to children, pesticides may also affect adult crop pickers, with particular hazards for pregnant women, since the pesticides have been linked with cancer, genetic mutation, birth defects, growth depression, and damage to the neurological, metabolic, blood, and liver systems.[62,95]

SELECTED INTERNATIONAL PERSPECTIVES
International organizations

There are several international organizations concerned with the welfare of women, both as paid and unpaid workers. The United Nations Commission on the Status of Women (UNCSW) is a working commission under the Economic and Social Council (ECOSOC). Its functions are to prepare recommendations and reports to ECOSOC on furthering women's rights in all aspects of life.

Three regional organizations, the Inter-American Commission of Women (IACW), or Comisión Interamericana de Mujeres (CIM) as it is known in Spanish, the United Nations Economic Commission for Africa (UNECA), and the United Nations Economic and Social Commission for Asia and the Pacific

(ESCAP) all basically have as their goals the training of women to participate more fully in productive society and to ensure their equal access of opportunity to participate.

More directly involved with workers is the International Labor Organization (ILO), which was established in 1919 and became, in 1946, the first specialized agency associated with the United Nations. Representatives of government, labor, and management participate in the ILO to achieve its goals of promoting economic and social stability, improved labor conditions and living standards, minimum standards for the workplace and for all workers, men and women, and the elimination of economic and social discrimination. The equality of treatment of women workers has been a publicly stated concern of the ILO since its inception, with recognition of the conflict between protective legislation and equality of opportunity, and the right of pregnant women to work, guaranteed in some countries since 1907.[42]

Hunt[44] notes that the ILO conventions "provide countries with a model position or conditions (of work) with which they can attempt to comply and to ratify as national policy." She states that "for a variety of complex social, economic, and political reasons the United States has ratified only seven conventions, all of them relating to seafaring, in contrast to 69 for the United Kingdom, 70 for Norway, and 72 for the Netherlands, many of them concerned with occupational safety and health. The narrowness of our (U.S.) views on maternity benefits and related issues is nowhere more dramatically emphasized than when we review the current and past practices of other countries, both industrial and agricultural."[44]

Safety standards in other industrialized countries are more stringent than in the United States. For example, 90 dB-A (decibel levels on the A weighting scale) is the accepted industrial standard in the United States, but 85 dB-A is the accepted standard in several central European countries. Considering that for every 6 dB-A increase, the sound power levels are doubled, this represents an appreciable difference. Safe microwave exposure levels are considered to be 0.5 in the United States and 0.05 in the USSR.[73]

Maternity benefits

Most significant for U.S. women workers are the maternity benefits available in other countries. Many countries guarantee as a right the transfer of a pregnant woman worker without lowering of pay or loss of seniority. Furthermore, many countries that refuse certain jobs to women workers to avoid fetal harm during pregnancy or contamination during breast-feeding guarantee womens' placement in jobs of equal earning capacity. The right of women to work is recognized, encouraged, and accepted.

Sweden. In Sweden a modification of maternity benefits occurred in January, 1974, with passage of the Parenthood Benefit. This provides that the parent who has custody of the newborn will receive a financial benefit that is paid for a maximum of 210 days per birth; parents may alternate custody and therefore receipt of the benefit during that period. Collective bargaining is common to all workers, and conditions such as housing, overtime, work hours, and night duty are all negotiated.[49] Pregnant women factory workers in Sweden can also be immediately transferred to lighter or safer jobs with seniority and pay ensured.[40] Of course there is still the problem of recognizing pregnancy prior to the incurrence of fetal damage. The maximum effort for safety and the well-being of mother and child is made, however.

People's Republic of China. In China the three-generational family structure, formally organized preschool activities, and the frequent provision of neighborhood child care after school assist the woman worker. Paid maternity leave is also the right of the woman worker.[82] As shown, the recognition of women's right to work and the expectation that they will work are accompanied by realistic social programs.

Polish People's Republic (Poland). Polish women workers enjoy similar benefits to those in China from standards established in the 1974 Labor Code. Paid maternity leave is 16 weeks for the first child with the opportunity for an additional unpaid 3 weeks' leave; job rights and salary are maintained. With a physician's recommendation, pregnant women can be moved to less taxing work with no salary loss.[40]

Union of Soviet Socialist Republics (USSR). Soviet women have maternity benefits that are among the most advanced and solicitous of maternal and fetal well-being. They are entitled to a total of 112 days of paid maternity leave, which is split into 8 weeks prenatally and 8 weeks postnatally. They may also return to work at the same salary and benefit level after an additional 1 year's unpaid leave. Specific hazardous jobs are generally prohibited to women workers, such as employment with chrome, coke ovens, and lead or benzene, but comparably paid opportunities exist. Furthermore, extensive research has been done and is continued by the USSR and other Eastern European countries on occupational hazards of all workers, male and female, pregnant and nonpregnant.[40]

•   •   •

Occupational hazards exist whether women, pregnant or otherwise, work in the home as housewives (almost always unpaid) or as paid employees. Societies that recognize the dual capacities of women's lives — reproduction and work — have established social programs to maximize the effectiveness of each and to minimize the hazards to each. Research regarding safety, enforcement of safe standards, and provision of day-care and maternity benefits maximizes not only the reproductive capabilities of women but also optimizes their productive labor; costs to society in terms of health, welfare, and lost productivity are minimized. With 4760 occupationally related deaths in 1976, and about 5.5 million occupational disabilities in 1977, U.S. workers are all in need of protection.[22]

SUGGESTED TOPICS FOR DISCUSSION, FURTHER RESEARCH, AND FIELD PROJECTS

1. How do days of work loss for disability compare between men and women in a sample of your local industries and offices? Does disability of women differ from men's when they enter predominantly male fields? Compare the causes of disability between men and women.

2. In planning a production schedule for an office or factory, what factors would you need to consider to adequately provide for women's dual role? Suggest how this could be achieved.

3. Participate in health education within the workplace. Suggested contact: Women's Occupational Health Resource Center, American Health Foundation, 320 E. 43rd Street, New York, N.Y. 10017.

4. Research labor force participation and income of women by marital status and number of children. What are the salary differentials between women and men who are heads of households? Suggested source: U.S. Department of Labor, Bureau of Labor Statistics; U.S. working women: a chartbook, bulletin 1880, Washington, D.C., 1975, U.S. Government Printing Office. Suggested contact: Women's Bureau, U.S. Department of Labor, telephone 202-523-6652.

5. What has been the impact of unionization on women's labor force participation? On women's occupational health? Research women's participation in labor unions. Has it differed historically from today?

6. What are the major occupations near where you live? What are the major health hazards of these occupations? What are their effects? Do the hazards differ between men and women employees? What steps are being taken to reduce these hazards?

7. Who was Karen Silkwood and what did she stand for? Why is her case important?

8. What factors are contributing to an increase of women in traditionally male skilled-worker fields such as carpentry and plumbing? Can we expect these factors to continue? What effects might this employment trend have on a specific occupation? What health hazards could women expect in these occupations? Would these differ from hazards experienced by men?

9. Select an occupation in which women comprise more than 40% of all workers and which is not discussed in the book. What percentage of workers in this field are women? What are the general characteristics of most of the women employed in this occupation? What are the health hazards? What kind of organizing, if any, is being done in this field to ameliorate conditions? What status does this occupation have?

10. Research the life and work of one of the early women who were interested in women's occupational health. What effect did her work have on women's occupational health? Are the effects of her work still being experienced today? How has the situation she was researching and working for changed since her day?

REFERENCES

1. American College of Obstetricians and Gynecologists (ACOG). Guidelines on pregnancy and work, National Institute for Occupational Safety and Health, no. (NIOSH) 78-118, Washington, D.C., 1977, U.S. Government Printing Office.

2. American Conference of Governmental Industrial Hygienists: Documentation of threshold limit values, Cincinnati, 1971, American Conference of Governmental Hygienists, P.O. Box 1937, Cincinnati, Ohio 45201.

3. American Society of Anesthesiology: Ad Hoc Committee on the Effect of Trace Anesthetics on the Health of Operating Room Personnel, Anesthesiology **41**:321-340, Oct., 1974.

4. Ames, B. N., et al.: Hair dyes are muta-genic: identification of a variety of mutagenic ingredients, Proc. Natl. Acad. Sci. U.S.A. **72**:2423-2427, June, 1975.

5. Angle, C. R., and McIntire, M. S.: Lead poisoning during pregnancy, Am. J. Dis. Child. **108**:436-439, Oct., 1964.

6. Baetjer, A.: Women in industry: their health and efficiency, Philadelphia, 1946, W. B. Saunders, Co.

7. Baker, E. L., et al.: Lead poisoning in children of lead workers: home contamination with industrial dust, N. Engl. J. Med. **296**:260-261, Feb. 3, 1977.

8. Baldwin, D.: Caution: office zone, Job Safety and Health **4**:4-12, Feb., 1976.

9. Blake, J.: Demographic science and the redirection of population policy, J. Chronic Dis. **18**:1181-1200, 1965.

10. Brandeis, E.: In Commons, J. R., et al.: History of labor in the U.S., vol. 3. Labor legislation, New York, 1918, Macmillan Publishing Co., Inc., pp. 462-463.
11. Bronson, G.: Pregnant women are told to avoid disinfectant in soaps, Wall Street Journal, June 28, 1978.
12. Brook, A.: Mental stress at work, The Practitioner **210**:500-506, April, 1973.
13. Bruere, M.: The triangle fire, Life and Labor **1**:137-141, May, 1911.
14. Burnett, C. M., and Menkart, J.: Hair dyes and breast cancer, N. Engl. J. Med. (letters) **229**:1253, Nov. 30, 1978.
15. Caldicott, H.: At the crossroads, New Age, Dec., 1977, reprinted by Environmental Action Reprint Source, 2239 E. Colfax, Denver, Colo. 80206, pp. 1-6.
16. Center for Disease Control: Increased lead absorption and lead poisoning in young children, Atlanta, 1975, Center for Disease Control.
17. Children's Bureau: Infant mortality in New Bedford, Mass., Infant Mortality Series 10, Pub. No. 68, Washington, D.C., 1920, Children's Bureau.
18. Conroy, A. E., II: Stop sale, use or removal order, Washington, D.C., Feb. 28, 1979, Environmental Protection Agency.
19. Corn, J. K.: Doctors afield: Alice Hamilton, M.D., and women's welfare, N. Engl. J. Med. **294**:316-318, Feb. 5, 1976.
20. Data on Consumer Product Injuries from Health United States, 1978, Washington, D.C., 1979, U.S. Department of Health, Education and Welfare.
21. Data of March, 1978, provided by Women's Bureau, U.S. Department of Labor, April, 1979, personal communication.
22. Data provided by Office of Occupational Safety and Health Statistics, Bureau of Labor Statistics, April, 1979, personal communication.
23. Data provided by Women's Bureau, U.S. Department of Labor. See also Ishikoff, M.: Jury awards Bowie man $905,000 in wife's traffic death, Washington Star, March 27, 1979.
24. Dolcourt, J., et al.: Lead poisoning in children of battery plant employees—North Carolina, Morbidity and Mortality Weekly Report **26**:321, Sept. 30, 1977.
25. Eddy, T. P.: Deaths from domestic falls and fractures, Br. J. Preventive and Social Medicine **26**:173-179, Aug., 1972.
26. Fatt, N.: Women's occupational health and

the women's health movement, Prev. Med. **7**:366-371, Sept., 1978.
27. Fielding, J. E.: Smoking and pregnancy, N. Engl. J. Med. **298**:337-339, Feb. 9, 1978.
28. Fink, G. E., editor: Labor unions, Westport, Conn., 1977, Greenwood Press.
29. Flexner, E.: Century of struggle, Cambridge, Mass., 1959, Belknap Press.
30. Freudenberg, N.: Alice Hamilton, Women & Health **1**:1-2, Sept./Oct., 1976.
31. Garfinkel, J., et al.: Possible increased risk of lung cancer among beauticians, J. National Cancer Institute **58**:141-143, 1977.
32. Gelfand, W. H.: Respiratory allergy due to chemical compounds encountered in the rubber, lacquer, shellac and beauty culture industries, J. Allergy **34**:374-381, 1963.
33. Green, M.: Gynecomastia and pseudo-precocious puberty following diethylstilbestrol exposure, Am. J. Dis. Child. **95**: 637-639, 1958.
34. Gronka, P. A., et al.: Mercury vapor exposures in dental offices, J. Am. Dent. Assoc. **81**:923, Oct., 1970.
35. Hamilton, A.: Do women in health industry need special health legislation? pamphlet no. 12, 1922, The Consumers' League of Connecticut, reprinted in The health of women and children, New York, 1977, Arno Press.
36. Hamilton, A.: Women workers and industrial poisons, U.S. Department of Labor, Bulletin of the Women's Bureau, no. 57, pp. 1-5, 1926.
37. Hamilton, A.: Exploring the dangerous trades, Boston, 1943, Little, Brown & Co.
38. HCP: a possible danger to gravidas, Modern Medicine **46**:24, Nov. 15-30, 1978.
39. Hopkins, H. C.: And now a word about your shampoo, FDA Consumer, March, 1975.
40. Hricko, A., with Brunt, M.: Working for your life: a woman's guide to job health hazards, Labor Occupational Health Program (LOHP), Berkeley, and Public Citizen's Health Research Group, Washington, D.C., 1976. (Available from LOHP, University of California, 2521 Channing Way, Berkeley, Calif. 94720.)
41. Hricko, A., and Marrett, C. B.: Women's occupational health: the rise and fall of a research issue, presented at the American Association for Advancement of Science Meetings, Jan. 28, 1975, New York.
42. Hunt, V. R.: Occupational health problems

of pregnant women, no. SA-5304-75, Washington, D.C., 1975, U.S. Department of Health, Education and Welfare.

43. Hunt, V. R.: Maternal and other health needs, report prepared at the request of the Joint Economic Committee of the Congress of the United States, H. H. Humphrey, chairman, Oct. 15, 1976.

44. Hunt, V. R.: Testimony on reproductive effects of lead exposure, presented at Occupational Safety and Health Administration, U.S. Department of Labor, Hearing on Occupational Exposure to Lead, March 17, 1977.

45. Infante, P.: Genetic risks of vinyl chloride, Lancet 1:734-735, April 3, 1976.

46. Ingersoll, B.: "DES intoxication"—feminized male workers, The Seattle Times, June 30, 1978.

47. Jelliffe, D. B., and Jelliffe, E. F. P.: Current concepts in nutrition. "Breast is best": modern meanings, N. Engl. J. Med. **297:** 912-915, Oct. 27, 1977.

48. Johnson, C. J., and VanDeusen, K.: Rates of congenital malformations in an area contaminated with plutonium, presented at the American Public Health Association Annual Meeting, Oct. 17, 1978, Los Angeles.

49. Johnsson, I.: How to improve the utilization of nurses and allied health support personnel: the Swedish model, Proceedings of the International Conference on Women and Health, (HRA) 76-51, Washington, D.C., June 16-18, 1975, Washington, D.C. 1975, Health Resources Administration, U.S. Department of Health, Education and Welfare.

50. Kemble, F. A.: Journal of a residence on a Georgian plantation in 1838-1839, London, 1863, Longman.

51. Kerr, L.: The prevention of occupational illness and injury: a reality, presented at the American Public Health Association Annual Meeting, Oct. 18, 1978, Los Angeles.

52. Kirkland, D. J., et al.: Chromosomal damage and hair dyes, Lancet 2:124-127, July 15, 1978.

53. Kline, J., et al.: Smoking: a risk factor for spontaneous abortion, N. Engl. J. Med. **297:** 793-795, Oct. 13, 1977.

54. Kmoike, Y., et al.: Fatigue assessment of key punch operators, typists and others, Ergonomics **14:**101-109, 1971.

55. Krekel, S.: Placement of women in high risk areas, presented at The Society for Occupational and Environmental Health, Conference on Women in the Workplace, June 17-19, 1976, Washington, D.C.

56. LaLeche League International, Inc. information sheets, Women & Health 3:24-28, Jan./Feb., 1978.

57. Lancranjan, I.: Genital system—men. In Occupational safety and health encyclopedia, vol. 1, Geneva, 1971, International Labor Organization.

58. Lancranjan, I.: Reproductive ability of workmen occupationally exposed to lead, Arch. Environ. Health **30:**396-401, Aug., 1975.

59. Lehmann, P.: Women workers: are they special? Job Safety and Health **3:**4-13, April, 1975.

60. Lehmann, P.: Protecting women out of their jobs, Science for the People **9:**30-33, Nov./Dec., 1977.

61. Love, M.: The health hazards of office work, Women & Health 3:18-23, May/June, 1978.

62. Love, T.: U.S. lets kids pick sprayed crops, The Washington Star, Nov. 23, 1978.

63. Maupin, J.: Labor heroines: ten women who led the struggle, 1974, Union Wage Educational Committee, P.O. Box 462, Berkeley, Calif. 94701.

64. McCann, M.: The impact of hazards in art on female workers, Prev. Med. **7:**338-348, Sept., 1978.

65. Mekky, S., et al.: Varicose veins in women cotton workers. An epidemiological study in England and in Egypt, Br. Med. J. **2:** 591-595, June 7, 1969.

66. Morton, W. E., and Ungs, T. J.: Cancer mortality in the major cottage industry, Women & Health **4:**345-354, Winter, 1979.

67. National Safety Council: Accident prevention manual for industrial operations, Chicago, 1969, National Safety Council.

68. Newhouse, M., et al.: A study of the mortality of female asbestos workers, Br. J. Ind. Med. **29:**134-141, April, 1972.

69. O'Brien, P.: Entire neighborhood dying; chemical dumping blamed, The Seattle Times, Nov. 23, 1978.

70. Occupational safety and health reporter, Bureau of National Affairs, p. 379, Aug. 21, 1975.

71. Palmer, A.: A morbidity survey of respiratory symptoms and functions among Utah

beauticians, Aug., 1975, National Institute of Occupational Safety and Health.

72. Palmer, A.: Respiratory disease in beauticians, Women & Health **1**:14-18, Sept./ Oct., 1976.

73. Reassessment of noise concerns of other nations, vol. I. Summary and selected topics, Washington, D.C., Aug., 1976, Environmental Protection Agency.

74. Radium poisoning, industrial poisoning from radioactive substances, Monthly Labor Review **28**:1200-1275, 1929.

74a. Report, a woman in that job, Job Safety and Health **2**:16, Feb., 1974.

75. Richards, B.: Pesticide—exposure warning overruled, The Washington Post, Nov. 23, 1978.

76. Rosen, G.: Early studies of occupational health in New York City in 1870's, Am. J. Public Health **67**:1100-1102, Nov., 1977.

77. Schneider, M.: Mercury: a health hazard associated with employment of women as dental assistants, presented at the Society for Occupational and Environmental Health, Conference on Women in the Workplace, June 17-19, 1976, Washington, D.C.

78. Scott, R.: Reproductive hazards, Job Safety and Health **6**:7-13, May, 1978.

79. Sex stereotyping: its decline in the skilled trades, Monthly Labor Review **97**:14-22, May, 1974.

80. Shafer, N., and Shafer, R. W.: Potential of carcinogenic effects of hair dyes, N.Y. State J. Med. **76**:394-396, 1976.

81. Shore, R. E., et al.: A case-control study of hair dye use and breast cancer, J. National Cancer Institute **62**:277-283, Feb., 1979.

82. Sidel, R.: New roles for women in health care delivery, conditions in the People's Republic of China, Proceedings of the International Conference on Women in Health, (HRA) 76-51, June 16-18, 1975, Washington, D.C., Health Resources Administration, U.S. Department of Health, Education and Welfare.

83. Smith, A. M.: Congenital Minamata disease (methyl-mercury poisoning and birth defects in Japan), presented at the Society for Occupational and Environmental Health, Conference on Women in the Workplace, June 17-19, 1976, Washington, D.C.

84. Smith, A. M.: Mercury poisoning and birth defects in Japan, Women & Health **3**:9-12, March/April, 1978.

85. Spyker, J.: Assessing the impact of low level chemicals on development, Fed. Proc. **34**:1836, Aug., 1975.

86. Steinberg, J.: Another Willow Island tragedy. Five women say 'sterilize the workplace, not workers,' Seven Days **3**, Feb. 23, 1979.

87. Stellman, J. M.: Women's work, women's health, New York, 1977, Pantheon Books.

88. Suffering toxicity for their art, Medical World News **18**:30, Nov. 28, 1977.

89. Tabershaw, I. R., and Gaffey, W. R.: Mortality of workers in the manufacture of vinyl chloride and its polymers, J. Occupational Med. **16**:509-518, Aug., 1974.

90. Ten workers found sterile—pesticide plant shut down, The Seattle Times, p. A. 18, Aug. 5, 1977.

91. Thériault, G., and Grand-Bois, L.: Mesothelioma and asbestos in the province of Quebec: 1969-1972, Arch. Environ. Health **33**:15-19, Jan./Feb., 1978.

92. Tokuhata, G. K., et al.: Fatal injuries attributed to consumer products in Pennsylvania, 1971, Public Health Reports **92**: 374-382, July/Aug., 1977.

93. Trebilcock, A. M.: OSHA and equal employment opportunity laws for women, Prev. Med. **7**:372-384, Sept., 1978.

94. United Nations: Demographic yearbook, New York, 1975, United Nations.

95. United Press International: Hair dye warning proposed, The Washington Post, Jan. 5, 1978.

96. U.S. Bureau of Labor: Report on condition of woman and child wage-earners in the U.S., Washington, D.C., 1910-1913, U.S. Government Printing Office. Prepared under direction of Charles P. Neill, Commission of Labor, 19 vols., 61st Congress, 2nd Session, Senate, DOC 645.

97. U.S. Department of Health, Education and Welfare: Man, medicine and work: historic events in occupational medicine, U.S. Public Health Service Pub. No. 1044, Washington, D.C., April, 1964.

98. U.S. Department of Labor: Infant mortality in Manchester, N.H., Infant Mortality Series 6, Children's Bureau Pub. 20, Washington, D.C., 1917.

99. U.S. Department of Labor: Asbestos in the office air, Job Safety and Health **4**:12-14, March, 1976.

100. Waller, J. A.: Non-highway injury fatalities. II. Interaction of product and human factors, J. Chronic Dis. **25**:47-52, Jan., 1972.

101. Ward, E.: Phosphorous necrosis in the manufacture of fireworks and preparation of phosphorus, U.S. Department of Labor Bulletin, no. 405, Washington, D.C., 1926.

102. Welch, R.: The causes of tenosynovitis in industry, Industrial Medicine **41**:16-19, 1972.

103. Women's Bureau, U.S. Department of Labor: 1975 Handbook on women workers, stock no. 029-016-0037-2, Washington, D.C., 1975, U.S. Government Printing Office.

104. Women's Bureau: Maternity standards, Washington, D.C., 1976, U.S. Department of Labor.

105. Women's Bureau: The earnings gap between women and men, Employment Standards Administration, U.S. Department of Labor, Washington, D.C., 1976, U.S. Government Printing Office; Current data from Bureau of Labor Statistics, U.S. Department of Labor, personal communications, March, 1979.

106. Women's Bureau: Personal communication, April 9, 1979.

107. Women's Bureau: Statement concerning PL. 95-555, April, 1979, U.S. Department of Labor.

108. Zuskin, E., and Bouhuys, A.: Acute airway responses to hair-spray preparations, N. Engl. J. Med. **290**:660-663, March 21, 1974.

ADDITIONAL READINGS

Ashford, N. A.: Summary of crisis in the workplace: occupational disease and injury. A report to the Ford Foundation, Cambridge, Mass., 1975, The MIT Press.

Baxandall, R., et al., editors: America's working women: a documentary history — 1600 to the present, New York, 1976, Vintage Books.

Bingham, E.: Proceedings of the Conference on Women and the Workplace, June 17-19, 1976, Washington, D.C., 1977, Society for Occupational and Environmental Health, 1714 Massachusetts Ave., N.W., Washington, D.C. 20036.

Corbett, T. H.: Operating room exposure: cancer, miscarriages, and birth defects, Women & Health **1**:11-14, Sept./Oct., 1976.

Corbett, T. H., et al.: Birth defects among children of nurse-anesthetists, Anesthesiology **41**:341-344, Oct., 1974.

Coye, M. J.: Organizing for health at the point of production: the role for science in occupational health, presented at the APHA Annual Meeting, Oct. 18, 1978, Los Angeles, Calif.

Curran, J.: Founders of the Harvard School of Public Health, New York, 1970, Josiah Macy Foundation.

Fabia, J., and Truong, D. T.: Occupation of father at time of birth of children dying of malignant diseases, Br. J. Preventive and Social Medicine **28**:98-100, 1974.

Goldsmith, F.: An occupational safety and health workbook, New York, 1977, Labor Safety and Health Institute, 381 Park Ave. S. (27th St.), New York, N.Y. 10016.

Hendershot, C. E.: Pregnant workers in the United States, Advance Data, no. 11, pp. 1-4, Sept. 15, 1977.

Henderson, W. J., et al.: Talc and carcinoma of the ovary and cervix, J. Obstet. Gynaecol. Br. Commonwealth **78**:266-272, March, 1971.

Hunt, V.: The health of women at work, bibliography, occasional papers, no. 2, 1977, Program on Women, Northwestern University, 619 Emerson St., Evanston, Ill. 60201.

Hunt, V. R.: Occupational radiation exposure of women workers, Prev. Med. **7**:294-310, Sept., 1978.

Hunt, V. R.: Work and the health of women, Cleveland, 1979, CRC Press.

International Labor Office, Washington Branch, 1750 New York Av., N.W., Room 330, Washington, D.C. 20006, various publications.

International Labor Organization (ILO): Encyclopedia of occupational health and safety, Geneva, 1971, International Labor Office, various publications.

Labor Occupational Health Program, University of California, 2521 Channing Way, Berkeley, Calif. 94720, telephone 415-642-5507, various publications.

Lehman, P., editor: Cancer and the worker, New York, 1977, The New York Academy of Sciences, 2 E. 63rd. St., New York, N.Y. 10021.

Newman, J. M.: Maternity standards, reprinted from *1975 Handbook on Women Workers,* 902-832, Women's Bureau Employment Standards Administration, U.S. Department of Labor, Washington, D.C., 1976, U.S. Government Printing Office.

O'Brien, M. W., and Page, J.: Bitter wages: the

Nader report on occupational health and safety, New York, 1973, Grossman Publishers.

OSHA—a means to improve the health of Americans, CCAHS Quarterly, pp. 1-8, Fall, 1974, Consumer Commission on the Accreditation of Health Services, 101 West 31st St., New York, N.Y. 10001.

Penney, J.: The hazards of hospital workers, Health Alert **3:**1-2, Oct., 1978.

San Francisco Women's History Group: What have women done? A photo essay on the history of working women in the United States, San Francisco, 1973, Banner Press.

Social issues. The dilemma of regulating reproductive risks, Business Week, Aug. 29, 1977.

Stellman, J., and Daum, S.: Work is dangerous to your health, New York, 1973, Vintage Books.

Stellman, J. M., guest editor: Forum: women's occupational health: medical, social, and legal implications, Prev. Med. **7:**281-293, Sept., 1978.

Stewart, A.: A note on the obstetric effects of work during pregnancy. Br. J. Preventive Medicine **9:**156-161, 1955.

The susceptibility of the fetus and the child to chemical pollutants, (supp.), Pediatrics **53:** 859, 1974.

Terlin, R.: A working woman's guide to her job rights, leaflet 55, 0-241-016 (24), Women's Bureau, Employment Standards Administration, U.S. Department of Labor, rev. 1975, Washington, D.C., 1977, U.S. Government Printing Office.

U.S. Bureau of Labor Statistics: Summary of the Report on Condition of Woman and Child Wage Earners in the United States, Dec., 1915, Washington, D.C., 1916, U.S. Government Printing Office.

U.S. Department of Health, Education and Welfare: A preliminary survey of the industrial hygiene problem in the United States, Public Health Bulletin, no. 259, Washington, D.C., 1940, U.S. Public Health Service.

U.S. Department of Labor: The industrial nurse and the woman worker, Washington, D.C., 1944, Women's Bureau.

Wallick, F.: The American worker: an endangered species, New York, 1972, Ballantine Books.

Wegman, D. H.: Occupational health hazards of women, presented at the American Association for the Advancement of Science, Jan. 28, 1975, New York, N.Y.

Wells, J. A.: Facts about women's absenteeism and labor turnover, Women's Bureau, Wage and Labor Standards Administration, U.S. Department of Labor, Aug., 1969, 0-361-490, Washington, D.C., 1969, U.S. Government Printing Office.

Wells, J. A.: Automation and women workers, Women's Bureau, Wage and Labor Standards Administration, U.S. Department of Labor, Feb., 1970, Washington, D.C., 1970, U.S. Government Printing Office.

Women's Bureau, U.S. Department of Labor: Protective legislation, Bulletin of the Women's Bureau, no. 66, Washington, D.C., 1929.

Women's Bureau: Mature women workers: a profile, Washington, D.C., 1976, Employment Standards Administration, U.S. Department of Labor.

The Women's Occupational Health Resource Center, School of Public Health, Columbia University, 60 Haven Ave., B-1, New York, N.Y. 10032, telephone 212-694-3464.

Yost, E.: American women of science, New York, 1943, Frederick Stokes Co.

Chapter 6

Health care for young women

Although adolescent health care is a growing specialty, there is still relatively little data on the general health status of teenagers. Adolescents have been widely regarded as healthy and have not been of priority to statisticians, planners, or providers. Specific health problems have been focused on by federal and voluntary agencies, but this highlighting has often obscured the general social, psychological, and physiological contexts within which such problems develop.

This is particularly true of most of the health problems of younger women (approximately 10 to 19 years of age) selected for discussion in this chapter: acne, pregnancy, VD, alcoholism and drug abuse, suicide, anorexia nervosa, smoking, prostitution, and accidents, injuries, and homicides. Each is affected, caused, or exacerbated by complex social factors. although these problems are of critical concern and viewed by many as being of epidemic proportions, teenagers are nonetheless also plagued by many conditions less likely to catch headlines.

Adolescence is a developmental stage generally beginning with the onset of development of secondary sex characteristics (puberty) and a physical growth spurt and ending with the assumption of an adult role, which usually includes a degree of economic independence. Although a chronological age, rarely agreed on by experts, is assigned to adolescence, for example 10 to 19 years, such an arbitrary division fails to consider the physiological, psychological, sociological, and cognitive changes that occur in developing humans and that may occur at widely varying ages. In 1978 there were an estimated 39.7 million adolescents, aged 10 to 19, in the United States; of these, 49.1% were females. In 1980, because of the lower birthrate, this number should be 38.4 million, with 49.1% being female.[22]

HISTORICAL BACKGROUND

In contemporary society when the changes of growth and puberty occur, roughly between ages 10 and 19, they are termed adolescence. In medieval times, adolescence was unclearly defined by function, dress, or behavior; some philosophers stated that it ranged from ages 14 to 28 or 35, but it was thought of in physiological rather than sociological terms. In the lower classes especially, today's familiar marks of adolescence were unknown; here there were no persons with few responsibilities for productive and economic contributions and who could attend extended schooling. As the life span extended and societies became more affluent, leisure time became a possibility. An age cohort that was exempt from productive labor could be supported. Childhood could also be a social not just a physiological reality.

Ariès states that military conscription contributed to the definition of adolescence. Strong young men were needed for military service, and an age grouping was identified. Schools also distinguished one age-group from another. Youth and adolescence came to be viewed as the hope of the society; society strived "to come to [adolescence] early and linger in it as long as possible."[8]

Until adolescence was recognized as part of the life of girls, they were taught to sew, paint, embroider, cook, and generally be productive at an early age. From Puritan New England there are records of many orders made to young seamstress girls, 5 to 7 years of age.[70] Girls were often indentured into household service and were expected to haul water, cook, and clean. The advent of public schools with their defined age-groups also contributed to establishing an adolescence for girls. As discussed later, the media, social expectations, laws, affluence, and, conversely, unemployment, have all contributed to maintaining this distinct age cohort.

GENERAL HEALTH STATUS OF ADOLESCENTS
Mortality

From the turn of the century until the 1930s, survival to adolescence was a major achievement. Deaths from tuberculosis, pneumonia, diphtheria, croup, and typhoid fever were common. Life expectancy was 47.3 years for someone born in 1900 as compared with 72.8 years for a person born in 1976. Infant mortality data (where available) suggest that 1 in 10 infants died in the first year of life, and even in 1930, 65 out of every 1000 babies born died before their first birthday; not until 1950 were infant mortality rates less than 30 per 1000 live births.[108]

Today adolescent mortality is at the lowest rate per 100,000 for the first 35 years of life. It is, however, still higher than it could be. Adolescents as a group (as do most of the rest of the population) die mostly from accidents; in 1976 about 50% of deaths among children aged 10 to 14 were from this cause, as were 59% of deaths among 15- to 19-year-olds. Motor vehicle accidents accounted for over a quarter of deaths from all causes in children past infancy, while 7% of all deaths were from drowning and 4% from fires.[108,p.52]

Ranking deaths from causes other than accidents shows some variation among female adolescents both by age and race. For example, the second and third causes of death in 1977 among young white women aged 10 to 14 were malignant neoplasms and congenital anomalies; the third cause for minority women was homicide. Among white females aged 15 to 19 suicide and homicide ranked third and fourth, while among minority females, homicides, malignant neoplasms, and suicides were second, third, and fourth, respectively (see Table 6-1).

Overall, death rates at all ages are higher for males than females; this is particularly true of accidents and homicides, which are double for males in some age-groups. Rates for diseases and pathological conditions are also generally higher among males, except for diabetes and anemia. Rates are extremely close for heart disease except among minority males and females aged 15 to 19, where heart disease causes twice as many deaths among males.

Table 6-1. Leading causes of mortality in persons aged 10 to 19, shown by numbers of deaths, 1977*

10 to 14 years

Cause of death	Total	White female	White male	Other female	Other male
All causes	6,745	1,962	3,487	439	857
Accidents	3,398	822	1,920	151	505
Malignant neoplasms	864	307	423	62	72
Congenital anomalies	304	114	142	24	24
Homicide	248	70	86	39	53
Suicide	188	23	146	7	12
Heart disease	186	69	70	24	23
Influenza and pneumonia	183	76	64	20	23
Cerebrovascular disorders and stroke	87	31	40	4	12
Benign neoplasms	53	23	23	3	4
Anemias	53	15	20	7	11
Diabetes	36	22	7	4	3

15 to 19 years

Cause of death	Total	White female	White male	Other female	Other male
All causes	21,443	4,847	13,209	1,023	2,364
Accidents	12,680	2,736	8,621	296	1,027
Homicide	1,897	276	754	201	666
Suicide	1,871	311	1,389	39	132
Malignant neoplasms	1,250	391	668	100	91
Heart disease	413	108	190	38	77
Congenital anomalies	350	122	181	17	30
Influenza and pneumonia	250	85	113	19	33
Cerebrovascular disorders and stroke	175	64	73	17	21
Anemias	74	20	19	19	16
Benign neoplasm	63	22	27	8	6
Diabetes	53	23	17	10	3

*Based on data provided by Donald Greenberg, Statistician, Mortality Statistics Branch, Division of Vital Statistics, National Center for Health Statistics, U.S. Department of Health, Education and Welfare, Washington, D.C.

Morbidity

Some adolescent morbidity is reflected in the mortality statistics in Table 6-1. For example, data from the National Center for Health Statistics show that about 4.6% of adolescents, about 1 out of 20, have cardiovascular problems. High blood pressure affects 4% of adolescent females,[59] and this has been significantly correlated to obesity and emotional well-being.[61]

Morbidity data, as all measures of health, are also affected by class. Class factors may lead to bias in the two principal modes of morbidity reporting among adolescents — physician assessed/reported, and self-reported subjectively experienced health, which Brunswick has termed ontological health.[18] Data that have been reported indicate that one third of 12- to 17-year-olds in a 1960s national survey had some kind of neuromuscular condition or joint abnormality and one third had a musculoskeletal defect (e.g., scoliosis). Twenty percent had some cardiovascular problem and 8% had significant neurological findings.[74] In 1964 Rogers and Reese[88] found that mental, weight, skin (particularly acne), vision, hear-

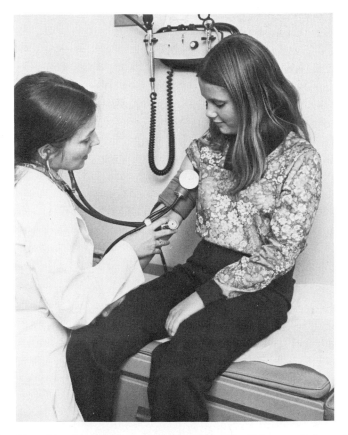

Fig. 6-1. Checking blood pressure. (Courtesy Health Sciences Information Service, University of Washington, Seattle.)

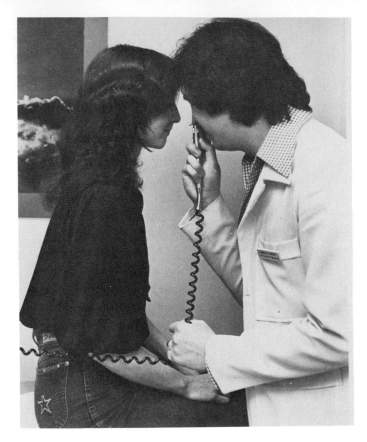

Fig. 6-2. Optical examination. (Courtesy Media Service, Child Development and Mental Retardation Center, University of Washington, Seattle.)

ing, and dental problems were common to adolescents. This was confirmed by Brunswick's data, also from the 1960s, which found respiratory tract disorders and neuromuscular and musculoskeletal problems as well as the cardiovascular and blood pressure problems mentioned earlier. Vision difficulties were more commonly reported in Brunswick's study by girls (23%) than boys (14%), and physicians reported a significant vision or eye problem for nearly 1 in 10 of the youths examined, irrespective of sex. Among young women ages 12 to 15 who were menstruating (17% in this age-group reported no menstruation), 3 in 10 reported that their periods were irregular and "produced problems which caused them to stay home and/or to go to bed."[20]

Kovar[59] reported in 1978 that 68% of all adolescents were affected by acne, 55% showed some sign of tooth decay, and 34% wore corrective lenses; of this latter group, 31% failed to reach the 20/20 level in vision testing when wearing their lenses.

Between 1966 and 1970, adolescents themselves reported that their health

Table 6-2. Selected measures of self-appraised health for adolescents aged 12 to 17, United States, 1966 to 1970*

Measure of self-appraised health	Both sexes (%)	Females (%)	Males (%)
Self-appraised health status			
Excellent	26.6	24.5	28.6
Very good	33.2	33.0	33.5
Good	35.7	37.3	34.1
Fair	4.2	4.9	3.4
Poor	0.4	0.4	0.4
Frequency of anxiety feelings			
Often	7.6	8.9	6.3
Sometimes	36.1	39.3	32.9
Rarely	36.0	34.9	37.1
Never	20.3	16.8	23.7
Preferred weight			
Thinner	32.9	48.4	17.9
About the same	48.0	40.8	55.0
Heavier	19.1	10.8	27.1
Preferred height			
Shorter	7.3	12.8	1.9
About the same	57.8	67.7	48.2
Taller	34.9	19.5	49.8
Reported a health problem	10.3	10.5	10.1

*Based on data from National Center for Health Statistics: Vital and Health Statistics, series 11, no. 147, April, 1975. (Data based on household interviews of a sample of the civilian noninstitutional population.)

was generally good; only 10% reported a health problem. This ranged from 7% of 12-year-olds to 13% of 17-year-olds. Slightly fewer adolescent females reported that their health was excellent (24.5%) than did adolescents as a group (26.6%); substantially more reported that they would prefer to be thinner (48.4%) than did all adolescents (32.9%). Preferences for being taller or shorter indicated frequent dissatisfaction with appearance (see Table 6-2).

Educational and communication impairments are another type of health problem for adolescents. The National Center for Education Statistics estimates that during 1974 and 1975 almost 8 million persons under 19 years of age suffered such a handicap, including speech impairments, learning disabilities, mental retardation, and emotional disturbances. These handicaps, although representing a broad interpretation of health, have implications for adolescent well-being equal to, if not greater than, most conventional medical conditions.[108]

Use of medical services

Ambulatory care. Of all the diseases affecting adolescents respiratory conditions cause more loss of days of school (61% of all school days lost in 1975 and 1976), more restricted activity, more days spent in bed, and greater use of medical services than does any other condition (25.6% of office visits by persons under 18 years in 1975 and 1976 — 33 million visits).[108]

Table 6-3. Visits by adolescents aged 12 to 17 to office-based physicians, United States, 1975 to 1976*

Sex and diagnosis	Total	12 to 15 years	16 to 17 years
Physician visits per person per year			
Both sexes	1.6	1.5	1.9
Females	1.7	1.5	2.2
Males	1.5	1.5	1.5
Percent distribution by principal diagnosis			
Females			
Illness	69.1	71.2	66.5
Injury	8.2	9.0	7.2
Examination and observation	21.1	18.5	24.5
Prenatal	6.3	3.0	10.5
Males			
Illness	60.6	61.9	58.3
Injury	16.8	16.3	17.7
Examination and observation	21.5	20.7	23.0

*From Kovar, M. G.: Public Health Rep. **94**:109-118, March/April, 1979.

For adolescents ages 12 to 17 other reasons for office visits included injuries (16%), skin conditions (14%), visual or hearing problems (10%), and infectious or parasitic diseases (10%). Adolescents themselves thought skin conditions were the only "problems."[59] (See Table 6-3.)

Many teenagers, however, seek care outside the traditional medical system or may not seek care at all. The 1960s survey showed that between 40% and 55% of all adolescents did not want to see a doctor for vomiting, overtiredness, nervousness, or loss of appetite.[59] Once visits to the pediatrician stop at about age 12, many adolescents do not see another physician until they marry, become pregnant, or become an adult. Visiting the family physician is disliked by many teenagers, particularly for problems relating to sexuality.

The anonymity and low charges provided by alternatives such as the Door in New York, Planned Parenthood, and free and community clinics are appealing to adolescents, although apparently not well used. Data from the 1974 Health Interview Survey show that during that year, of persons under 18 years, 69% went to a physician; of these, 62% went to a private physician in an office, 21% went to a hospital outpatient or emergency department, and 5% went to a free-standing clinic. Some persons used all three settings.[108]

Until age 16 more boys than girls visit the physician; this is primarily because of injuries, discussed later. By the age of 16 to 17, girls make more visits than boys. Prenatal care accounts for part of this shift; 11% of all visits made by young women aged 16 to 17 years to private physicians in 1975 and 1976 were for prenatal care.[108]

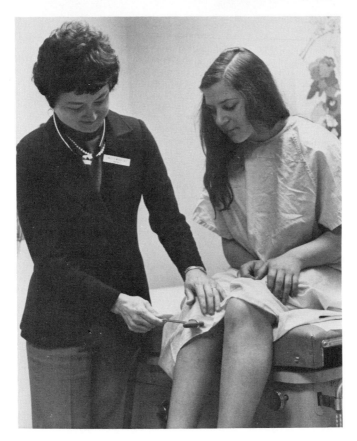

Fig. 6-3. Checking reflexes. (Courtesy Media Service, Child Development and Mental Retardation Center, University of Washington, Seattle.)

Hospitalization. For adolescents 12 to 17 years of age, days spent in hospital during 1975 and 1976 were mainly for respiratory conditions (8%), injuries (23%), mental problems (11%), digestive conditions (11%), and pregnancy and delivery (13%).[61] The leading diagnosis, however, of all hospitalized adolescents aged 10 to 14 in 1977 was hypertrophy of tonsils and adenoids; this held true when data were analyzed within each sex. Male adolescents aged 15 to 19 in 1977, though, were most often hospitalized for intracranial injury, whereas for females in that age-group, hospitalization was principally for delivery without mention of complications (see Table 6-4).

Institutionalized adolescents. The U.S. Bureau of the Census reported that in 1976 there were slightly fewer than 152,000 children and youths under 18 years of age in institutions for medical or protective care (see Table 6-5).[106] Kovar notes that most of these children were admitted for medical (38%) or family (31%) reasons, such as family being unable to care for the child. Mental retardation was the most common condition among those admitted for medical reasons; this diagnosis

Table 6-4. Leading diagnoses of all patients discharged from nonfederal short-stay hospitals, 1977*†

	All	Female	Male
10 to 14 years			
All discharge diagnoses	969	454	514
Hypertrophy of tonsils and adenoids	101	64	37
Appendicitis	61	25	36
Intracranial injury excluding skull fracture	45	12	33
Fracture of upper limbs	37	10	27
Congenital anomalies	30	11	19
Diseases of ear and mastoid process	24	11	12
Fracture of lower limb except neck of femur	28	8	20
Pneumonia	25	12	12
15 to 19 years			
All discharge diagnoses	2394	1603	790
Delivery without mention of complications	390	390	0
Delivery with complications	147	147	0
Hypertrophy of tonsils and adenoids	99	75	24
Abortion	90	90	0
Appendicitis	70	35	36
Diseases of oral cavity, salivary glands, jaws, and esophagus	69	51	18
Complications of pregnancy	57	57	0
Intracranial injury excluding skull fracture	64	20	44
Fracture of lower limb except neck of femur	41	8	32
Dislocation without fracture	45	14	31
Laceration and open wounds (except eye, ear, and head; includes multiple lacerations)	36	9	28

*Based on data provided by Gloria Gardocki, Survey Statistician, Hospital Care Statistics Branch, National Center for Health Statistics, U.S. Department of Health, Education and Welfare, Washington, D.C.
†Numbers rounded to nearest thousand.

accounted for 12% of all children in institutions. Nervous disorders and mental illness were the second and third most common reasons for medical admissions.[108]

Most adolescents who receive mental health care do so on an outpatient basis. In 1975 the National Institute of Mental Health estimated that for children and youths under 18 years of age, 25,252 were admitted to state and county mental hospitals, 15,426 to private mental hospitals, 42,690 to the inpatient psychiatric units of general hospitals, and 12,022 to residential treatment centers for emotion-

Table 6-5. Institutionalized population under age 18, United States, 1976*

	Total number	Percent
	151,530	100.0
All females	64,750	42.7
All males	85,410	57.3
White females†	51,760	44.8
White males†	63,580	55.2
All other females†	12,990	37.3
All other males†	21,820	62.7

*Based on data from U.S. Bureau of the Census: Current population reports, series P-23, no. 69, Washington, D.C., June, 1978, U.S. Government Printing Office.
†"White" and "other" categories do not equal total, since total includes those of unknown color.

ally disturbed children. These admissions represented about 15% of the total psychiatric admissions (both inpatient and outpatient) for 1975.[95]

GOVERNMENT PROGRAMS AND LEGISLATION
Historical background

Formally expressed interest in the rights and welfare of children began at the turn of the century and was marked by the first of the decennial White House conferences on children. The 1909 meeting, entitled the White House Conference on the Care of Dependent Children, focused on the need for a home life (foster or child's own) for all children. The financial feasibility of this and the child's "rights" were the motivating concepts rather than a home's advantages to healthy psychosocial development.

From this conference came the Children's Bureau, established finally on April 9, 1912. The motivation for its establishment came in large part, according to Richmond, from the belief that the United States "ought to do as much for child care and research as the Department of Agriculture was doing for hogs."[87] Its energetic first chief, Julia Lathrop, promptly began collecting needed data on infant mortality and forced the nation to consider diverse aspects of child welfare.

The second White House conference in 1919 reflected the activities of the Children's Bureau and focused not only on the need for a sound home life but also on employment rights of children, special needs of selected groups of children (e.g., the handicapped), and the need to protect children from the effects of war. At this conference minimum standards concerning employment, education, and health of both mothers and children were established.

By the third White House conference in 1930 the emphasis had shifted to collecting facts on the physical and mental development of children. President Hoover stated the importance of providing protection and stimulation for normal children in addition to those with special needs.

Inequalities of opportunity for all children and youth—who were specifically included—were the focus of the fourth White House conference in 1939. Migrants, minorities, and low-income groups were discussed, and the overall integration of children into a democracy was the theme. Recognition came of the relationship between social problems and child development.

In 1950 the White House Conference on Children and Youth focused on how to achieve healthy emotional growth for children to ensure a healthy nation. This theme was expanded in the sixth White House conference in 1960, which promoted the concept of the realization of full potential for all children and youth.

By the seventh conference in 1970, the complexities of needs for children and youth led to dividing the conference into two sessions. The first in December, 1970, dealt with children aged 0 to 13; the second in April, 1971, addressed youth aged 14 to 24. Under Richard Nixon the conference stressed the importance of developing a sense of patriotism. Practical concerns were also discussed, such as the need for child care for children of working mothers, health insurance, experimental schools, and solutions for social problems affecting children.[41]

Contemporary programs

Many federal and state programs were influenced by these conferences and by the social climates that they reflected. Many of these, which directly concerned health, also involved women (mothers) and are discussed in Chapter 3.

There are numerous other federal programs functioning specifically for children and youth, however. Those which concern health include Child Welfare Services Programs, Indian Social Services, Child Welfare Assistance Programs, Appalachian Child Development Program, National School Lunch Program, Handicapped Children's Program, Mental Health Children's Services, Childhood Lead-Based Paint Poisoning Control, Runaway Youth, Child Development – Child Abuse and Neglect Prevention and Treatment, Youth Research and Development, and Child Support Enforcement.

In addition, there are programs in education (e.g., Handicapped Innovative Programs, such as Deaf-Blind Centers and Right to Read, and Elimination of Illiteracy), employment (e.g., Apprenticeship Outreach, Federal Employment for Disadvantaged Youth – Summer), income maintenance (e.g., Aid for Dependent Children), and food and nutrition (e.g., food stamps and other school food programs). Other programs such as those for family planning benefit many teenagers although not specifically intended for them (see Chapter 3).

The largest publicly supported health program for children is Medicaid; in fiscal year 1976 over half (54%) of the public expenditures for health care of children and youth under 19 years came from Medicaid. The 2.5 million Medicaid dollars spent were comprised of $1.4 million from the federal government and $1.1 million from state and local governments. Kovar notes that Maternal and Child Health Services programs (Title V of the Social Security Act, see Chapter 3) spent approximately $500 million in 1976, "which was substantially less than the $800 million spent by the Department of Defense for dependent minors of military personnel."[108] An additional $876 million came from other programs, approximately $35 million of which came from Medicare funds for about 1900 enrollees under 19 years. Most of these had end-stage renal disease (see Chapter 3).

Children and Youth Projects are part of the Maternal and Child Health Services funded under the Social Security Act, Title V, Section 205. Specifically meant for preschool and school age children (although the minimum and maximum age limits are sometimes flexible depending on need), these projects provide broad-based primary care, including family planning services. Begun in 1965, these programs serve children and youth living in low-income areas. They are financed by project grants to the states, which select the site of the program; they are frequently run by prestigious teaching hospitals, although some are operated by city or county health departments. In 1978, 578,880 children and youth were served by these projects, and a similar-sized population is expected to have been served in 1979.

Crippled Children's Programs, also funded under Title V, serve handicapped children and youth from birth to 21 years. In 1978, 606,000 were served, and 649,000 are estimated for 1979. Neither this nor the children and youth projects maintain sex-specific data.[81]

Legislation

Of particular concern to adolescents, especially young women, is the ability to obtain health services without parental consent. Most of the laws on consent to medical care deal with minors' rights to services for venereal disease (VD), drug dependency, alcoholism, pregnancy, dental care, general medical care, and hospitalization. Access to services without parental consent varies within each state and ranges from permitting minors 12 years and over to obtain VD treatment to prohibiting anyone under age 18 from obtaining an abortion without parental consent. Most states specifically prohibit those under 18 from donating blood for compensation without parental consent, and their right to agree to sterilization without parental consent is unclear. In almost all states married minors and minors who are parents may consent to all types of care for themselves or for their children.[43]

Access to birth control services is particularly important for young women. In one study, *Improving Family Planning Services for Teenagers,* it was reported that as of June, 1976, only 23 states and the District of Columbia had granted those under 18 the right to obtain birth control services without parental consent. In some states, although parental consent was not required for older teens, it was required for those under 15 who sought contraceptive services. Thus the very young, most fearful of parents "finding out," were the least likely to obtain the services desperately needed.[102] By May, 1978, a state-by-state analysis showed that 26 states and the District of Columbia specifically permitted minors access to contraceptive services without parental consent.[83] In 25 states and the District of Columbia those under 18 could obtain abortions without parental consent.[43] Parental consent as a condition of service in federally funded family planning programs was ruled unconstitutional in 1976.

However, the 1976 study on *Improving Family Planning Services for Teenagers* found that poorly defined or undefined laws in many states, or the social climate, frequently resulted in practices that effectively denied minors access to medical care, including birth control and abortion services. In these situations, clinics were found to have employed the following strategies: requiring "parents' signatures," which were never verified; prescribing pills or diaphragms and not

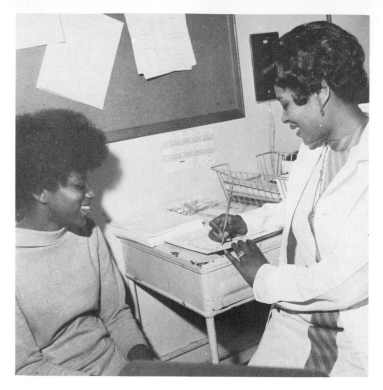

Fig. 6-4. Counseling. (Courtesy National Union of Hospital and Health Care Employees, Local 1199.)

intrauterine devices because insertion of the latter can be regarded as a surgical procedure; requiring "cooling off" periods for teen patients, which consisted of a counseling session and a suitable period for thought, after which treatment was provided; allowing only physicians to treat teens; or simply refusing to treat teens even with parental consent.[102]

The parents of minors can be held liable for their children's health care expenses, and, although this rarely occurs when teens initiate requests for contraceptive or abortion services, fear of exposure to parents through billing may curb teenagers' willingness to seek needed care. Although data are not sex-specific, one study found that teenagers themselves wanted and could be expected to assume some financial responsibility for their contraceptive services, since "substantial numbers of adolescents do have some disposable income, either from allowances or from earnings." The study noted that a sliding fee scale would be equitable, but clinics must still be prepared to absorb the total costs of caring for about one out of five of those under 18 and to subsidize the remainder of their teen clients.[100] These findings affirm that current cuts in Medicaid funds for abortions are likely to affect teenagers particularly. Recent legislation, Public Law 95-626, contains measures designed to provide pregnancy prevention programs and maternity care.

One other legal aspect that affects teenagers is age of consent for sexual inter-course. This is determined to be age 16 in the majority of states, but a recent New Jersey Criminal Code modification lowered the age of consent to 13;[13] at the same time, intercourse between even younger children was legalized if there was less than 4 years' difference between their ages. Although the ruling to restore the age of consent to 16 has been introduced, promoters of the lowered age said it was done in the interests of keeping the law current with the sexual behavior of teen-agers (see later discussion on pregnancy).

Contemporary social factors

Government programs and legislation frequently have little effect on the health and welfare of teenagers in the face of overwhelming social influences. These social forces are frequently divorced from studies of adolescent health and, instead, personality types, motivational factors, family and individual value sys-tems are studied as providing causes and explanations for problems.

Social factors strongly affect the young.[133,96] Teenagers are particularly influ-enced by commercial pressures of advertising, televison, the movie and record industries, and clothing and cosmetic manufacturers, and by social expectations of "normal" adolescent turbulence. Adolescents are a powerful consumer market, and their fears of not being accepted are reflected in advertisements for smoking, cosmetics, products such as toothpaste, mouthwash, and deodorant, and clothes. (Joseph Califano, former secretary of the U.S. Department of Health, Education and Welfare, began a campaign in 1978 to get 10% of cigarette manufacturers' advertising budget spent on *dissuading* teenagers from smoking.) Rock stars and the media provide role models of behavior involving fast cars, sex, violence, and drugs. Much teenage irresponsibility, short of major vandalism, is put down to "getting it on" or "being cool," and the causative nature in social factors is not explored or stopped. Young women especially are constantly being pressured regarding the need to be sexy and appealing, and to get a boyfriend.

Poverty continues to be a major social factor affecting adolescent well-being. Despite government programs and laws for immunization, hundreds of thousands of children are not immunized. Four times more children and youth in low-income families reported that their health was fair or poor than did middle-income chil-dren; low-income children lose more school days and have more days of re-stricted activity than do others.[108]

Family disruption can be particularly difficult for adolescents. Increasingly, children are raised in families with only one parent, and while this is not in and of itself a negative force, social burdens such as poverty, unemployment, and general exhaustion in the single parent can make it so. One estimate states that almost half of all children born in 1977 will spend some part of their childhood with only one parent.[37] Although estimates of the early 1900s show about 29% of children had only one parent[10] (usually because of maternal mortality), social conditions that facilitated extended family living, household help, and early adolescent employ-ment helped to mitigate some of the disruption.

Today about 16% of children live with their mothers only,[37] and in 1976, 52% of families headed by women were in poverty.[105] Three times as many black children in families headed by women live in poverty as do black children of families where fathers are also present. For white children the figures are 42.7% and 7.1%, respectively.[104]

Perhaps the most significant social factor affecting adolescent well-being, however, is access to employment. As of April, 1979 (note this is during the school year), 814,000 males aged 16 to 19 and 756,000 females aged 16 to 19 were in the labor force. Of these, 16.8% of males were unemployed, as were 16.2% of females; 34.5% of blacks and "others" (sex unspecified) were unemployed in this age-group.[23] Although a job will not cure disease, it may provide support for medical care, access to health insurance and, in providing a sense of productivity and achievement, do much toward preventing pregnancy, alcoholism, drug abuse, boredom, which can be a factor in precipitating the former problems, and general ennui.

SPECIFIC HEALTH PROBLEMS
Acne

As noted earlier, one of the main reasons adolescents visit the physician is to obtain treatment for skin conditions; for many adolescents, skin problems are "the only" problem.

Acne, as adolescent seborrhea is known, is related to the hormonal changes of puberty and the development of secondary sex characteristics, although the nature of the relationship is unclear. Usually occurring from approximately ages 13 to 18, acne can cause extreme agony to adolescents, who are beginning to develop socially, because of its unappealing appearance and potential disfigurement. The National Center for Health Statistics reported that in 1975 and 1976 nearly 1 in every 10 adolescents of both sexes under 15 years of age visited the physician for infections and inflammations of the skin. The rates of office visits to physicians specifically for acne by older adolescents, those aged 15 to 24 years, were 77.6 per 1,000 for males and 114.3 per 1,000 for females.[108]

Adolescent diets, which typically have an excess of starches and sugars and a low amount of water, may exacerbate acne in some persons; the emotional stress experienced by most adolescents may similarly exacerbate it. Adolescents in general, and young women in particular because of the sex appeal connotations, are extremely susceptible to the marketing of acne-cure products, nearly all of which provide little to no relief beyond that which can be achieved by washing with water.

Pregnancy

Despite numerous attempts by studies and theories to do so, no cause of teenage pregnancy (beyond the obvious) has been defined.* Young teenage women who become pregnant come from diverse socioeconomic backgrounds, represent a range of personality types, and have had varied social experiences. One researcher has stated that pregnancy is the only difference between pregnant and nonpregnant teens.[38]

---

*References 2, 51, 53, 55, 58, 62, 82, 85.

In 1977, 441,455 first babies were born to young women 19 years and under. Of these, 10,833 were born to women under 15 years of age; although about 50% more than in 1966, this figure represents a continuation of the decrease after a 1975 peak of 11,976.[75] (See Chapter 1 for a 10-year perspective.)

The most obvious reason for the high number of teenage pregnancies lies in the number of teenagers having intercourse. Estimates (given the difficulty in obtaining reliable information) of sexually active teenagers indicate that by 1976, 41% of unmarried 17-year-old women reported that they had had sexual intercourse at least once. This was an increase of 52% from the 27% figure for the same age-group in 1971. For 15-year-old girls, the increase was from 14% in 1971 to 18% in 1976.[117] Frequency of intercourse varies, and Kovar reports that of the 15- to 17-year-olds who had had intercourse, 20% reported doing so only once; of those who reported having had intercourse three times or more in the previous 4 weeks, 46% had had more than one partner. Although proportionately more black adolescent females aged 15 have experienced intercourse than have white females (38% compared with 14%), the increase in sexual experience during 1971 to 1976 has been proportionately higher among whites.[60]

Although data are extremely scarce on sexual activity of young women under age 15, it is estimated that about 10% of 13-year-olds have experienced intercourse, and a study among mainly white middle-class teenagers in one midwestern city showed the rate of 14-year-old females who had experienced intercourse had increased from 10% in 1971 to 17% in 1973.[60,103,111]

Approximately 10% of females 15 to 19 years of age (the group principally studied) become pregnant each year, and about 6% give birth, for a total of 600,000 births. Of girls younger than 15, about 30,000 become pregnant annually, and nearly 13,000 give birth. Two thirds of the adolescent women are unmarried.[3] Some of the pregnancies, about 100,000, end in miscarriage. Many other teenagers seek abortion as the solution to their pregnancies, and this in part explains the decline in births (see Chapter 1) among women 19 years of age and younger at the same time that their sexual activity has increased. Data from 1976 suggest that over 50% of pregnancies among those under 14 are terminated by abortion, as are about one third among those aged 15 to 19 years. Overall, about one third of the abortions annually in the United States are obtained by teenage women.[25]

About 94% of all young women who give birth keep their babies at home, 3.5% give up their children for adoption, and 2.5% send the child to relatives or friends for care. When the teenagers are unmarried, 87% keep their babies, 8% select adoption, and 5% give their babies to friends or relatives. More than half of all out-of-wedlock births in the United States annually are to teenagers. Of young women who do marry, about 40% of those under 17 presumably do so because of pregnancy, since the date of birth indicates premarital conception. Among 18- and 19-year-olds, about 21% of births are premaritally conceived; this is to be compared with 5% of births among 20- to 24-year-olds.[116]

For most adolescent women, both pregnancy (66%) and births (50%) are unintended.[116] However, the majority of young women do not seek contraceptive services until they have an established sexual relationship.[26,93,97] This reluctance may stem from refusal to admit to oneself that sexual activity is planned, unwilling-

Table 6-6. Never-married women aged 15 to 19 who correctly perceived the time of greatest pregnancy risk within the menstrual cycle, by age, race, and sexual experience, 1976 and 1971*

Age	All races			White						Black					
	Total	Experienced	Not experienced	Total		Experienced		Not experienced		Total		Experienced		Not experienced	
	(%)	(%)	(%)	%	Number	%	Number	%	Number	%	Number	%	Number	%	Number
1976															
15 to 19 years	40.6	47.3	36.9	43.9	1194	53.2	365	39.8	829	23.5	646	24.0	405	22.8	241
15 years	29.5	33.5	28.6	30.5	272	40.5	37	28.9	235	22.7	132	17.6	51	25.9	81
16 years	33.5	42.8	30.3	39.8	289	50.8	65	36.6	224	18.0	133	17.4	69	18.8	64
17 years	47.0	51.7	43.7	48.0	271	51.0	98	46.2	173	26.6	139	28.4	95	22.7	44
18 years	49.2	52.7	46.3	52.6	215	57.0	93	49.2	122	22.3	139	23.1	104	20.0	35
19 years	48.6	46.7	51.1	56.5	147	59.7	72	53.3	75	29.1	103	29.1	86	29.4	17
1971															
15 to 19 years	37.6	41.6	36.1	40.2	2624	50.2	562	37.5	2062	16.0	1333	16.3	681	15.8	652
15 years	28.6	32.8	28.0	29.5	640	41.4	70	28.1	570	16.1	341	14.4	104	16.9	237
16 years	34.0	35.3	33.7	36.7	659	41.4	111	35.8	548	15.4	319	15.6	147	15.1	172
17 years	38.7	41.6	37.6	42.7	644	51.8	141	40.2	503	16.3	295	16.8	173	15.6	122
18 years	44.5	46.7	43.2	48.9	395	56.2	128	45.3	267	15.0	227	16.9	142	11.8	85
19 years	48.5	45.8	50.8	54.6	286	55.4	112	54.0	174	18.5	151	17.4	115	22.2	36

* Reproduced with permission of Zelnik, M., and Kantner, J. F.: Fam. Plann. Perspect. **9**:55-71, March/April, 1977.

ness to appear less spontaneous, and lack of access to services, as well as from ignorance. Many adolescent females do not know when they are fertile[114] (see Table 6-6). In addition, one study of available educational and informational materials found that "almost none deal with such subjects as the early symptoms of pregnancy, how to get a pregnancy test, the alternative of abortion, the possibility of miscarriage, and how to get a job, child care, and educational counseling, as well as medical care and economic help."[5] Although about 1 million adolescents receive birth control through organized programs and another 500,000 rely on a private physician, an estimated 2 million sexually active adolescents receive no services.[27,102]

Most adolescents presume contraception is the girl's responsibility, although this changes with age. Little is known of male motivation to use contraceptive measures (even among adults) but public acknowledgment of, research into, and programs to defeat the double standard and promote shared responsibility are very slowly developing.[9,36,89]

Projecting to 1984, Teitze[99] estimates on the basis of current rates that of the approximately 2 million girls who turned 14 in 1978, about 21% will have experienced at least one live birth by their twentieth birthday. By age 20, about 15% will have obtained one legal abortion and about 6% will have had at least one miscarriage or stillbirth.

It has been argued that contrary to popular descriptions, teenage pregnancies are endemic rather than epidemic,[50] and certainly a 10-year perspective (see Chapter 1) would suggest an ongoing occurrence. Whether pregnancies are epidemic or endemic, however, young women bear babies at high physical and social cost to themselves and their infants. Adolescent pregnancies are characterized by increased health risk to the mother and to the infant, and by costly social consequences of lost social, educational, vocational, and economic opportunities.[3,29,39,47]

Although some studies have found that teenagers with adequate prenatal care suffer fewer complications than do women over 40,[11] the reality is that many teenagers receive scant prenatal care.[75] The majority of studies report, therefore, that young women have increased maternal death risk (as much as 60% higher) and increased incidence of toxemia, anemia, labor difficulties, and cephalopelvic disproportion. Young women under 15 years of age are particularly at risk for these latter two conditions, since their physical development is insufficiently advanced to cope with pregnancy, labor, and delivery.

Adolescents give birth to babies who are much more likely to be of low birth weight. In 1977, 15% of babies born to mothers under age 15 weighed less than 2500 grams (5.5 pounds.)[75] (See Table 6-7). Low birth weight continues to be a major, if not the major, cause of infant mortality. About 6% of first babies born to women under age 15 die in their first year; babies of 15-year-olds face a risk of dying double that of babies of 20- to 24-year-old mothers.[3] Inadequate nutrition of teenagers is a contributing factor.

Young mothers face economic deprivation throughout their lives.[32] Most (8 out of 10 women who become mothers at age 17 or younger) do not complete their high school education,[69] thereby reducing employment opportunities. Welfare

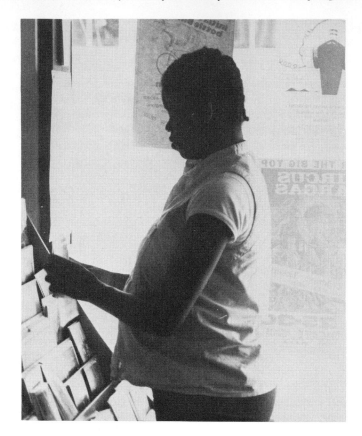

Fig. 6-5. Young motherhood.

Table 6-7. Percent of low–birth weight infants by age of mother and race: United States, 1977*†

All races‡		White		Black	
Mothers	Low birthweight infants (%)	Mothers	Low birthweight infants (%)	Mothers	Low birthweight infants (%)
All ages	7.1	All ages	5.9	All ages	12.8
Under 15 years	15.0	Under 15 years	11.3	Under 15 years	12.7
15 to 19 years	9.8	15 to 19 years	7.9	15 to 19 years	14.6
15 years	12.0	15 years	9.0	15 years	15.9
16 years	11.1	16 years	9.2	16 years	14.6
17 years	10.3	17 years	8.4	17 years	14.9
18 years	9.7	18 years	8.0	18 years	14.4
19 years	8.8	19 years	7.1	19 years	14.3

*Based on data from National Center for Health Statistics: Vital Statistics Report **27**, Feb. 5, 1979.
†Low birth weight is defined as less than 2500 g (5 pounds 8 ounces).
‡Includes races other than white and black.

dependency is likely, and at least 50% of out-of-wedlock children become welfare beneficiaries.[68,115] In one study it was found that the incidence of poverty among primiparous mothers between ages 13 and 15 was 2.6 times greater than among mothers aged 20 and over. Marital instability among teenagers is two to three times higher than among those aged 20 and over.[67]

The problems of poverty, divorce, lack of education, few employment opportunities, and immaturity may cause such psychological disruption that adolescent mothers become more at risk to commit child abuse. These conditions may be aggravated by failure to achieve expected adult status through pregnancy, and failure to obtain anticipated love and devotion from the infant. Although causal relationships between mother's age at birth and child abuse have been suggested, the social conditions outlined that characterize young motherhood are more likely to be causative.[57,79] The association between the two reemphasizes the need for school programs for adolescent mothers.[42,72,92] job training, financial support, education about and improved access to contraceptive services,[52,98] and prevention of pregnancy among adolescents.[15]

Frequently overlooked, too, is the role of the male and the need to involve the partners in contraceptive, parenting, vocational, and economic counseling. Recent court decisions that have awarded custody of babies born out-of-wedlock to their young fathers require additional societal efforts to ensure optimal opportunities for the children.

Most important in preventing adolescent pregnancy is the need to provide satisfying alternatives to adolescents. Jekel concludes:

As with older women, fertility reduction will occur only when there are meaningful, personally fulfilling alternatives to childbearing . . . teenagers may be the last group to hold fully to the national image that a woman is proved and fulfilled through childbearing and that the number of children sired is somehow a measure of manhood.[50]

Venereal disease

Increases in sexual activity have led to increased incidence of sexually transmitted diseases among adolescents. Although 1977 data suggested that the rate may have stabilized (see Tables 6-8 and 6-9) and to be slowly declining, it rose again in 1978. Venereal diseases are cited as being of epidemic proportions. From 1956 to 1976 the incidence of gonorrhea among girls aged 10 to 14 increased 148% and among 15- to 19-year-old females, 289%. Even among girls 9 years of age and younger gonorrhea incidence increased 141%. Since 1976, rates in all age-groups have not risen as rapidly, but this may simply reflect attainment of a maximum reporting rate, rather than a slowing of the actual rate.

Adolescent girls report higher rates of gonorrhea than do boys. For girls, the effects are particularly hazardous, since the disease may progress to pelvic inflammatory disease (PID), which when inadequately treated even once, is estimated to result in permanent sterility in from 15% to 40% of the patients.[60] PID is also associated with some forms of arthritis in females. Women and men may frequently not know they are infected because symptomless gonorrhea occurs in both. Known to occur in women, symptomless gonorrhea was only recently recognized to occur in about 60% of all males who actually have the disease.[45]

Table 6-8. Reported cases of gonorrhea, 1956 to 1978*

Year	Number			Rate per 100,000 population		
	Females	Males	Total	Females	Males	Total
10 to 14 years						
1956	1935	496	2431	28.7	7.1	17.7
1960	2068	1190	3258	24.8	13.8	19.2
1973	6203	2330	8533	60.6	21.9	40.9
1974	6515	2373	8888	64.2	22.5	42.9
1975	7443	2199	9642	74.4	21.1	47.2
1976	6919	2240	9159	71.2	22.2	46.2
1977	7162	2394	9556	76.1	24.5	49.8
1978	6996	2162	9158	76.8	22.8	49.3
15 to 19 years						
1956	20,938	24,223	45,161	372.0	462.9	415.7
1960	23,000	30,649	53,649	347.1	480.9	412.7
1973	124,773	108,221	232,994	1234.5	1075.2	1155.0
1974	138,331	111,788	250,119	1351.2	1094.8	1223.1
1975	151,109	115,504	266,613	1462.4	1121.5	1292.2
1976	150,740	110,760	261,500	1445.8	1061.5	1253.6
1977	147,887	104,586	252,473	1422.0	1003.2	1212.4
1978	153,227	101,701	254,928	1481.7	977.6	1228.9

*Based on data provided by Kathy Dry, Statistical Assistant, Venereal Disease Control Division, Center for Disease Control, Atlanta, May, 1979. The Center for Disease Control estimates that approximately 50% of the actual cases are reported.

Table 6-9. Reported cases of primary and secondary syphilis, 1956 to 1978*

Year	Number			Rates per 100,000 population		
	Females	Males	Total	Females	Males	Total
10 to 14 years						
1956	54	13	67	0.8	0.2	0.5
1960	105	30	135	1.3	0.4	0.8
1973	146	74	220	1.4	0.7	1.1
1974	170	71	241	1.7	0.7	1.2
1975	150	70	220	1.5	0.7	1.1
1976	120	64	184	1.2	0.6	0.9
1977	91	55	146	1.0	0.6	0.8
1978	90	54	144	1.0	0.6	0.8
15 to 19 years						
1956	636	527	1163	11.3	10.1	10.7
1960	1274	1303	2577	19.2	20.4	19.8
1973	1989	1880	3869	19.7	18.7	19.2
1974	1964	2029	3993	19.2	19.9	19.5
1975	1833	1886	3719	17.7	18.3	18.0
1976	1714	1890	3604	16.4	18.1	17.3
1977	1306	1566	2872	12.6	15.0	13.8
1978	1316	1716	3032	12.7	16.5	14.6

*Based on data provided by Kathy Dry, Statistical Assistant, Venereal Disease Control Division, Center for Disease Control, Atlanta, May, 1979. The Center for Disease Control estimates that approximately 50% of the actual cases are reported.

Primary and secondary syphilis rates have also shown a similar pattern of increasing, declining, and then more slowly increasing, at least for 15- to 19-year-old females (see Table 6-9). Easier to treat than gonorrhea, syphilis can also cause particular harm in women, causing neurological damage or death to their unborn babies.

Alcoholism and drug abuse

Since World War II, teenage drinking has steadily increased, although it appeared to level off in the 1970s, particularly among younger adolescents (see Table 6-10). Nonetheless, students have reported that alcohol is easy to obtain in schools,[77] and in one survey of the high school class of 1977, over 90% reported having tried alcohol at least once; 71% reported having used alcohol in the previous 30 days.[54] Adolescents typically began drinking in 1978 at age 12.6 years as compared with 13.4 years in 1966. Among twelfth graders, four out of five drink; of these, two out of every five boys and one out of every five girls reported a drinking problem. Joseph Califano, then Secretary of the Department of Health, Education and Welfare, noted that in 1975, 20% of all high school students report-

Table 6-10. Percentages of adolescents aged 12 to 17 who were current drinkers, United States, 1972 to 1977*†

Selected characteristics	Percent			
	1972	1974	1976	1977
TOTAL PERCENTAGE OF CURRENT DRINKERS	24	34	32.4	31.2
Age				
12 to 13 years	16	19	19	13
14 to 15 years	21	32	31	28
16 to 17 years	35	51	47	52
Sex				
Female	21	29	29	25
Male	27	39	36	37
Race				
White	24	37	34	33
Nonwhite	19	21	23	23
Region				
Northeast	28	44	42	35
North Central	28	33	38	35
South	15	21	21	24
West	28	46	32	36
Population density				
Large metropolitan area	24	44	38	36
Other metropolitan area	28	27	33	30
Nonmetropolitan area	20	28	26	27

*From Abelson, H. I., et al.: National Survey on Drug Abuse: 1977, Rockville, Md., 1977, National Institute on Drug Abuse.
†In 1977 "current drinker" was defined as one who had drunk in the past 7 days. From 1974 to 1977 "current drinker" was defined as one who had drunk in the past month.

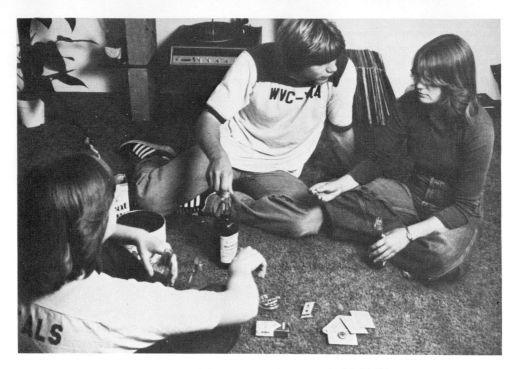

Fig. 6-6. Social pressures. (Courtesy Keith Hall.)

ed being intoxicated at least once a week.[24] Other data report that at least one out of four teenagers in grades 7 to 12 drink at least weekly, and 2.4% drink daily; 10% consume the equivalent of 5 to 12 drinks per session per week. The differential between teenage girls and boys who drink had narrowed from 17% in the mid-1960s to 7% by the mid-1970s.[107]

Adolescent drinking is slightly higher in the West and rates are lower in the South. One California study in Orange County (south of Los Angeles) showed that of children aged 7 to 11 who were polled, 6% were already showing signs of alcoholism.[4] A 1975 study among New York State high school students under 16 years showed that of the more than 26,000 respondents, over one third reported being drunk more than three times in the past year: about 6% reported blackouts. Rates among males and females did not differ significantly.[33]

Among black adolescents, one study showed that for girls, drinking significantly correlated with early pregnancy, whereas among boys, drinking correlated with smoking. Samples were small but suggest that alcohol was used to cope with stress.[21] In the Orange County survey, age and grade were found to be the highest predictors of drinking status; other predictors were the cultural variables of drug use and peer group use of alcohol.[4] Nearly all studies have found correlations between the incidence (frequency and quantity) of parents' drinking and that of their children.[107]

Table 6-11. Percentages of adolescents aged 12 to 17 who used marijuana and/or hashish in the past month, United States, 1971 to 1977*

Selected characteristics	Used in past month					Significance of 1976 to 1977 change‡
	1971†	1972†	1974	1976	1977	
TOTAL YOUTH AGED 12 TO 17	6	7	11.6	12.4	16.1	S
Age						
12 to 13 years	2	1	2	2	4	NS
14 to 15 years	7	6	12	13	15	NS
16 to 17 years	10	16	20	22	29	NS
Sex						
Female	5	6	11	10	13	NS
Male	7	9	12	14	19	NS
Race						
White	§	8	12	12	17	S
Nonwhite	§	2	9	10	12	NS
Region						
Northeast	9	7	14	14	21	NS
North Central	5	7	11	15	19	NS
South	2	4	6	7	7	NS
West	11	14	19	17	22	NS
Population density						
Large metropolitan area	9	§	14	18	22	NS
Other metropolitan area	7	§	11	10	16	NS
Nonmetropolitan area	3	§	10	9	10	NS

*From Abelson, H. I., et al.: National survey on drug abuse: 1977, Rockville, Md., 1977, National Institute on Drug Abuse.
†Marijuana only
‡S = Significant at 0.05 level; *NS* = not significant.
§Data not available.

Data on drug use are also complicated by the difficulty in obtaining honest responses. Although adolescent females' drug use is slightly lower than that of adolescent males, it is still substantial and appears to be increasing. Highest drug use is in the West, but it is only slightly greater than in the Northeast and North Central regions. Large metropolitan areas report the highest percentage of drug users, although one study has shown that the incidence of heroin addiction shifted in the 1970s from larger to smaller cities (see Tables 6-11 and 6-13).[46]

A study of high school graduating classes of 1977 reported that 56% of students (about 6.9 million) had tried marijuana, and this represented a 19% increase since 1975. Most of the increase had occurred among metropolitan whites. Many adolescents, however, may begin marijuana use between ages 15 and 17 and discontinue use with maturity and employment. About 1.4 million adolescents reported currently using marijuana, although the data are questionable because users of illegal drugs are more apt to drop out of school and, therefore, not be sampled. Use of hard drugs such as hallucinogens, inhalants, opiates, and cocaine did not appear to have increased substantially from 1975 to 1977; about 36% reported having tried these drugs. Specifically, about 990,000 adolescents said they had tried cocaine and 200,000 reported using it currently.[1,54,60,65]

Among black adolescents, drug use has been recently examined. Although young black male and female adolescents use legal drugs nearly equivalently, illegal drug use was found to be higher in males. Adolescent females experimented with marijuana more frequently than did males but were less likely to continue its use. On the other hand, young black women used heroin with greater frequency than did males; this was the only drug use, including alcohol, that followed this pattern.[19]

Smoking

The number of teenage smokers increased by 50% between 1958 and 1977; the rate of teenage girls who smoked doubled during this time period. From a longitudinal perspective, the Center for Disease Control estimated that among all adolescents aged 13 to 19, 2.2 million smoked (14%) in 1955, 3.5 million (14%) in 1965, and 6.0 million (20%) in 1975.[76] In addition, in the late 1970s about 100,000 children under age 13 were smokers. Encouragingly, overall adolescent smoking may be declining, since the numbers of adolescent cigarette smokers had declined by 1977 from their peak in 1974 (see Table 6-12).[24,56,60]

Table 6-12. Percentage of adolescents aged 12 to 17 who were current smokers, United States, 1971 to 1977*†

Selected characteristics	Percent				
	1971	1972	1974	1976	1977
TOTAL PERCENTAGE	15	17	25	23.4	22.3
Age					
12 to 13 years	5	4	13	11	10
14 to 15 years	17	16	25	20	22
16 to 17 years	23	32	38	39	35
Sex					
Female	14	17	24	26	22
Male	16	17	27	21	23
Race					
White	‡	‡	25	22	23
Nonwhite	‡	‡	26	28	18
Region					
Northeast	18	16	27	22	24
North Central	14	19	27	24	26
South	9	17	22	25	20
West	22	16	27	21	19
Population density area					
Large metropolitan area	16	16	27	25	25
Other metropolitan area	15	19	22	22	23
Nonmetropolitan area	14	16	27	24	19

*From Abelson, H. I., et al.: National survey on drug abuse: 1977, Rockville, Md., 1977, National Institute on Drug Abuse.
†In 1977, 1974 and 1976, "current smoker" was defined as one who had smoked within the past month. In 1971 and 1972 "current smoker" was defined as one who smokes at the present time.
‡Not tabulated.

Smoking among young women is particularly troublesome because of its links with low–birth weight infants.[30] In 1968 about 9% of girls aged 12 to 18 years, as opposed to 17% of boys of the same age, were regular smokers (smoked at least once a week). By 1972 girls smoked 85% as much as boys; by 1974 the difference in smoking rates had narrowed to 15.3% of adolescent girls and 15.8% of adolescent boys.[94]

Family smoking patterns strongly influence adolescent smoking. Adolescents with two parents who smoke are twice as likely to smoke as those with nonsmoking parents; this rises to four times as likely to smoke when a teenager has both a parent and an older sibling who smoke. Although about 60% of teenage girls reported they have tried to quit smoking, smoking appears to be part of a wider behavior pattern. The Gallup Index notes that about 25% of adolescent females who smoke report marijuana use as well, compared with 3% of nonsmokers; about one third of smokers report drinking to get drunk in contrast to 4% of nonsmokers. One third of teenage smokers state that they hate school as compared with 16% of nonsmokers, and the smoker is more apt to be a C or D student in contrast to the nonsmoker student, who is more likely to get high grades. About 31% of smokers report having had sexual relations in contrast to 8% of nonsmokers.[94]

In 1926 the National Congress of Parents and Teachers (PTA) adopted a resolution urging action to eliminate smoking by minors,[86] yet today, many schools have smoking lounges. The tobacco industry, which spends one-half million dollars annually on advertising, and strong peer pressure to smoke encourage about 4000 teenagers daily to become regular cigarette smokers.[24] Both the Gallup Index and surveys sponsored by the U.S. Department of Health, Education

Table 6-13. Use of specified substances by adolescents aged 12 to 17, United States, 1977*

Substance	Percent who had ever used				Percent who had never used
	Total	Past month	Past year, not past month	Not past year	
Legal substances					
Alcohol	52.6	31.2	16.3	5.0	46.5
Cigarettes	47.3	22.3	†	†	48.6
Illicit drugs					
Marijuana or hashish or both	28.2	16.1	5.7	6.4	71.8
Inhalants	9.0	0.7	1.5	6.9	91.0
Hallucinogens	4.6	1.6	1.5	1.5	95.4
Cocaine	4.0	0.8	1.8	1.4	96.0
Heroin	1.1	0.0	0.6	0.7	98.9
Other opiates	6.1‡	0.6	2.8	2.3	92.8‡
Prescription drugs, nonmedical use					
Stimulants	5.2	1.3	2.4	1.1	94.8
Sedatives	3.1	0.8	1.2	1.1	96.9
Tranquilizers	3.8	0.7	2.2	0.6	96.2

*From Kovar, M. G.: Public Health Rep. **94:**109-118, March/April, 1979.
†Not available.
‡Includes Methadone.

and Welfare have found that most adolescents believe that alcohol and drugs, legal and illegal, are harmful.[78] Societal forces (including parents' substance use) are such that, as Table 6-13 demonstrates, teenagers believe the rewards outweigh the risks.

Prostitution

Teenage prostitution is possibly an endemic problem; recent attention suggests it may be epidemic. Few data exist on the numbers of teenage prostitutes, but arrests listed in the Uniform Crime Reports suggest that teenage prostitution, both male and female, is on the rise. In 1977 there were 3315 arrests of adolescents under 18 years of age for prostitution. At the same time, there were 185,447 runaways under 18 arrested.[28] Since prostitution is the primary source of support for runaways and it is estimated that there were as many as one million runaways in 1977, prostitution probably far exceeds the arrest rate.

In Seattle, Washington, and Minneapolis, Minnesota, studies of teenage prostitutes are in progress.[49]* Preliminary data from the Seattle study show that teenage prostitutes are either runaways or relatively economically comfortable young women seeking pin money for records, shows, and clothes. All the young women in the study have passed through Juvenile Court, where they were interviewed and determined to be prostitutes on the basis of their own statements as to whether they have had one or more sexual experiences for money. Nonprostitutes serve as controls. About 60% of the prostitute sample have actually been arrested for O & A (offering and agreeing to an act of prostitution). The study samples (106 prostitutes, 93 controls) show no significant differences in general characteristics on the basis of preliminary data. In the study, 54.8% came from average income families, but only 24.6% had parents who lived together. Many (72.9%) had been placed outside their family home, some in several other homes; the most frequently cited reason for leaving the original home was physical abuse. The majority (55.8%) did not attend school, and 79.4% had a history of school suspensions, usually for nonattendance.

The Seattle study found that in the prostitute sample, 30.2% were enrolled in school and 10.4% were working at the time of first prostitution; for most (51.9%) the first act occurred in a motel/hotel room, and for 24.5% sex took place on the street. Most (53.7%) of the prostitutes worked 4 to 7 days per week, and 53.8% reported having a pimp at some time during their street experience.

Significant differences between the nonprostitute and prostitute groups were that prostitutes were more likely to claim that they enjoyed sex; had sexual relations at an earlier age (average age, 14.6 years); reported that sexual activity was a factor in their relationships with their parents; had friends of both sexes serving time; used contraception (although 41.5% of the prostitutes and 66.7% of the controls used none, and the difference was largely due to condom use required by the prostitutes); had sexual problems; and were involved in arrests for carrying con-

---

*One by Enablers, 100 W. Franklin, Minneapolis, Minn. 55404, the other at the University of Washington, Seattle.

cealed weapons, curfew violations, and for using false identification, whereas the control groups were more likely to be involved in auto theft and trespassing. Prostitutes also stated willingness to use hard drugs. In Seattle, adolescent white girls generally work at prostitution during the day, whereas adolescent black girls work at night.

Money and material goods were reported by 71.7% of the prostitutes as being the best feature of their work; abuse from customers (35.8%) and police harrassment (18.9%) were the two most frequently reported negative aspects. The study has found that parents of prostitutes may also get involved through being conned into paying for "street protection" for their daughters. Further study and data are needed for compilation of final statistics.[63]

Suicide

For 1976, National Institute of Mental Health Statistics report that 1560 adolescents 15 to 19 years old committed suicide. Experts estimate, however, that a more accurate count is about 5000 annually, since adolescent suicides are frequently mistaken for accidents or are disguised as such by families. Since the 1950s, adolescent suicides have increased by 200% with a 40% increase from 1970 to 1975.[24,65]

While adolescent boys most often resort to hanging or shooting themselves, adolescent girls most frequently take overdoses of pills or jump from heights.[24] Many more females attempt suicide than do males, however, and between 200,000 and 400,000 suicide attempts are made by adolescents annually. In 1977 suicide was the eighth leading cause of death among white females aged 10 to 14 and the seventh among black females in the same age-group. Among 15- to 19-year-old white and black females, it was the fourth leading cause of death (see Table 6-1). A recent study confirmed the suspected under reporting of suicide statistics and noted from New York City records that white suicides are probably underestimated by 40% and black suicides by 80%. For black females aged 18 to 24, suicide is believed to be underestimated by 96%.[113]

Suicides occur among all socioeconomic groups, and, except in rare cases, depression seems to be the one single characteristic in common. Feelings of no self-worth, fear of failure at school and job, and feelings of apathy and hopelessness have been expressed by those who attempt suicide. Frequently adolescents who commit suicide are those who appear to have "everything." Waldron and Eyer[112] in reviewing increased mortality from suicide note correlations between increased divorce, decreased adolescent marriage, increased adolescent pregnancy, increased unemployment, and increased alcohol and drug use. Causal relationships are suggested but not proved.

Factors specific to suicide among adolescent girls are unclear. Pregnancy or belief that they were pregnant was found to be a relatively common factor in one study,[48] whereas another found a pattern of family histories that were "chaotic, excessively mobile."[91] Some of the girls reported rejection by boyfriends, but suicidal reactions have been noted as usually being a repetition of similar reactions to perceived familial rejections.[90] Failure to conform to socialization expectations by obtaining good grades and being popular, appealing to boys, and pretty have also been suggested.[101] Whatever the causes, adolescent females are estimated to have the highest per capita rate of known suicide attempts with the lowest lethality rate; estimates range from 8 to 50 attempts per actual suicide.[91]

Anorexia nervosa

Anorexia nervosa is willfull self-starvation, sometimes to the point of death. It is a condition that nine times out of ten strikes teenage girls; frequently the girls are from middle-class homes and seem to have "everything." Incidence rates of anorexia nervosa are unknown but are believed to be rapidly increasing; one study of middle-class England cites an incidence of 1 per 200 girls.[17] About 5% to 15% of anorexics in psychiatric treatment have died.

Anorexia nervosa was described historically (seventeenth century)[14] and was believed to be endocrinological; contemporary thinking classifies it as psychological. Adolescent girls are believed to be more prone to anorexia nervosa in part because of the dramatic body changes experienced at puberty. Palazzoli notes that "the anorexic is trying to grow up, to get free from the family, but paradoxically she does it by fighting the threatening image of the swollen, invaded adult body—and so ends up clinging to childhood."[80]

Anorexic girls are almost always amenorrheic, perhaps as a response to the lack of nutrition; some girls, however, have been reported to have become amenorrheic prior to the onset of anorexia nervosa. Most think that they are exceedingly beautiful and are obsessed with the appearance of any fat on their bodies. Anorexics delight in dieting but also think constantly of food. They may go on eating binges but train themselves to vomit at will. Many consume laxatives compulsively. Most have high energy levels and are in generally good health until starvation finally takes over.[14] Most therapists agree that family involvement is essential in treating anorexics, who generally were "ideal, good kids" prior to the onset of their disease. Although length of hospitalization and therapy methods vary, there is agreement that the demands for love, caring, and attention and the unwillingness to mature that characterize these young girls may require extensive behavior modification by both the adolescent and her family.[16]

Accidents, injuries, and homicides

As noted in Table 6-1, accidents of all types are the leading cause of death for adolescents of all ages. Under this classification motor vehicle accidents comprise the largest portion. During the 1960s the rates of motor vehicle accidents increased by over 25%, and by 1976, 36% of all adolescents aged 12 to 17 who died, did so as the result of car accidents. Other accidental deaths were by drowning (6%), suicide (5%), and homicide (6.5%).[60] In 1977, the under-25 age-group accounted for 48% of all car fatalities; of these, 73% were male and 27% were female.[109]

Teenage drinking is clearly involved in car accidents. In Massachusetts, traffic fatalities involving "drunken" teenagers nearly tripled after the drinking age was lowered to 18 in 1973;[12] similar statistics in other states are prompting a trend to raise the drinking age to 21 years. Regardless of their own behavior, young women, because of the social custom of boys driving girls, are placed at particular risk of being passengers in cars where the driver is drunk or is perhaps "showing off." Death is not the only tragic outcome of car accidents; in 1976, for every adolescent killed in a car accident, 43 others were injured, many permanently.[24]

Recent studies also show the number of accidents that occur in school-related settings. In a 1-year survey of high schools and college sports programs, over 1 million injuries and 14 deaths were reported. Most of these injuries (326,000) occurred from playing football. Women suffered 235,000 injuries, for a rate of 54 per 1000. This contrasts with 825,000 injuries of men, for a rate of 72 per 1000.[73]

A 2-year study of girls' high school athletic programs found that three times as many injuries occurred during practices than in competitive events. Although over one third of the injuries required a physician's services, 59% of the injured had returned to full athletic activity within a week. Most of the injuries were sprains and strains.[34]

A study of one school district (Bellevue in Washington State) used past experience to project annual injuries for the entire state. In 1 year, in students from kindergarten through twelfth grade, 36,400 accidents are projected. Of these, 13,916, or 38.2%, will occur to girls; of the total, 17,429 (47%) will require a physician, hospitalization, or a dentist.[7]

One reason for the rate of injuries may be teenagers' lack of physical fitness. Sedentary life-styles, cars, and poor nutrition have contributed to the fact that one out of every six youngsters aged 10 to 17 is "weak or uncoordinated enough to be classed as physically underdeveloped by the standards of the President's Council on Physical Fitness and Sports."[24] Califano further noted in 1978 that "each year schools discover countless apparently healthy teenage girls who cannot run a city block without stopping to rest."[24]

Injuries in school may also occur from discipline. In 1976 at least 1.5 million corporal punishment incidents occurred. This number probably is much too low because the nonresponse rate to the data collection system of the Office for Civil Rights was extremely high; data from New York City, Chicago, and Philadelphia were not reported.[110] In addition, at least two nation-wide organizations, End Violence Against the Next Generation, Inc. (EVAN-G)* and the National Committee to Abolish Corporal Punishment in Schools (NCAPCS),† monitor school corporal discipline and note as further evidence of physical injury to children the numbers of lawsuits and school board deliberations on excessive and abusive beatings, both for discipline and from teachers' lack of emotional control. There are no national sex-specific data on corporal discipline, but studies indicate that most abusive discipline occurs to little boys and teenage girls as a result of both social and sexual factors.[6,66] (In 1976 the disciplinary actions of suspension and expulsion in elementary and secondary schools occurred to 671,195 boys and 293,728 girls. The total was at least 1,628,929, which includes actions in which the sex is not stated.)

Although child abuse in schools is seldom reported,[35] national attention is

---

*977 Keeler Ave., Berkeley, Calif. 94708.
†549 Parkhurst, Dallas, Texas 75218.

beginning to focus on child abuse, both physical and emotional, in the home and community.[40,44,66,71] Sexual abuse in the home most frequently is against adolescent girls; the mother sometimes knows, but for complex reasons takes no action. Defining the consequences of such abuse for the physical and psychological health of adolescent girls is beyond the scope of the chapter, but it is significant that among the teenagers studied in regard to prostitution, in Seattle, both prostitutes and nonprostitutes, 37.4% had been sexually molested as children and 32.6% were either physically or emotionally forced into their first sexual experience. Of the prostitutes, 11.3% had had their first intercourse with an incestual partner in comparison with 3.3% of the nonprostitutes.[63]

Violent deaths (homicides) among adolescents most frequently occur, and are rising, among black males. Homicides among adolescent females are also increasing (see Table 6-1) and are among the leading causes of death. Studies have shown that the rise in homicide is related to alcohol consumption, impulsive rage, unemployment, and a general disregard for societal institutions.[112] Nationally, about 10% of homicides involve romantic triangles and lovers' quarrels, and this type of homicide increased by 25% during the 1960s.[112] About 9% of all homicide victims nationally are adolescents aged 15 to 19, and this age-group accounts for 19% of the homicide arrests.[96]

SELECTED INTERNATIONAL PERSPECTIVES
Pregnancy

Adolescent pregnancy is a worldwide phenomenon. Sometimes the result of cultural factors that promote early marriage and childbearing while women are still in their teens, adolescent pregnancy may also, as in the United States, be a response to a perceived lack of alternatives.[84]

Data from some developing nations show the percentages of live births to women aged 15 to 19 during the 1970s. These range from 3.5% in Egypt to 17.7% in Jamaica. In contrast, 1% of births in Japan were to adolescents, as were 9% in West Germany. In the United States, 17% of live births were to adolescents.[169] Further data are given in Table 6-14. Regardless of the country, teenage mothers and infants face the same risks as do those in the United States. Frequently, however, these risks are exacerbated by extreme poverty, poor sanitation, and absence of prenatal care. For example, data published in 1975 show that in Chaco Province in the Argentine, 133.5 babies per 1000 live births died; in El Salvador, 116.6 babies per 1000 live births died. These data are to be contrasted with infant mortality rates during that period of about 15.0 per 1000 in the United States.[75]

Adolescent mortality

Although data are not sex specific, accidents and suicide continue to be the leading causes of adolescent mortality in several nations besides the United States. The particularly high number of adolescent suicides in Japan is believed to be related to the extraordinary competitive pressures to gain admission to academic institutions at all levels (see Table 6-15).

Accidents and suicide are also among the leading causes of adolescent death

Table 6-14. Number of births per 1000 females aged 15 to 19, selected countries, 1970s*

Country	Rate	Country	Rate
Japan	5	Greece	39
USSR	16	Israel	41
Netherlands, Spain	17	Italy	43
Switzerland	19	United Kingdom, Norway	44
Ireland	20	Czechoslovakia	46
Denmark	28	Australia	54
France	29	Hungary	57
Belgium	30	United States	58
West Germany, Sweden	31	Romania	61
Portugal	33	New Zealand	63
Canada	36	East Germany, Bulgaria	72

*Based on data from Alan Guttmacher Institute: 11 Million teenagers, New York, 1976, Planned Parenthood Federation of America, Inc.

Table 6-15. Leading causes of adolescent mortality by frequency, selected nations, 1973*†

Country	Motor vehicle accidents	Other accidents	Suicide	Malignant neoplasm
Japan	3369	1608	1850	‡
Canada	1917	866	421	‡
England, Wales, Scotland, and Northern Ireland	1380	484	200	330

*Based on data provided by Otero, M., United Nations Statistical Office, May, 1979.
†Rates unavailable.
‡Not among top 4 causes.

in New Zealand. Although not sex specific, rates for females are stated to be lower in all categories than those for males.[31] Similar social pressures obtain in New Zealand as in the United States, and the relatively high alcohol consumption rate among adolescent New Zealanders undoubtedly contributes to the extremely high rate of traffic fatalities. Deaths from motor vehicle accidents are almost double among Maoris (10.0 per 10,000) than Pakehas (whites, 5.2 per 10,000). Over the last four decades adolescent suicide among Pakehas has changed relatively little from a 1930s rate of 0.7 to a 1972 rate of 0.8 per 10,000. For Maoris, the rate has dropped from 2.5 per 10,000 in the 1930s to 0.2 in 1972.[31] Increased employment opportunities and efforts to reestablish Maori culture and family life may be contributory. Homicide is not a leading cause of death in any age or ethnic group in New Zealand. The most dramatic shift in all mortality rates has occurred among Maoris whose 1940s rate for adolescent death from tuberculosis was 64.1 (Pakehas 3.0). By the 1950s the Maori rate was 12.0 per 10,000 (Pakehas 0.6), and by 1972 both races had no mortality in the age-group from this disease.

•　　•　　•

Adolescent morbidity and mortality as discussed in this chapter demonstrate the importance of establishing life-styles and behavior patterns that will promote adolescent well-being. The complex nature of adolescence in United States society, where adolescents are neither children nor adults with adult responsibilities yet have many adult "rights," including the "right" to death and disease from traditionally adult causes, demands an urgent evaluation of the social values and roles that create this conflict. The high mortality and morbidity rates from accidents, homicides, suicides, heart disease, and stroke need to be substantially reduced by both individual behavioral changes and by the public demanding a reduction in social pressures (e.g., advertising, images projected by television) that promote harmful health habits and attitudes.

Without acknowledgment and control of the forces in our society that contribute to adolescent health problems, government and medical efforts will be largely wasted and the inevitable outcomes specifically discussed in this chapter—pregnancy, early sexual experiences, VD, alcoholism and drug abuse, smoking, prostitution, anorexia nervosa, and accidents—will continue to impede the growth of our young people.

SUGGESTED TOPICS FOR DISCUSSION, FURTHER RESEARCH, AND FIELD PROJECTS

1. What are the issues in the provision/nonprovision of birth control and sterilization for mentally retarded adolescent females? What are the relevant laws in your state? (Suggested initial reference: Hamilton, J.: The retarded adolescent: a parent's view, Fam. Plann. Perspect. 8:257, Nov./Dec., 1976.)

2. Research the girls' athletics programs in your local school district. What programs are available? What percentage of girls participate? How many injuries and physical disciplinary actions have occurred within your local school district? What is the distribution of these among males and females?

3. Select a government program that benefits adolescents. How does an adolescent qualify for the program? What are its benefits? Does the program contribute to maintaining the condition it attempts to alleviate? What factors contribute to the success/lack of success of the program? What, if any, services are provided by the private sector?

4. Research your local state laws regarding the provision of health services to adolescents without parental consent. What are the specific laws regarding provision of contraceptive, abortion, sterilization, and VD services?

5. Develop a school nutrition program for adolescents. What should a school policy be on "junk foods" sales in schools? What health education tools could you use to educate adolescents about nutrition? What are the political factors that influence national, state, and local policies regarding school nutrition?

6. What social factors most affect teenage women's health status? Do these factors similarly affect adolescent males? How could the negative effects of these factors be counteracted in a health education program for adolescent women?

7. Select a cause of hospitalization of adolescents. How does incidence of this condition differ by sex and race? Is this a condition also found in adults? If not, why not? Do aspects of adolescent life-style cause this condition?

8. What elements should be included in a comprehensive care program for pregnant teenagers? Research the available services for pregnant teens within your school district. What services are available in the community? Research the rates of teenage pregnancy in your area. What is the outcome for mother and child of most of these pregnancies?

9. Are there any differences between the reasons for and the characteristics of suicide incidence among adolescents and adults? What services are available in your area to address the problem of adolescent suicides?
10. What are the effects of employment status on adolescent health?

REFERENCES

1. Abelson, H. I., et al.: National survey on drug abuse: 1977. Main findings, vol. 1, No. (ADM) 78-618, Rockville, Md., 1977, National Institute on Drug Abuse.
2. Abernethy, V.: Illegitimate conception among teen-agers, Am. J. Public Health **64:** 662-665, July, 1974.
3. Alan Guttmacher Institute: 11 Million teenagers, New York, 1976, Planned Parenthood Federation of America, Inc.
4. Alibrandi, T.: Young alcoholics, Minneapolis, 1978, CompCare Publications.
5. Ambrose, L.: Misinforming pregnant teenagers, Fam. Plann. Perspect. **10:**51-57, Jan/Feb., 1978.
6. Amiel, S.: Child abuse in schools, Northwest Medicine **71:**808, Nov., 1972.
7. Amiel, S.: Report to Washington State Board of Health, Seattle, Washington, Feb. 14, 1979.
8. Ariès, P.: Centuries of childhood. A social history of family life, translated by Baldick, R., New York, 1962, Vintage Books.
9. Arnold, C. B.: The sexual behavior of inner city adolescent condom users, J. Sex Research **8:**298-309, 1972.
10. Bane, M. J.: Here to stay, American families in the twentieth century, New York, 1976, Basic Books, Inc., Publishers.
11. Battaglia, F. C., et al.: Obstetric and pediatric complications of juvenile pregnancy, Pediatrics **32:**902-910, Nov., 1963.
12. Beck, M., and Malamud, P.: A new prohibition for teenagers, Newsweek, p. 38, April 2, 1979.
13. Beck, M., et al.: A law that makes sex legal at 13, Newsweek, p. 36, May 7, 1979.
14. Blum, S.: Children who starve themselves, The New York Times Magazine, Nov. 10, 1974.
15. Brann, E. A., et al.: Strategies for the prevention of pregnancy in adolescents, Atlanta, 1978, Center for Disease Control.
16. Bruch, H.: Perils of behavior modification in treatment of anorexia nervosa, J.A.M.A. **230:**1419-1422, 1974.
17. Bruch, H.: The golden cage: the enigma of anorexia nervosa, Cambridge, Mass., 1978, Harvard University Press.
18. Brunswick, A. F.: Indicators of health status in adolescence, Int. J. Health Serv. **6:** 475-492, 1976.
19. Brunswick, A. F.: Black youth and drug use behavior. In Beschner, G. M., and Friedman, A. S., editors: Youth drug abuse: problems, issues and treatment, Lexington, Mass., 1979, D. C. Heath & Co., Lexington Books.
20. Brunswick, A. F., and Josephson, E.: Adolescent health in Harlem. II, Am. J. Public Health 62(suppl.):1-62, Oct., 1972.
21. Brunswick, A. F., and Tarica, C.: Drinking and health: a study of urban black adolescents, Addict. Dis: An International Journal **1:**21-42, 1974.
22. Bureau of the Census: Projections of the population of the United States: 1977-2050, Current Population Reports, Series P-25, no. 704, July, 1977.
23. Bureau of Labor Statistics: Personal communication, May, 1979.
24. Califano, J.: Keynote address presented at the Conference on Adolescent Behavior and Health, Division of Health Science Policy, National Academy of Sciences, Washington, D.C., June 26-27, 1978, No. (IOM) 78-004.
25. Center for Disease Control: Abortion surveillance 1976, Atlanta, Aug., 1978, Family Planning Evaluation Division, Center for Disease Control.
26. Cutright, P.: The teenage sexual revolution and the myth of an abstinent past, Fam. Plann. Perspect. **4:**24-31, Jan./Feb., 1972.
27. Dryfoos, J. G., and Heisler, T.: Contraceptive services for adolescents: an overview, Fam. Plann. Perspect. **10:**223-233, July/Aug., 1978.
28. Federal Bureau of Investigation: Crime in the United States, 1977, Uniform Crime Reports, Washington, D.C., 1978, U.S. Government Printing Office.
29. Fielding, J. E.: Adolescent pregnancy revisited, New Engl. J. Med. **299:**893-895, 1978.
30. Fielding, J. E., and Yankauer, A.: The pregnant smoker, Am. J. Public Health **68:**835-836, Sept., 1978.
31. Foster, F. H., editor: Trends: health and health services, Wellington, New Zealand,

1975, National Health Statistics Centre, Department of Health.

32. Freedman, D. S., and Thornton, A.: The long-term impact of pregnancy at marriage on the family's economic circumstances, Fam. Plann. Perspect. **11:**6-21, Jan./Feb., 1979.

33. Freudenberg, N.: Social and economic threats to adolescent health, presented at the American Public Health Association Meeting, Oct. 18, 1978, Los Angeles.

34. Garrick, J. G., and Requa, R. K.: Girls: sports injuries in high school athletics, J.A.M.A. **239:**2245-2247, 1978.

35. Gil, D. G.: Violence against children, Cambridge, Mass., 1970, Harvard University Press.

36. Gilbert, R., and Matthews, V. G.: Young males' attitudes toward condom use. In Redford, M. A., editor: The condom: increasing utilization in the United States, San Francisco, 1974, San Francisco Press.

37. Glick, P. C., and Norton, A. J.: Marrying, divorcing, and living together in the United States today, Population Bulletin **32:**3-39, 1977.

38. Gordon, S.: Family planning education for adolescents. In Park, R., and Westoff, C., editors: Aspects of growth policy, Commission on Population Growth and the American Future Research Reports, Vol. 6, Washington, D.C., 1972, U.S. Government Printing Office.

39. Green, C. P., and Potteiger, K.: Teenage pregnancy: a major problem for minors, Washington, D.C., Aug. 1977, Zero Population Growth.

40. Greene, N. B.: A view of family pathology involving child molest—from a juvenile probation perspective, Juvenile Justice, p. 28, Feb., 1977.

41. Grotberg, E. H.: Child development. In E. H. Grotberg, editor: 200 Years of children, U.S. Office of Child Development, No. (OHD) 77-30103, Washington, D.C., 1977, U.S. Government Printing Office.

42. Hansen, H., et al.: School achievement: risk factor in teenage pregnancies? Am. J. Public Health **68:**753-759, Aug., 1978.

43. Health Law Center: Hospital law manual, consent to medical or surgical procedures. I. Germantown, Md., May, 1978, Aspen Systems Corp.

44. Hett, E. J., and Fish, J. E.: Some descriptive characteristics of abusive families evaluated at Kansas University Medical Center, J. Clin. Child Psychol. **8:**7-9, Spring, 1979.

45. Holmes, K. K.: Personal communication, April, 1978.

46. Hunt, L.: Recent spread of heroin use in the United States, Am. J. Public Health **64:** (suppl.) 16-23, Dec., 1974.

47. Hunt, W. B.: Adolescent fertility: risks and consequences, Popul. Rep. [J.] **10:**157-175, July, 1976.

48. Jacobs, J.: Adolescent suicide, New York, 1971, Wiley Interscience.

49. James, J., principal investigator: Study on entrance into juvenile prostitution, University of Washington, Seattle, 1977-1980.

50. Jekel, J. F., and Klerman, L. V.: Teenage fertility: an epidemic or endemic problem? presented at the American Public Health Association Annual Meeting, Oct. 19, 1978, Los Angeles.

51. Jekel, J. F., et al.: Factors associated with rapid subsequent pregnancies among school-age mothers, Am. J. Public Health **63:**769-773, Sept., 1973.

52. Jekel, J. F., et al.: Induced abortion and sterilization among women who become mothers as adolescents, Am. J. Public Health **67:**621-625, July, 1977.

53. Johnson, C. L.: Adolescent pregnancy: intervention into the poverty cycle, Adolescence **9:**391-402, 1974.

54. Johnston, L. D., et al.: Drug use among American high school students: 1975-1977, No. (ADM) 78-619, Rockville, Md., 1977, National Institution on Drug Abuse.

55. Juhasz, A. M.: The unmarried adolescent parent, Adolescence **9:**263-272, 1974.

56. Kelson, S., et al.: The growing epidemic. A survey of smoking habits and attitudes towards smoking among students in grades 7 through 12 in Toledo and Lucas County public schools—1964 and 1971, Am. J. Public Health **65:**923-938, Sept., 1975.

57. Kinard, E. M., and Klerman, L. V.: Early parenting and child abuse: are they related? presented at the American Public Health Association Annual Meeting, Oct. 18, 1978, Los Angeles.

58. Klerman, L.: Adolescent pregnancy: the need for new policies and programs, J. Sch. Health **45:**263-267, 1975.

59. Kovar, M. G.: Adolescent health status and health-related behavior, presented at the Conference on Adolescent Behavior and

Health, Division of Health Science Policy, National Academy of Sciences, June 26-27, 1978, Washington, D.C., No. (IOM) 78-004.

60. Kovar, M. G.: Some indicators of health-related behavior among adolescents in the United States, Public Health Rep. **94:** 109-118, March/April, 1979.

61. Kovar, M. G., et al.: Adolescent health indicators, presented at the American Public Health Association Annual Meeting, Oct. 18, 1978, Los Angeles.

62. Luker, K.: Taking chances: abortion and the decision not to contracept, Berkeley, 1975, University of California Press.

63. Mackenzie, S., Research Analyst, University of Washington, Seattle, Wash.: Study on entrance into juvenile prostitution, personal communication, April, 1979.

64. Madison, D. L.: Organized health care and the poor, Med. Care Rev. **26:**783-807, Aug., 1969.

65. Manber, M. M.: Adolescents, Med. World News **20:**41-51, April 2, 1979.

66. Maurer, A., guest editor: Violence against children, J. Clin. Child Psychol. **2:**1-58, Spring, 1975 (3rd printing, copyright 1973).

67. McCarthy, J., and Menken, J.: Marriage, remarriage, marital disruption and age at first birth, Fam. Plan. Perspect. **11:**21-30, Jan./Feb., 1979.

68. Moore, K., et al.: The consequence of early childbearing: an analysis of selected parental outcomes using results from the national longitudinal survey of young women, Washington, D.C., 1977, The Urban Institute.

69. Moore, K. A., and Waite, L. J.: Early childbearing and educational attainment, Fam. Plann. Perspect. **9:**220-225, Sept./Oct., 1977.

70. Morgan, E. S.: The Puritan family: religion and domestic relations in seventeenth century New England, New York, 1966, Harper & Row, Publishers, Inc.

71. Morgan, S. R.: Psycho-educational profile of emotionally disturbed abused children, J. Clin. Child Psychol. **8:**3-6, Spring, 1979.

72. Murdock, C. G.: The unmarried mother and the school system, Am. J. Public Health **58:**2217-2224, Dec., 1968.

73. National Center for Education Statistics: Athletic injuries and deaths in secondary schools and colleges, 1975-1976, Washington, D.C., Feb., 1979, U.S. Government Printing Office.

74. National Center for Health Statistics: Children and youth. Selected health characteristics. United States 1958 and 1968, Vital and Health Statistics, PHS Pub. No. 1000, series 10, no. 62 PHS, Washington, D.C., 1971, U.S. Government Printing Office.

75. National Center for Health Statistics: Final natality statistics, 1977, Monthly Vital Statistics Report **27** (supp.):1-27, Feb. 5, 1979.

76. National Clearinghouse for Smoking and Health: Adult and teenage cigarette smoking patterns — United States, Morbidity and Mortality Weekly Report, **26:**160, May 13, 1977.

77. National Institute of Education: Violent schools — safe schools: the safe school study report to the Congress, Vol. 1., Washington, D.C., Jan. 1978, U.S. Government Printing Office.

78. National Institutes of Health: Teenage smoking: national patterns of cigarette smoking ages 12 through 18, in 1972 and 1974, No. (NIH) 76-931, Bethesda, Md., 1976, U.S. Government Printing Office.

79. Ory, M. G., and Earp, J.: The influence of teenage childbearing on child maltreatment: the role of intervening factors, presented at the American Public Health Association Annual Meeting, Oct. 18, 1978, Los Angeles.

80. Palazzoli, M. S.: Self-starvation: from individual to family therapy in the treatment of anorexia nervosa, New York, 1978, Jason Aronson.

81. Pardee, R., Office of Maternal and Child Health, U.S. Department of Health, Education and Welfare: Personal communication, April, 1979.

82. Pauker, J.: Girls pregnant out of wedlock, J. Operational Psychiatry **1:**15-19, 1971.

83. Paul, E. W., et al.: Pregnancy, teenagers and the law, 1976, Fam. Plann. Perspect. **8:** 16-21, Jan./Feb., 1976.

84. Piotrow, P. T., editor: Mothers too soon, Draper World Population Fund Report, No. 1, Washington, D.C., Autumn, 1975, Population Crisis Committee.

85. Plionis, B. M.: Adolescent pregnancy. Review of the literature, Social Work **20:**302-307, 1975.

86. The PTA and comprehensive health education. From challenge to action, Focal Points, Atlanta, Jan., 1979, Center for Disease Control.

87. Richmond, J. B., and Weinberger, H. L.: Session II. Program implications of new knowledge regarding the physical, intellectual, and emotional growth and development and the unmet needs of children and youth. II, Am. J. Public Health **60** (supp.): 23-73, April, 1970.

88. Rogers, K. D., and Reese, G.: Health studies—presumably normal high school students. I. Physical appraisal, Am. J. Dis. Child. **108**:572-600, 1964.

89. Scales, P.: Males and morals: teenage contraceptive behavior amid the double standard, The Family Coordinator **26**:211-222, July, 1977.

90. Schrut, A.: Some typical patterns in the behavior and background of adolescent girls who attempt suicide, Am. J. Psychiatry **125**:1, 1968.

91. Schrut, A., and Michels, T.: Adolescent girls who attempt suicide—comments on treatment, Am. J. Psychother. **23**:243-251, 1969.

92. Services for and needs of pregnant teenagers in large cities of the United States, 1976, Public Health Rep. **93**:46-54, Jan.-Feb., 1978.

93. Settlage, D. S. F., et al.: Sexual experience of younger teenage girls seeking contraceptive assistance for the first time, Fam. Plann. Perspect. **5**:223-226, July/Aug., 1973.

94. Smoking in America: public attitudes and behavior, The Gallup Opinion Index, Report No. 155, June, 1978.

95. Snapper, K. J., and Ohms, J. S.: The status of children 1977, Office of Human Development Services, No. (OHDS) 78-30133, Washington, D.C., 1978, U.S. Government Printing Office.

96. Somers, A.: Violence, television and the health of American youth, N. Engl. J. Med. **294**:811-817, 1976.

97. Sorenson, R. C.: Adolescent sexuality in contemporary America, New York, 1973, World Publishers.

98. Thomas, B. C.: The maturing teenage mother, Women & Health **4**:147-158, Summer, 1979.

99. Tietze, C.: Teenage pregnancies: looking ahead to 1984, Fam. Plann. Perspect. **10**: 205-207, July/Aug., 1978.

100. Torres, A.: Teenage income and clinic fees, Fam. Plann. Perspect. **8**:263–266, Nov./Dec., 1976.

101. Treffert, D. A.: Why Amy didn't live happily ever after, Prism **2**:63-67, Nov., 1974.

102. Urban and Rural Systems Associates (URSA): Improving family planning services for teenagers, Office of the Assistant Secretary for Planning and Evaluation/Health, U.S. Department of Health, Education and Welfare, Washington, D.C., June, 1976, U.S. Government Printing Office.

103. U.S. Bureau of the Census: Estimates of the population of the U.S. by age, sex, and race: 1970-1975, Current Population Reports, series P-25, no. 614, Washington, D.C., Nov., 1975, U.S. Government Printing Office.

104. U.S. Bureau of the Census: Money, income, and poverty status of families and persons in the U.S., 1976, Current Population Reports, series P-60, no. 107, Washington, D.C., 1977, U.S. Government Printing Office.

105. U.S. Bureau of the Census: Population profile of the U.S., 1977, Current Population Reports, series P-23, no. 66, Washington, D.C., 1978, U.S. Government Printing Office.

106. U.S. Bureau of the Census: 1976 Survey of institutionalized persons, a study of persons receiving long-term care, Current Population Reports, series P-23, No. 69. Washington, D.C., June, 1978, U.S. Government Printing Office.

107. U.S. Department of Health, Education and Welfare: Alcohol and health reports to Congress, Washington, D.C., 1974 and 1978, U.S. Government Printing Office. Cited in *The Young Drinkers: Teenagers and Alcohol,* Miami, 1978, Health Communications, Inc., 7541 Biscayne Blvd., Miami, Fla. 33138.

108. U.S. Department of Health, Education and Welfare: Health, United States, 1978, No. (PHS) 78-1232, Washington, D.C., 1978, U.S. Government Printing Office.

109. U.S. Department of Transport, Region X: Personal communication, April, 1979.

110. Valez, L., Office for Civil Rights, U.S. Department of Health Education and Welfare: Personal communication, May 11, 1979.

111. Vener, A. M., and Stewart, C. S.: Adolescent sexual behavior in middle America revisited: 1970-1973, J. Marriage and the Family, **36**:728-734, Nov., 1974.

112. Waldron, I., and Eyer, J.: Socioeconomic causes for the recent rise in death rates for 15-24 year olds, Soc. Sci. Med. **9:**383-396, 1975.

113. Warschauer, M., and Monk, M.: Problems in suicide statistics for whites and blacks, Am. J. Public Health **68:**383-388, April, 1978.

114. Whelan, E. M., and Higgins, G. K.: Teenage childbearing, extent and consequences, Washington, D.C., Jan., 1973, Child Welfare League of America, Inc., Consortium on Early Childbearing and Childrearing.

115. Zackler, J., and Brandstadt, W.: The teenage pregnant girl, Springfield, Ill., 1975, Charles C Thomas, Publisher.

116. Zelnik, M., and Kantner, J. F.: The resolution of teenage first pregnancies, Fam. Plann. Perspect. **6:**74-80, Spring, 1974.

117. Zelnik, M., and Kantner, J. F.: Sexual and contraceptive experience of young unmarried women in the U.S., 1971 and 1976, Fam. Plann. Perspect. **9:**55-71, March/April, 1977.

ADDITIONAL READINGS

Adams, J. B., and Hatcher, R. A.: The perplexing problem of teenage pregnancies, Urban Health **6:**26-27, 48-49, March, 1977.

Alan Guttmacher Institute: Special issue. Teenagers U.S.A., Fam. Plann. Perspect. **8:**148-208, July/Aug., 1976.

Alan Guttmacher Institute: Special issue on teenage pregnancy, Fam. Plann. Perspect. **10:**148-208, July/Aug., 1978.

American Academy of Pediatrics, Committee on Youth: Drug abuse in adolescence, Pediatrics **44:**131-141, July, 1969.

Baldwin, W. H.: Adolescent pregnancy and childbearing: growing concerns for Americans, Population Bull. **31:**1-36, 1976.

Brunswick, A. F.: Health needs of adolescents: how the adolescent sees them, Am. J. Public Health **59:**1730-1745, Sept., 1969.

Brunswick, A. F., and Collette, P.: Psychophysical correlates of elevated blood pressure: a study of urban black adolescents, J. Human Stress **3:**19-31, Dec., 1977.

Brunswick, A. F., et al.: Who sees the doctor? A study of urban black adolescents, Soc. Sci. Med. **13A:**45-56, 1979.

Castleman, M.: HEW proposes campaign against teen pregnancy, In These Times, p. 19, Feb. 1-7, 1978.

Center for Disease Control: Surveillance summary. Unintended teenage childbearing—United States, 1974, Morbidity and Mortality Weekly Report **27:**131-132, April 21, 1978.

Cottman, G.: Baby dolls, West Magazine, Los Angeles Times, Nov. 21, 1971.

Edwards, M.: Teenage parents, Seattle, June, 1978, Penny Press.

Fischman, S. H., and Palley, H. A.: Adolescent unwed motherhood: implications for a national family policy, Health and Social Work **3:**31-46, Feb, 1978.

Furstenburg, F. F.: Unplanned parenthood: the social consequences of teenage, childbearing, New York, 1977, The Free Press.

Gallagher, J. R., et al.: Medical care of the adolescent, ed. 3, New York, 1976, Appleton-Century-Crofts.

Girls Clubs of America, Inc.: Today's girls, tomorrow's women, Wingspread Conference, Racine Wisc., 1978, Girls Clubs of America, Inc.

Goldsmith, S.: San Francisco's teen clinic: meeting the sex education and birth control needs of the sexually active schoolgirl, Fam. Plann Perspect. **1:**23-26, Oct., 1969.

Gordon, J. S.: Caring for youth: essays on alternative services, Alcohol, Drug Abuse, and Mental Health Administration, no. (ADM) 78-557, U.S. Department of Health, Education and Welfare, Washington, D.C., 1978 U.S. Government Printing Office.

Gordon, J. S., director: Final report to the President's Commission on Mental Health of the Special Study on Alternative Mental Health Services, Division of Special Mental Health Programs, Washington, D.C., Feb., 15, 1978, National Institute of Mental Health.

Gordon, S., and Conant, R.: You, New York, 1975, Quadrangle Press.

Hertz, D. G.: Psychological implications of adolescent pregnancy: patterns of family interaction in adolescent mothers-to-be, Psychosomatics, **18:**13-16, Jan./Feb./March, 1977.

Howard, M.: Only human: teenage pregnancy and parenthood, New York, 1975, Seabury Press.

International Medical News Service: Consistency of effective contraceptive use increases dramatically among unwed teens, Ob-Gyn News, June 1, 1977.

Jacobson, H. N., et al.: Long-term effects of a nutrition education program for pregnant adolescents as measured by a new nutritional analysis program, New Brunswick, N.J., 1976, New Brunswick Public School District.

Jekel, J. F., et al.: Reasons for hospitalization of adolescent women in the U.S. — 1971, presented at the American Public Health Association Meetings, Oct. 18, 1978, Los Angeles.

Jessor, R., and Jessor, S. L.: Problem behavior and psychosocial development, New York, 1977, Academic Press, Inc.

Kandel, D.: Adolescent marijuana use: role of parents and peers, Science, 181:1067-1070, 1973.

Keniston, K., and The Carnegie Council on Children: All our children, the American family under pressure, New York, 1977, Harcourt Brace Jovanovich, Inc.

Lancet, M., et al.: Sexual knowledge, attitudes and practice of Israeli adolescents, Am. J. Public Health 68:1083-1089, Nov., 1978.

Levenkron, S.: The best little girl in the world, Chicago, 1978, Contemporary Books.

Lieberman, E. J., and Peck, E.: Sex and birth control: a guide for the young, New York, 1975, Schocken Books.

Minuchin, S., et al.: Psychosomatic families: anorexia nervosa in context, Cambridge, Mass., 1978, Harvard University Press.

Moore, K. A., and Caldwell, S. B.: The effect of government policies on out-of-wedlock sex and pregnancy, Fam. Plann. Perspect. 9:164-169, July/Aug., 1977.

National Research Council: Toward a national policy for children and families, Washington, D.C., 1976, National Academy of Sciences.

Newberger, E. H., et al.: Child health in America, toward a national public policy. Milbank Memorial Fund Quarterly 54:249-298, Summer, 1976.

Nolte, A.: Perspectives on adolescent health: a book of readings, Dubuque, Iowa, 1965, William C. Brown Book Co.

Oliver, L. I.: The association of health attitudes and perceptions of youths 12-17 years of age with those of their parents, United States, 1966-1970, Vital and Health Statistics, series 11, no. 161, (HRA) 77-1643, Washington, D.C., March, 1977, National Center for Health Statistics.

Osofsky, H.: Teen-age out of wedlock pregnancy; some preventive considerations, Adolescence 5:151-167, 1970.

Pediatric Clinics of North America: Symposium on adolescence, Meiks, L. T., and Green, M.,

consulting editors, Philadelphia, 1960, W. B. Saunders Co., vol. 7, pp. 1-232.

Salber, E. J., and Abelin, T.: Smoking behavior of Newton school children — 5-year follow-up, Pediatrics 40:363-372, Sept., 1967.

Shelton, J. D.: Very young adolescent females in Georgia: has abortion or contraception lowered their fertility? Am. J. Public Health 67:616-620, July, 1977.

Smith, P. B.: The medical impact of an antepartum program for pregnant adolescents: a statistical analysis, Am. J. Public Health 68:169-170, Feb., 1978.

Society for Adolescent Medicine, P.O. Box 3462, Granada Hills, Calif. 91344.

Stickle, G., and Ma, P.: Pregnancy in adolescents: scope of the problem, Contemporary OB/Gyn 5:85-91, June, 1975.

Stokes, B.: Teenage pregnancy, global epidemic, Washington Post, May 6, 1978.

U.S. Department of Health, Education and Welfare Social and Rehabilitation Service: The story of the White House Conferences on Children and Youth, Washington, D.C., 1967, U.S. Government Printing Office.

U.S. Department of Health, Education and Welfare: Food for the teenager during pregnancy, no. 017-026-00062-3 (pamphlet), Washington, D.C. 1977, U.S. Government Printing Office.

U.S. Department of Health, Education and Welfare: Smoking among teenagers and young women no. (NIH) 77-1203, Washington, D.C., 1977, U.S. Government Printing Office.

Ventura, S. J.: Teenage childbearing: United States, 1966-1975, Monthly Vital Statistics Report 26(supp.):1-15, Washington, D.C., Sept. 8, 1977, National Center for Health Statistics.

Williams, D. A., et al.: Teen-age suicide, Newsweek, pp. 74, 77, Aug. 28, 1978.

Wishik, S. M.: Commentary — should our children pay for the cigarette commercials? Pediatrics 31:535-537, 1963.

World Health Organization: Health needs of adolescents, WHO Technical Report Series, no. 609, Geneva, 1977, World Health Organization.

Zelnik, M., and Kantner, J. F.: Contraceptive patterns and premarital pregnancy among females aged 15-19 in 1976, Fam. Plann. Perspect. 10:135-142, May/June, 1978.

Chapter 7

Impact of technology on women's health care

Since World War II all medical care in the United States has been increasingly affected by the growth of the medical-industrial complex. The tremendous resources of the medical industry (over $9 billion within the drug industry alone in 1977) have produced new devices, drugs, equipment, and techniques and continuously varied modifications of each.

Senate hearings[325,326,part 15] and the literature[63,100,Chapter 5] confirm the unprecedented potential for profits from the medical-industrial complex, and these in turn fuel its growth. Other growth factors include third-party coverage, the widespread use of expensive diagnostic and preventive screening tests, and the creation of both physician and consumer demand. Widely accepted today, much medical technology nonetheless remains of dubiously proved benefit.[18,118] At issue are the appropriate utilization of such innovations and whether there are benefits to human life that outweigh the health risks and enormous financial costs.

All health care recipients have experienced the growth of technology, but women have been particularly affected. One main focus has been on women's reproductive capacity, which, as a clearly defineable health need, is easily targeted for technological management. Discussed in this chapter are specific examples of prime concern.

CONTRACEPTION
Historical background

Women have been limiting their fertility since earliest recorded history for a wide range of economic, social, political, and physiological reasons. Various methods such as use of sponges, pessaries, herbs, potions, amulets, coitus interruptus, abortion, infanticide, and prayer have been tried.[14,71,142]

Throughout the world the history of contraceptive use has been, and continues to be, marked by legal, medical, and social impediments. For example, condoms had been publicized by Annie Besant in England in the 1870s,[17] as had the diaphragm developed in 1882 by Dr. Aletta Jacobs of the Netherlands. But the medical profession in Europe and the United States almost uniformly refused to distribute contraceptive information or devices until the 1930s.[117] Poignant pleas for assistance were published in *Mother England* in 1929 by Marie Stopes, English birth control activist. In this volume Stopes printed letters from women de-

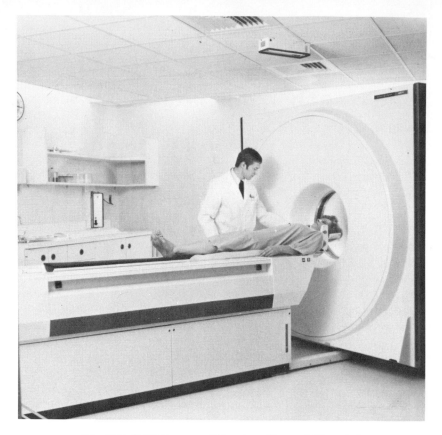

Fig. 7-1. CAT Scanner. (Courtesy General Electric.)

scribing human suffering the medical profession chose not to alleviate, as demonstrated by the following quotations:

Now the doctor has advised me to have no more family but did not give us a remedy.

The Matron of the Maternity Home said I must not have any more but she never told me how to avoid it and what's the good of telling a person it is more than their life's worth to have any more without telling them how to avoid it [sic].

I am 35 years of age and have up to the present given birth to seven children, six of which are living, so that I do not think I am asking advice before I have at least done my duty as a woman . . . My husband . . . is very lustful . . . I would like to satisfy his desires yet I am terrified at the thought anytime he comes near me.[12]

Similar miseries were expressed to Julia Lathrop, founding chief in 1912 of the Children's Bureau. Working to improve the welfare of women and children in the United States, Lathrop responded to those who beseeched her for information. Letters such as the following[13] are on file in the Library of Congress and attest to the desperation and misery in women's lives:

Dear Madame:

I need advice. I am a farmers wife. Do my household duties and a regular field hand too. The mother of 9 children and in family way again. I am quarlesome [sic] when tired and fatigued. When I come out of the field to prepare dinner my husband and all the children gets in my way. I quarrel at them for being in my way. I tell them I will build them a fire if they are cold. I also threaten to move the stove out on the porch. What shall I do? My husband won't sympathise with me one bit but talks rough to me. If I get tired and sick of my daily food and crave some simple article, should I have it. I have helped make the living for 20 years. Should I benied [sic] of a few simple articles or money either.

Does it make a mother unvirtuous for a man physician to wait on her during confinement; is it safe for me to go through it without aid from anyone? Please give me some advise. There isn't any midwives near us now. I am not friendless but going to you for advise to keep down gossip.

Contraception slowly became available in the United States after the opening of Margaret Sanger's birth control clinic in 1916, and the growth of the birth control movement (see Chapter 8). In addition to physician reluctance, another major obstacle in the United States was the Comstock Law, which had originated in 1873 with Anthony Comstock and the New York Society for the Suppression of Vice. This law, which equated contraception with obscenity, effectively forbade the sale or distribution of contraceptive devices. Although its effectiveness was eventually eroded, the last major legal victory for contraception came in 1936 when the U.S. Circuit Court of Appeals affirmed the legality of importing contraceptive appliances from abroad. In the now famous case of *The United States* vs. *One Package*, tested by Dr. Hannah Stone, the Court ruled the federal birth control statute was not intended "to prevent the importation, sale, or carriage by mail of things which might intelligently be employed by conscientious and competent physicians for the purpose of saving life or promoting the well-being of their patients."[124]

Many states followed this federal lead and thus freed physicians and medically supervised agencies to prescribe contraception. Only in Connecticut and Massachusetts, where legal difficulties arose, was the Comstock Law in existence until 1965 and 1966, respectively. Physician reluctance and legal barriers also retarded research. It was not until the 1950s with the reintroduction of the intrauterine device (IUD) derived from the Graefenberg ring[272] and the development of the birth control pill[326,parts 15-17] ("the Pill"), that women had access to methods other than variations of ancient techniques.

Contemporary contraceptives

Criteria for judging the acceptability of a contraceptive method are (1) that the rate of pregnancy is low, (2) that it is esthetically acceptable and not associated with coitus, (3) that it is safe, (4) that it has minimal side effects, (5) that it is relatively inexpensive, and (6) that there are no environmental requirements for its use, for example, a clean water supply.

When judged according to these criteria, the Pill and the IUD were viewed as having provided women with nearly ideal contraception. The technology of the IUD and subsequent variations, including those combined with copper,[25] and of the Pill and later hormonal variations such as Depo-Provera, were hailed as breakthroughs in fertility control; these methods were soon in widespread use (see Table 7-1).

Although the methods indisputably meet the above criteria, particularly that of effectiveness (see Table 7-2), and therefore have the potential to relieve age-old anxieties of women and men, the safety of such technology is at issue. For many women these technologies have indeed brought the ability to control their fertility, an essential ingredient in economic equality; for many others they have also produced new anxieties, morbidities, and deaths. Although not all women experience all side-effects, the extensive discussions of the benefits and risks of the Pill merit careful evaluation.* Following are the adverse reactions reported to date: blood clots, stroke, death, hypertension, elevated blood levels of serum cholesterol and triglycerides, abnormalities of the breast (including tumors and cysts), breast tenderness, diabetic reactions and diabetes, viral infections, vaginal yeast infections, loss of hair, loss of libido, edema, cervical erosion, changes in cervical secretions, endometriosis, adenosis, diseases of the liver (including tumors), gastrointestinal disorders, nausea and vomiting, headache, migraine, hyperthyroidism, skin disorders (including rashes and "butterfly syndrome"), obesity, gallbladder disease (including gallstones), vitamin deficiencies, changes in vision and eye pressure, arthritis, depression and personality changes, infertility (after discontinuing the Pill), and birth defects to the fetus (heart and limb malformations).† Recent research confirms that many of these risks are magnified for women who smoke and/or are over 30.[157,314] In addition, when the Pill is taken in combination with other medications, additional complications from drug reactions may occur.[195]

Currently there are about 100 different types of intrauterine devices (IUDs) in use. Unlike the mechanism of the Pill, which alters the hormonal balance to suppress ovulation, the fertility control mechanism of the IUD is still not understood. This technological innovation has provided women with another contraceptive of low financial cost that is unrelated to coitus and relatively effective. IUDs are readily inserted, and in the Third World, paramedics are trained to insert them, as are some women's health care specialists in the United States. However, in the United States, IUD insertion is done mainly by physicians.

The technology of the IUD has had negative effects on women's health, but, as with the Pill, these are not experienced by all women. Common to all types of IUDs are the following complications and side effects: pelvic infections, septic abortions sometimes resulting in death, perforation of the uterine wall, pain, bleeding, embedding and/or fragmentation of the IUD, expulsion (pregnancy may then occur), and ectopic pregnancy.‡

One brand of IUD, the Dalkon Shield, has also been the subject of a class action suit. As of January, 1976, 17 women had died from septic abortions associated with IUD use.[77,255] The Dalkon Shield has since been withdrawn from the

---

*References 64,65,156,215,218,288, 289,291,321, 329.
†References 1,24, 32, 50, 59, 75, 133, 158, 196, 201, 206, 207, 251, 274, 276, 299.
‡References 2, 30, 48, 49, 74, 135, 169, 226, 272, 313, 340.

Table 7-1. Number of currently married women aged 15 to 44 and percent distribution by contraceptive status, United States, 1973 and 1976*

Contraceptive status	Total†		White		Black		Hispanic origin‡	
	1976	1973	1976	1973	1976	1973	1976	1973
Number in thousands§								
All women	27,185	26,646	24,518	24,249	2,144	2,081	1,673	1,676
Percent distribution								
Sterile couples								
All sterile couples	30.2	23.8	31.0	24.0	24.3	22.7	20.5	21.6
Nonsurgical	1.9	0.9	1.9	0.8	2.6	1.9	1.5	0.7‖
Surgical	28.3	22.9	29.1	23.1	21.7	20.8	19.0	20.9
Noncontraceptive	9.0	6.5	9.0	6.6	8.8	6.2	7.8	5.2
Female	8.2	6.3	8.2	6.3	8.7	6.1	7.0	5.2
Male	0.8	0.2	0.8	0.3	0.0	0.0	0.9‖	-
Contraceptive	19.3	16.4	20.1	16.5	12.9	14.6	11.2	15.7
Female	9.6	8.6	9.6	8.2	11.0	13.6	7.0	10.7
Male	9.7	7.8	10.5	8.4	1.9	1.0	4.2	5.0
Fecund couples								
Noncontraceptors								
Pregnant, postpartum, seeking pregnancy	13.4	14.2	12.8	14.2	16.6	14.0	20.8	18.9
Other nonusers	7.7	8.7	7.2	7.8	13.5	17.9	10.5	9.7
Contraceptors								
All methods	48.6	53.2	49.0	54.0	45.4	45.3	48.1	49.8
Oral contraceptive pill	22.3	25.1	22.5	25.1	22.0	26.3	20.7	22.9
Intrauterine device	6.1	6.7	6.1	6.6	6.1	7.6	10.4	8.7
Diaphragm	2.9	2.4	3.0	2.5	1.8	1.2	2.4	1.8‖
Condom	7.2	9.4	7.4	9.9	4.5	3.2	6.1	7.0
Foam	3.0	3.5	2.9	3.5	3.8	3.0	3.5	1.8‖
Rhythm	3.4	2.8	3.5	2.9	1.4	0.7	3.1	2.1
Withdrawal	2.0	1.5	2.0	1.6	1.8	0.4	1.1‖	2.2
Douche	0.7	0.6	0.5	0.5	2.7	1.8	0.1‖	0.6‖
Other	0.9	1.3	0.9	1.3	1.2	1.0	0.5‖	2.7

*From National Center for Health Statistics: Advance Data, no. 36, Washington, D.C., Aug. 18, 1978, U.S. Government Printing Office.
†Includes white, black, and other races.
‡Women of Hispanic origin are included in the figures for white and black women if they were identified as such by the interviewer.
§In the 1973 figures, estimates of the number of women included cases for which contraceptive status was not ascertained but was imputed. Only those cases in which contraceptive status was ascertained are included in the 1976 figures.
‖Figure does not meet standards of reliability or precision.

Table 7-2. Type of exposure to the risk of conception among continuously married

| Type of exposure | Years of marriage | | | | | | |
| | Less than 5 | | | | 5 to 9 | | |
	1975	1973	1970	1965	1975	1973	1970
Total number in study	1041	1090	1010	600	703	882	853
Percent distribution							
Using contraception	71.3	68.9	61.7	58.5	76.7	75.0	69.2
Not using contraception	28.7	31.1	38.3	41.5	23.3	25.0	30.8
Pregnant, postpartum, or							
trying to get pregnant	23.2	25.0	29.6	34.5	17.4	18.5	19.7
Sterile and other nonuse	5.5	6.1	8.7	7.0	6.0	6.5	11.1
Number of contraceptive users	742	748	623	351	539	661	590
Percent distribution of							
contraceptive methods							
Wife sterilized	0.8	1.9	0.3	0.0	11.7	9.4	3.9
Husband sterilized	0.7	0.6	1.0	0.3	10.0	9.0	4.2
Pill	64.8	64.1	57.1	53.3	38.6	39.4	42.9
IUD	8.1	9.7	8.5	1.4	14.5	14.5	11.4
Diaphragm	4.3	2.6	3.5	4.6	3.3	3.2	4.2
Condom	12.0	11.4	9.8	14.8	11.7	10.3	13.6
Withdrawal	1.8	1.6	1.4	2.8	1.7	2.1	1.4
Foam	3.4	4.3	8.2	4.8	4.6	8.2	8.8
Rhythm	1.8	2.0	5.0	8.5	2.2	2.2	4.7
Douche	0.4	0.2	1.8	3.7	0.2	0.4	1.0
Other	2.0	1.5	3.4	5.7	1.5	1.3	3.9

*From Westoff, C. F., and Jones, E. F.: Fam. Plann. Perspect. 9(4), July/Aug., 1977. Reprinted
†Blacks were reluctantly excluded from the reinterview because the original 1970 sample of blacks
many analyses.

market, although it remains inserted in unknown numbers of women, particularly in Third World countries.

Contraceptive technology is developing continuously, and the market for it is expected to reach $310 million annually by 1987.* There are several new innovations, many of which have adverse reactions. A hormone-releasing IUD, Progestasert, has been developed but has been cited in the Medical Letter as causing increased bleeding and abdominal pain without increase in pregnancy prevention as compared with other IUDs.[255] Birth control by immunization is expected to be available in 10 years. The vaccine will contain antibodies that will block fertilization by attaching themselves to an egg and repelling sperm cells.[223]

Depo-Provera, a contraceptive injected every 3 to 6 months, is estimated to be used already by 3 to 5 million women worldwide, yet as of 1979 it was unapproved for use in the United States by the Food and Drug Administration (FDA). It was the subject of congressional hearings on August 8, 1978, in which the United States Agency for International Development (USAID) and various interna-

---

*Reported in *The Nation's Health*, p. 8, Dec., 1978.

white women, National Fertility Study, 1965 to 1975*†

	Years of marriage										
	10 to 14				15 to 19				20 to 24		
1975	1973	1970	1965	1975	1973	1970	1965	1975	1973	1970	1965
632	731	731	571	553	710	626	636	400	493	564	405
85.9	80.8	75.4	73.7	85.9	71.6	67.9	70.6	79.5	67.8	65.4	62.2
14.1	19.2	24.6	26.3	14.1	28.4	32.1	29.4	20.5	32.2	34.6	37.8
6.2	8.0	8.5	7.4	2.9	3.0	4.5	5.5	1.5	1.8	1.6	3.0
7.9	11.2	16.1	18.9	11.2	25.4	27.6	23.9	19.1	30.4	33.0	34.8
543	594	551	421	475	513	425	449	318	337	369	252
20.6	15.3	7.4	7.1	27.8	13.3	13.4	9.1	30.2	18.8	13.6	8.3
22.7	15.1	7.8	5.2	23.8	18.7	12.2	5.8	25.5	18.2	15.4	8.7
25.2	22.4	28.1	20.7	15.8	22.0	20.7	10.5	10.4	16.0	14.6	8.7
9.0	11.2	8.2	0.7	5.1	6.4	4.0	1.1	3.8	2.2	2.7	0.0
1.7	3.9	6.4	10.5	4.0	5.7	8.2	13.8	7.5	6.1	8.1	17.1
8.8	17.1	16.0	25.9	9.5	19.2	19.1	25.8	12.6	21.6	18.4	23.8
1.1	1.5	3.3	4.5	3.4	3.9	2.8	5.1	2.5	3.3	3.5	6.3
4.4	6.6	6.7	3.6	2.9	2.2	4.2	1.3	1.9	3.7	3.0	0.8
3.5	4.6	8.2	13.5	4.0	6.2	9.2	12.9	3.1	6.6	10.6	13.5
0.4	0.5	1.6	3.3	0.6	1.0	3.1	4.7	0.6	0.8	5.1	5.2
2.6	1.9	6.4	5.0	3.2	1.5	3.1	9.8	1.9	2.5	4.9	7.5

with permission.
had serious biases and the numbers in each 5-year marriage cohort would have been too small for

tional family planning agencies sought to have the FDA ruling overturned to permit use of the contraceptive in the United States and its distribution by USAID abroad. Experts noted there were about 70 countries that have approved the use of Depo-Provera.[174,249,252,278]

Another innovation is a Silastic hormonal contraceptive that is implanted under the skin and may provide contraceptive protection for as long as 5 to 7 years. Among side effects known to date are amenorrhea and intermenstrual bleeding.[12,223] The popular press has also reported that Swedish researchers are developing a hormonal nasal spray that would work on the pituitary to suppress ovulation.[180]

Nonhormonal innovations include contraceptive zinc-medicated sponges,[10] spermicidal foam tablets,[296] and spermicidal wax tablets[82] that are inserted into the vagina. It is claimed that these contraceptives have minimal or no side effects, but the claims to effectiveness are not definitive.[238]

One result of these technological developments has been to ignore the more traditional, but less potentially hazardous, birth control methods. Widely regarded as less reliable than other contraceptives, condoms,[248] cervical mucus testing,[91] cervical caps,[315] and diaphragms[250] have received scant promotion to encourage their correct usage and therefore increase their effectiveness and esthetic appeal. Diaphragms, for example, when properly fitted, retained in place for 6 to 8 hours, and used with jelly, are estimated to be at least 98% effective.[314] Continuing research also shows that women have inadequate knowledge of their fertility cycles, which is essential for reliable barrier method use[254] (also see Chapter 8).

Barrier methods are frequently cited in the literature as being particularly unsuited for younger women, yet one study of over 2000 young, mostly never-married women showed that only about 2% had had an accidental pregnancy and more than 80% continued to use their diaphragms after the first year.[184]

The scientific appeal of complex technological innovations has also hindered research into more simple methods, potentially safer for women. In fiscal year 1978, for example, out of $61.1 million budgeted by the Center for Population Research, National Institute of Child Health and Human Development, for contraceptive research, only $175,000 was spent on barrier method research.

The rapidity of development of these technological advances has also diffused pressure to develop a male contraceptive. In fiscal year 1978, $966,000 was spent on this approach compared with $6 million for female contraceptive development. Similarly, $2.1 million was spent for evaluation studies on male

Table 7-3. Birth- and birth control method–related deaths per 100,000 women per year*

Regimen and type of death	15 to 19 years	20 to 24 years	25 to 29 years	30 to 34 years	35 to 39 years	40 to 44 years
No birth control, birth related	5.3	5.8	7.2	12.7	20.8	21.6
Abortion only, method related	1.0	1.9	2.4	2.3	2.9	1.7
Pills only/nonsmokers						
Birth related	0.1	0.2	0.2	0.4	0.6	0.4
Method related	0.6	1.1	1.6	3.0	9.1	17.7
TOTAL	0.7	1.3	1.8	3.4	9.7	18.1
Pills only/smokers						
Birth related	0.1	0.2	0.2	0.4	0.6	0.4
Method related	2.1	4.2	6.1	11.8	31.3	60.9
TOTAL	2.2	4.4	6.3	12.2	31.9	61.3
IUDs only						
Birth related	0.1	0.2	0.2	0.4	0.6	0.4
Method-related	0.8	0.8	1.0	1.0	1.4	1.4
TOTAL	0.9	1.0	1.2	1.4	2.0	1.8
Barrier methods only, birth related	1.1	1.5	1.9	3.3	5.0	4.0
Barrier methods, plus abortion, method related	0.1	0.3	0.4	0.4	0.4	0.2

*From Tietze, C.: Induced abortion: 1979, ed. 3, New York, 1979, The Population Council. Reproduced with permission.

contraceptives as compared with $4.5 million on evaluating female contraceptives.[345] Several explanations are offered for the rejection of the findings of some early studies on male contraception and the current relative lack of interest in it. These include the belief in the contraceptive responsibility of women, the sex of the researchers, the complexity of the spermatogenesis process, and the unwillingness of men to accept side effects such as decreased libido. Also cited is the early influence of Margaret Sanger and Mrs. Stanley McCormack, who, in their determination to give women a means to control their own fertility, respectively encouraged and in large amount financed Dr. Gregory Pincus in his development of the Pill.[33]

It is perhaps the combination of pressing need for fertility control and huge profit possibilities that lead to potentially the most damaging effect of technology: hasty release of innovations without adequate and comparative risk assessment (see Table 7-3). The Pill was released on the basis of studies of only 132 Puerto Rican women who had taken the Pill for more than 1 year and 718 other women who had taken it for less than 1 year. Although five of the women died, they were not examined during their illnesses by study physicians, nor were autopsies performed.[326] The Dalkon Shield was marketed after studies on only 82 patients with an average test period of only 5.5 months.[77] In contrast, a recent report notes that the drug company Upjohn, also a manufacturer of Depo-Provera, has a new synthetic birth control liquid for dogs that "has been more than 90 percent effective in preventing pregnancies in 5 years of tests on more than 2,000 dogs."[15] A previous drug was withdrawn from the market in the mid-1960s "after a number of dogs developed an infection of the uterus."[15]

ESTROGENS
Historical background

In the late 19th century, research was first undertaken to identify hormones and to determine which organs were responsible for their manufacture. Estrogen, or the estrus hormone, commonly known as the female sex hormone, was identified in the early 1920s. Following early laboratory synthesis of estrogens, in 1938 a synthetic estrogen compound known as diethylstilbestrol (DES) was formulated. Inexpensive to prepare, orally administerable, and almost as potent as natural estrogen, DES was readily accepted for several purposes.[335] Subsequently other estrogens were manufactured, including those used in oral contraceptives and for estrogen replacement therapy. The latter term generally refers to the use of conjugated natural estrogens containing principally sodium estrone sulfate for relief of menopausal symptoms. This conjugated estrogen is marketed chiefly by Ayerst as Premarin. Currently there are numerous uses for estrogens, including to correct estrogen deficiency associated with primary ovarian failure, to treat amenorrhea and female hypogonadism, to control uterine bleeding, to dry up breast milk in the postpartum period, and to prevent pregnancy when used in the "morning-after" pill.[290] The *National Disease and Therapeutic Index* estimates that 91 million estrogen prescriptions are written annually.[227] The extent of use of Premarin and DES (discussion follows) has been estimated in the literature: in 1976 the FDA estimated that 5 million women were taking Premarin for menopausal symptoms,[284] although this number is believed to have dropped substantially since adverse publicity. This figure did not include other brands of menopausal estrogens, nor the numbers of women taking estrogens for other purposes. Estimates of the number of women for whom DES was prescribed between 1943 and 1970 as an antimiscarriage drug range from 500,000 to 6 million,[332] although most reports suggest 2 million women were affected.

Diethylstilbestrol (DES)

The ready availability and early reports of its efficacy[301,302] rapidly led to widespread use of DES as an antimiscarriage drug. Because proved efficacy before marketing of a new drug was not required by Congress until 1962,[164] DES remained unproved until 1953.[73] Even though clinical trials then showed that the drug was not effective for this purpose, its use as an antimiscarriage agent nonetheless continued until 1971.

In 1970 and 1971 the first reports appeared in the literature of a rare cancer — clear cell carcinoma of the vagina — in women 15 to 22 years of age.[131,136] Herbst et al. noted that previously in the world literature there were only three cases of this cancer in women under the age of 35. The initial clusters of women were studied, and maternal DES therapy was found to be a common factor.[138,139,269,270] The DES given to their mothers to prevent miscarriage had crossed the placenta; transplacental carcinogenesis in humans had occurred. Of the approximately 250 persons with this cancer identified to date, 22% have died. Many other DES daughters have developed adenosis, a condition in which the cells of the vagina and cervix are not fully developed and which may be precancerous.

Currently this inadequately tested and unnecessarily used technological innovation is estimated to have produced a prevalence rate of clear cell adenocarcinoma of the vagina or cervix ranging from 1.4 per 1000 exposed DES daughters to 1.4 per 10,000.[183] Young women affected are advised to do some or all of the following, depending on diagnosis: seek semiannual colposcopic iodine staining, have cytology and biopsy examinations for the rest of their lives,[271] and avoid all further contact with estrogens. Many others will never know that they are DES daughters because they are dependent on practitioners researching 20-year-old records and notifying their mothers. For others, the cost of the examination may prove prohibitive. If diagnosed as cancerous, a young woman may face surgery, chemotherapy, or irradiation, each with its own potentially damaging effects.

A new study has shown also that DES daughters have a higher incidence of misshapen uteri and that their ability to carry a pregnancy to term may be impaired.[234] An ongoing 5-year study of DES daughters in four medical centers has noted that there were significant variations in the amount of exposure to DES, which may affect incidence of adenocarcinoma and other abnormalities.[183]

At present there is controversy about the effects of DES ingestion on the mothers. The women who participated, unknowingly (see later), in the clinical trial that produced the 1953 data have been contacted and assessed for incidence of cancer of the breast, endometrium, ovary, colon, cervix, and "other" body part. The researchers in the follow-up study claim that there is no statistically significant difference[27] between the 32 cancers found in the 693 DES-exposed women (4.6%) and the 21 (3.1%) in the 668 unexposed women, but this is contested by other authorities,[346] particularly when the women under age 50 are compared. For all exposed mothers, however, there is guilt, anxiety, and anger about their use of DES.

Emerging evidence also suggests that there may be effects of DES on the sons of exposed mothers. Some findings suggest abnormal semen and anatomical lesions of the male genital tract, but at present there is no definitive association with testicular cancer and/or reduced fertility.[26,108,109]

The administration of DES in the face of insubstantial evidence of safety and the firm evidence of its inefficacy has engendered several suits. Recently a class action suit was filed against the University of Chicago, where the 1951 to 1952 clinical trials were performed and in which the women were unknowing participants, and against Eli Lilly & Co., a leading DES supplier. Previous suits generally have not been decided in favor of the plaintiffs, usually because the DES ingested could not be traced to one specific company that could be held liable; the informed consent issue of this suit may eventually provide some redress for the women affected.[266]

Menopausal estrogens

One aspect of the aging process for women is the cessation of the menstrual cycle, referred to as menopause. On the average, menopause occurs at age 49, at the same time that other physiological changes of the aging process such as drying skin and loss of bone mass are also occurring. Little is definitively known about menopause and whether certain conditions are indeed menopausal or merely part of the aging process. Little is also known about the direct psychological effects of menopause on women as compared with the effects of sociopsychological events such as "empty-nest" syndrome and husband's retirement, which may occur simultaneously with menopause.[21,212]

This dearth of accurate information has provided a source for negative attitudes and reliance on technological solutions. Conditioned to think of themselves as childbearers, sex partners, and, above all, feminine, women have easily believed that menopause meant the end of their femininity and appeal. Such sentiments are echoed in medical texts, where menopause is frequently described (even by women physicians) as a deficiency disease with dire health consequences.[33,162,212] A comment in 1973 reported in the *Journal of the American Medical Association* and in the popular press summarized this attitude. Dr. Frances P. Rhoades, then president of the American Geriatric Society, was reported as stating that "menopause is a chronic and incapacitating deficiency disease that leaves women with flabby breasts, wrinkled skin, fragile bones, and a loss of ability to have or enjoy sex."[92]

In the 1960s, help was offered for this dismal specter through the technology of estrogen replacement therapy. Although such therapy had been a practice since the 1930s, a new drive was spearheaded by Dr. Robert Wilson, head of a foundation financed by Ayerst, manufacturers of Premarin, the major menopausal estrogen. In his book *Feminine Forever* Wilson discusses women who are the "pioneers" in estrogen replacement therapy:

The women in this pioneer group are different in one vital aspect from any other woman since the beginning of the human race: They will never suffer menopause.

Instead of being condemned to witness the death of their own womanhood during what should be their best years, they will remain fully feminine — physically and emotionally — for as long as they live.

You may have passed them on the street or seen them on the bus. You may have met them at a party, in church, or at the club. Perhaps one of them is working at your office. You can't tell unless you know their age.

But when you find a women of 50 looking like 30, or a woman of 60 looking — and acting — like 40, chances are that she is one of the lucky ones who have benefited from the new techniques of menopause prevention.

The outward signs of this age-defying youthfulness are a straight-backed posture, supple breast contours, taut, smooth skin on face and neck, firm muscle tone, and that particular vigor and grace typical of a healthy female. At fifty, such women still look attractive in tennis shorts and sleeveless dresses.

To the emotionally mature women, this physical attractiveness is rarely an end in itself. Rather, it is a subtle psychological means by which she relates to the world around her. While this quality may not be directly erotic, its charm usually derives from a woman's sexual self-confidence. And now, thanks to recent medical advances, it is possible for any woman to retain her sexual appeal along with her sexual vitality throughout later life. By retaining these functions she also safeguards the less direct and more elusive aspects of her total femininity.[343]

Such appeals to women's age-old fears were successful, and by 1975, prior to much-publicized reports of the adverse effects of menopausal estrogen, Ayerst's annual Premarin sales reportedly exceeded $70 million.[232] Many women report beneficial effects from this particular technology. The data, however, suggest that if there are benefits, they come at a cost.* Links between estrogen use and cancer have appeared in the literature since the 1940s, and early studies suggested that although there may be an increased incidence of endometrial cancer (of the lining of the uterus), estrogens appeared to offer protection against breast cancer.[105,123] Although there is still some question regarding the cancerous effects on the breast of menopausal estrogens, the links between these drugs and endometrial cancer are firmly established.

On the basis of the studies cited, the FDA suggests that, depending on the duration and dosage of estrogen, the annual incidence of endometrial cancer in estrogen users is 4 to 8 per 1000 women, and that these women face a three to eleven times greater risk of endometrial cancer than do women who do not take estrogens.[94,120] These estimates have been validated[116] despite an attempt to assert that there was a bias.[148,153] A more recent study examined the incidence of endometrial cancer during the period following the 1975 studies, a period in which there was also a substantial decline in the number of replacement estrogen prescriptions. During this period a sharp downward trend was noted in endometrial cancer

---

*References 94, 147, 204, 300, 304, 333, 334, 349.

incidence, which suggests that the increased risk of endometrial cancer from estrogen decreases quickly when the drug is discontinued.[163]

Controversy as to whether the benefits of estrogen replacement therapy outweigh the risks still exists, however. Prescribed for hot flashes, nervous disorders, symptoms of senility, genital atrophy, dry vaginas, aging skin, and osteoporosis (bone loss), estrogen is listed by the FDA as "probably effective" for prevention of the latter. In addition, estrogen is suggested by other researchers to be effective in ameliorating vasomotor instability (hot flashes) and in relief or prevention of urogenital epithelium atrophy.[194,278]

The technology of menopausal estrogens has also had the effect of offering a quick palliative for physiological problems, which may be more psychosocial in origin and which may in fact simply be a stage of the aging continuum. The availability of estrogen has highlighted menopause as a treatable problem and has squelched research efforts into appropriate nutritional or exercise regimens that may ease temporary discomforts for menopausal women and prevent osteoporosis.

Despite, or because of, the controversy and the mounting negative evidence, hard-sell marketing efforts continue, as demonstrated by a December 17, 1976, memo between Ayerst and Hill & Knowlton, a New York public relations company, whose memo delineated their strategies to downplay the negative medical aspects of estrogen use while conducting a "general exposition on the menopause." That their efforts are successful beyond actual menopausal needs is apparent.[165,192,280] The FDA reports that less than half of the approximately 1.5 million women who enter menopause in a single year visit a physician with menopausal complaints, and since only a portion of these have major vasomotor symptoms, "the annual use of orally administered estrogens equal to 6 million patient years, is far in excess of that required for short-term management of the menopausal syndrome."[94]

OBSTETRICAL PROCEDURES
Historical background

Technology of a sort has always been a part of childbirth. In nonindustrialized societies, birth is surrounded by specific practices, rules, and rituals[273]; in highly industrialized societies, births are surrounded by machines, instrumentation, and rituals involved in their use. In spite of, or because of (depending on one's viewpoint), these things, women have in the main successfully delivered their babies.

In earlier centuries, when a difficult obstetrical case occurred, rituals were of little use; women and babies were mutilated or died. Even after the advent of the universities in the thirteenth century and more formalized training, aid remained at a minimum for poor and rich alike. For example, when Beatrice d'Este (1475-1497) an Italian noblewoman, experienced atrocious labor pains in her third pregnancy on New Year's Day, 1494, her attendants offered a variety of remedies. Midwives suggested she swallow the white of an egg with a few bits of scarlet silk in it; sit over a pot of boiling water; tie the duke's cap to her abdomen; swallow a potion of hot spirits cooked with stubs of deer's antlers and cochineal, and offer an incantation about the eagle stone under her right armpit and a lode stone under her left. Her husband was urged to eat a piece of wolf's meat while another incantation was said. The court *medicus* (doctor), Marliani, was called and said he could do nothing. Another *medicus* suggested 3 ounces of river snails with muskat nuts and red brayed coral; yet another *medicus* suggested adding cow's dung to the snail mixture; still another advocated phlebotomy but was contradicted by another who said that Mars was in the constellation of Cancer and therefore phlebotomy was contraindicated. Beatrice's husband, Duke Ludovico, called all the attendants and the clergy fools and went to the chapel to pray. Beatrice died.[152]

By the eighteenth century, complicated obstetrical management had advanced; cesarean section was understood and used, although with high mortality.[348] The fetal positions had been defined by the skilled French midwife Louyse Bourgeois (1563-1636),[69] and a teaching manikin of the female torso had been developed (and preceded that of William Smellie of England) by another French midwife, Angelique Marguerite le Boursier du Coudray (1712-1789).[89]

Although instruction for all attendants in obstetrics in parts of Europe did improve, technology such as cesareans and forceps (see Chapter 4) soon became the province of male physicians only. This pattern persisted in the United States and became particularly marked in the early twentieth century, when the strongest efforts were made to abolish the practice of midwifery.[72]

Initially the increase in technology did little for maternal and infant mortality, however. According to data from states with birth registration, maternal mortality was 717.9 per 100,000 live births from 1915 to 1919 and continued above 300 per 100,000 until 1941. Until 1965 it was over 30 per 100,000 (see Chapter 1). Infant mortality was estimated to be 1 in 10 live births at the turn of the century, dropping to 65 per 1000 by 1930 to 24.7 by 1965, and an estimated 13.7 in 1978.[330]

Maternal mortality did gradually decline after the 1940s (see Chapter 1), and medical efforts focused on the further reduction of infant mortality. Post–World War II affluence, the "baby boom," and the medical-industrial complex combined to foster the growth of baby-saving technologies, a marketable commodity with wide public appeal.

Current obstetrical technology*

Clearly some obstetrical technologies help some people, but their responsibility in reducing infant mortality is debatable.[18,54,230,239] Futhermore, use of one technology frequently requires the use of another to alleviate or complement the effects of the first. The complex forces that foster technology operate independently of the woman and her baby, and she comes to participate in their use without her truly informed consent. Specific obstetrical technologies in widespread use to be considered are electronic fetal monitoring, oxytocin challenge test, induction of labor, amniocentesis, diagnostic ultrasound, and cesarean section.

Electronic fetal monitoring (EFM). EFM is used to provide continuous data on the fetal heart rate during labor; data may be obtained externally (indirect) or in-

---

*Much of this discussion is drawn from Marieskind, H. I.: An evaluation of Caesarean section in the United States, Washington, D.C., 1979, Department of Health, Education and Welfare.

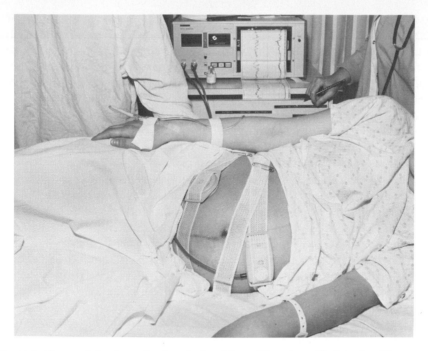

Fig. 7-2. External fetal monitoring during labor. (Courtesy Christopher Sherman.)

ternally (direct), and for either method the woman lies basically flat and station-ary. External monitoring uses two instruments placed on the mother's abdomen by a belt: a tocodynamometer to indicate the frequency and duration of uterine contractions, and an ultrasonic transducer to measure fetal heart rate. Believed superior because of improved accuracy, internal, or direct, monitoring obtains data on the fetal heart rate by means of a uterine catheter inserted into the uterus between the fetus and the uterine wall and by a spiral electrode attached to the presenting part (usually the scalp) of the fetus. Both methods register their mea-surements on a machine that provides a printout of the fetal heart rate. Both meth-ods measure the strength of uterine contractions and the amount of oxygen (which affects heart rate) reaching the fetus. Because for these monitoring methods, women must assume the supine position, which is widely believed to promote de-livery complications, a new variation of monitoring, telemetry, has been devel-oped. This would provide the same readings by means of a small transmitter strapped to the patient's thigh and would allow her to ambulate. Although not yet widely in use, telemetry is hailed as the device of the future.[3] It is estimated, although unverified, that almost all obstetrical services in the United States have at least one EFM device, and that probably over half of all patients are moni-tored.[258] It is becoming the prevailing practice for most institutions that have EFM to try to monitor as close to 100% of patients as possible. It is debatable, however, whether EFM should be used for both high- and low-risk pat-ients.[154,220,230,240] Physician acceptance of EFM is high.[134]

Most studies report on the advantages of EFM.* An extensive literature review of the costs and benefits of EFM was recently published[19]; both it and other sources cite five principal criticisms: accuracy of the recordings is questionable, the information received through EFM beyond that from traditional auscultation (monitoring by stethoscope) is of questionable value in affecting infant outcome, EFM may cause complications, EFM adds costs for little benefit, and EFM may contribute to an increase in cesarean sections.

There have been four attempts by prospective controlled clinical trials to prove causality between use of EFM and improved infant outcome; three have found no differences in perinatal outcome from the use of EFM,[131,132,172] and the one which did find a superior outcome has methodology which is open to question.[264] In the first study by Dr. Albert D. Haverkamp and colleagues at Denver General Hospital, 483 high-risk women were randomly assigned to an auscultation (monitoring by stethoscope) group and to an EFM group. For the outcome measurements of neonatal death, Apgar scores, cord blood gases, and neonatal nursery morbidity, there were no recorded differences, although there were more cesareans in the monitored group.[131]

Haverkamp and colleagues also completed a second study in which 690 high-risk women were randomly assigned to three groups: auscultated, electronically monitored, and electronically monitored with fetal scalp blood sampling. All women were attended by individual study nurses, and again there was no difference in perinatal outcome. An increase in cesarean section in the monitored groups was found although it was less in the group with monitoring and scalp sampling combined. In a 9-month follow-up study completed February 1, 1978, on 512 of these patients, no differences in motor or mental development of the babies were detected.[132] The third study, conducted by Dr. Ian Kelso and colleagues at the Jessop Hospital for Women in Sheffield, England, randomly assigned 504 low-risk patients to two groups: EFM and auscultation. No differences in perinatal outcome were recorded, although more cesareans in the monitored group than in the nonmonitored group occurred. A study for indications showed that three of the cesareans in the auscultated group and four in the monitored were for fetal distress.[172]

The fourth study, conducted in Melbourne, Australia, by Dr. Peter Renou and colleagues, randomly assigned a total of 350 high-risk patients to each of two groups: control (auscultation) and intensive care (EFM and fetal scalp blood sampling). An improvement in perinatal outcome in the intensive care group was measured by means of Apgar scores, neurological sequellae, and cord gases. A higher incidence of cesarean section was also recorded in this group, but when the incidence of routine repeat cesareans was subtracted, the difference was not significant. The presence of these patients with repeat cesareans, in addition to other methodological problems, seriously impaired this study.[264]

Complications from EFM arise for both mother and infant. Data suggest that

---

*References 5, 22, 23, 31, 51, 53, 80, 102, 103, 112, 114, 143-146, 151, 166, 181, 186, 190, 198, 217, 243-245, 259, 260, 263, 282, 283, 287, 297, 320.

for both, the chances of infection appear to be increased. This is because amniotomy (rupture of the membranes) is frequently performed to insert the electrode and catheter* and because use of EFM may prompt more vaginal examinations. There are contradictory reports on this, however.[107,126] Damage to the fetal head may also occur after amniotomy because the protective cushion of the amniotic fluid is lost; this may in itself cause fetal distress.[43,44,242,286] Maternal hemorrhage, minor lacerations from improper insertion of the uterine catheter,[275] and gonococcal sepsis secondary to EFM[310] have all been reported. Abscesses and cellulitis are the most frequent infant complications.† Cerebral spinal fluid leakage, damage to the lower eyelids of the baby, tear of a fetal vessel,[88] fatal neonatal sepsis,[318] and scalp lacerations have also been recorded from improper electrode catheter placement or improper scalp puncture for fetal scalp sampling.[229] Furthermore, the supine position necessary for EFM,[42,309] called the worst possible for delivery, may also cause fetal distress either by cutting the blood supply to the infant and/or by causing maternal discomfort. Mothers have also reported psychological stress from the monitor, which is perceived as an interference,[275,305] and possibly this may cause confusion of the tracings.[186]

Other costs of monitoring are monetary.[19] An electronic fetal monitor currently costs between $6500 and $7500, and central equipment to monitor several mothers in labor costs three to four times that amount.[200] It is estimated that costs of the monitor therefore add between $35 and $100 to each delivery. That these monitors are profitable is evidenced by their sales, which are said to have totaled $25 million in 1976 and are expected to reach $40 million by 1986.[98]

Oxytocin challenge test (OCT). The oxytocin challenge test (OCT), or "stressed monitoring," is another obstetrical intervention designed to detect a baby who will be compromised by or who will not survive labor and vaginal delivery. In this test, an attempt is made to duplicate labor by inducing uterine contractions by administering intravenous Pitocin (synthetic oxytocin). The test is performed between 31 and 44 weeks. The progression of labor is simulated by increasing the dosage until contractions are at a frequency of three every 10-minute period, with simultaneous monitoring of the fetal heart so that placental insufficiency can be detected and fetal welfare assessed. An OCT is regarded as positive when the fetal heart rate (FHR) has three successive late decelerations; in a negative test there are no ominous changes in FHR. As with much obstetrical technology, the OCT was originally designed for high-risk women under any of the following conditions: a postmature baby (after 42 weeks from estimated date of conception "a notoriously inexact measure"),[110] meconium staining, intrauterine growth retardation, or previous stillbirths. However, the OCT has gradually become part of routine obstetrical practice and is joined by other tests for placental insufficiency, for example, estriol studies and human placental lactogen tests.

This is an example of one technology leading to use of another; the use of

---

*References 104, 106, 185, 187, 339, 344.
†References 87, 115, 209, 236, 237, 247, 311.

Pitocin, documented as producing stronger and more rapid than usual contractions, may prevent the fetus from restoring its oxygen supply as rapidly as it does with a normal contraction. The fetus is challenged, the EFM records the stressed FHR and although interpretation of FHR patterns and the appropriate course of action are not definitive, cesarean section becomes the therapy of choice. The lack of specificity of the OCT is demonstrated by studies in which women and infants with positive OCTs have, nonetheless, tolerated labor and vaginal delivery well;[96,97] as many as 25% of women and infants with positive OCTs have experienced labor without complications.[85]

Induction of labor. Induction of labor means to force labor to start. This is usually achieved by use of oxytocin given intravenously. Induction may be medically indicated (therapeutic), about which there is general consensus,[41,170] or elective.[129,171,316,342] Therapeutic induction may be for Rh incompatibility, postmaturity, and maternal diabetes; elective inductions may be for convenience, and the FDA recently banned the use of oxytocin for this purpose.[257] Although there are staunch advocates of induction for improved fetal outcome,[58,317] other physicians are cautious,[29,235] since in either case there is the risk of respiratory distress syndrome (RDS) if an immature fetus is delivered.

Studies suggest that medical judgment is not the paramount factor[266] determining the use of induction, since its use appears to vary with the days of the week. Race may also be a factor in its use; one large study showed the rate among

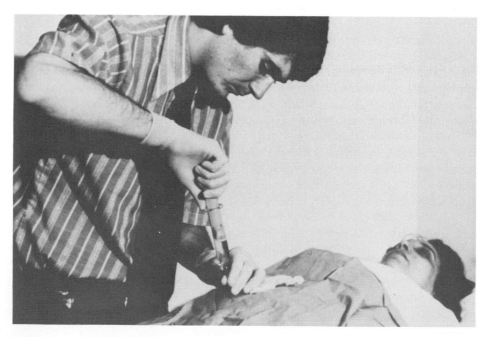

Fig. 7-3. Amniocentesis. (Courtesy Health Sciences Information Services, University of Washington, Seattle.)

white women to be double that among blacks;[233] this may, however, be more indicative of socioeconomic status.

As in the OCT, induction by oxytocin produces stronger and faster contractions, which may stress the infant. If the induction fails but the membranes have already ruptured and the cushion for the fetal head is lost, fetal stress also may occur. The risk of infection, high at any time with induction, is heightened when it fails. Another technology is then involved, since cesarean section becomes the therapy of choice in these circumstances. Another complication and another cause for use of cesarean section may come from the intensity of the contractions, which can rupture the uterus. Some women whose labor is induced also need additional pain-relieving medications, and as these cross the placenta, they may depress the system of the infant, who then shows a deceleration of heart rate on the monitor—an indication for surgical intervention.

Amniocentesis. Amniocentesis (a procedure in which amniotic fluid is removed from the uterus and sampled for genetic abnormalities) came into well-publicized use as a diagnostic technique in the early 1970s and can, with the availability of abortion, be a boon to a pregnant older woman or a woman concerned with the genetic heritage of her infant, and in determining fetal maturity through a lecithin/sphingomyelin ratio. Although widely acclaimed as safe, it is not without risk to mother and child.[55,130] Reported risks include fetomaternal hemorrhage,* fetal or maternal injury,[175] placental hemorrhage,[85] isoimmunization in the Rh-negative mother, and death to the fetus[28,205] in the event of transplacental hemorrhage associated with second trimester amniocentesis.

Diagnostic ultrasound. Diagnostic ultrasound is recognized "for the considerable contribution (it) can make to diagnosis,"[173] but the effects of it on the fetus are unknown. Although the FDA reports that preliminary animal studies do suggest abnormalities, no effects have been shown to date on the human fetus.[323] A particular hazard of this technology, however, is that ultrasound, when it is used as a tool for judging fetal growth and maturity after 20 weeks[188] can given an assessment of fetal age that is inaccurate by 5 to 6 weeks.[188] A physician may intervene surgically, believing in the accuracy of the test and therefore believing the fetus to be mature. There is a risk that the fetus will be born with respiratory distress syndrome.[83] Estimates are that about 17% of obstetrical services in the United States use diagnostic ultrasound and that about one third of all births occur in hospitals where it is used. There are also reports of routine use of ultrasound during prenatal care.[323]

Cesarean section. According to data from the National Hospital Discharge Survey (NHDS), the rate of cesarean sections has increased by 198% during the years 1968 to 1978 (see Table 7-4). For the same years the birth rate declined by 17%. The Hospital Record Study projected a rate of 13.9% for 1978, but the NHDS reported that 15.2% of deliveries were by cesarean that year.

The reasons for this rise in technological intervention in birth are complex, and I have extensively analyzed them elsewhere.[207a] Although no one factor can

---

*References 37, 67, 113, 193, 219, 277.

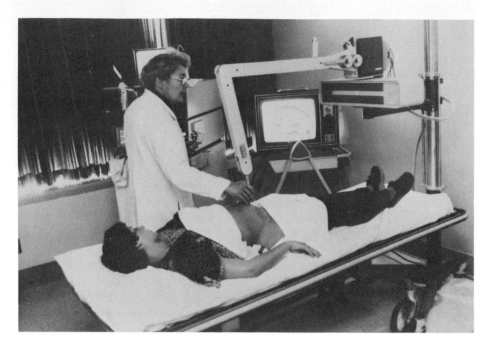

Fig. 7-4. Ultrasound. (Courtesy Health Sciences Information Services, University of Washington, Seattle.)

Table 7-4. Cesarean sections as a percentage of all deliveries, United States, 1968 to 1977*

Year	Number of cesarean sections (000)	Number of deliveries (000)	Cesarean sections (%)	Change in number of cesarean sections (%)	Change in number of deliveries (%)
1968	172	3346	5.1		
1971	194	3337	5.8	+13.7	−0.3
1972	227	3224	7.0	+20.7	−3.4
1973	246	3093	8.0	+14.3	−4.1
1974	286	3122	9.2	+15.0	+0.9
1975	328	3048	10.8	+17.4	−2.3
1976	378	3126	12.1	+12.0	+2.6
1977	455	3331	13.7	+13.2	+6.6
1978	510	3361	15.2	+10.9	+0.9

*Based on data from National Center for Health Statistics: National Hospital Discharge Survey, 1968–1977, Washington, D.C., 1977.
Data for 1969 and 1970 are unavailable because the data collection system was altered.

be pinpointed, several factors do combine interdependently and continue to keep the rate increasing.

Although each factor in this increased use of an old, possibly ancient, surgical technology, affects women differently, the overall effect of the increase is to make cesarean section a routine, expected, "normal" procedure. The many groups that provide support to cesarean parents perform a valuable service, but demonstrate the current routine nature of the use of cesarean section. Issues addressed by the group include the importance of the use of the term cesarean "birth" as opposed to "section," familial support for parents during the surgery, assistance for parents with rooming-in, breast-feeding, and the longer postpartum period, and support for the mother to overcome guilt feelings for not having delivered vaginally. All these goals are important, but they avoid the fundamental issue: is the increase in cesareans contributing to improved maternal and fetal outcome? Based on nation-wide data, the factors for this rise are presented here in order of significance for reasons of clarity, but this approach at times obscures the interaction one factor may have with another.

In my study the most frequent reason given by physicians for the increase in the cesarean section rate was fear of a malpractice suit if a cesarean was not per-formed and the outcome was a "less than perfect infant." Although studies of malpractice suits by the National Association of Insurance Commissioners,[224] the American College of Obstetricians and Gynecologists (ACOG), and ACOG District II[8] in New York do not support this fear, the incidence of even one or two claims combines with other factors to favor this particular technological develop-ment. The effect on women is that a cesarean becomes "defensive obstetrics," standard medical practice, and therefore a routine procedure for any deviation from the norm.

The Professional Activity Study (PAS) data in 1974 demonstrated that re-peat procedures comprise about one third of the indications for cesarean section in the United States and Canada. This policy of routine repeat cesarean is the second highest contributing factor to the current rate. In the 1974 PAS study, for example, only 358 females (0.9%) of a total 120, 684 had a vaginal delivery fol-lowing a previous cesarean.[199]

Despite abundant evidence both in the United States and abroad that vaginal deliveries can be successfully accomplished when the conditions warranting the first cesarean no longer exist,[211,216,222,268,285] few physicians go against standard obstetrical practice by adopting the policy of a trial of labor, fearing claims of mal-practice in the event of an adverse outcome. For women the effect is adherence to Cragin's 1916 dictum: "once a Caesarean, always a Caesarean."[66] Cornell Uni-versity Medical College for example, which for many years has had a policy of not routinely doing repeat cesarean sections, notes that fear of suits has led to a shift in the policy, with the result that the cesarean section rate has gone from 7% in 1965 to 24% in 1978.[99]

Physician training appears to be the next most important contribution to the cesarean section rate increase. During the course of data collection, a frequent reason given by physicians (and supported in the literature) for the section rate increase was that residents were not trained in normal obstetrics and were ill-prepared to manage labor. Two sources gave several examples of little to no training in many areas, including auscultation by stethoscope, external cephalic version, and vaginal breech deliveries, but in contrast, reported extensive training in usage of EFM, ultrasonic monitoring, scalp sampling, and cesarean surgery for any labor abnormalities.[114,261,347]

The fourth factor in the rate of cesarean section is that throughout the nation, physician focus has shifted from the mother to the infant—to obtaining a perfect product. As discussed earlier, the literature frequently noted and physicians stated that they believed that the increased use of cesarean section plus the widespread utilization of EFM are largely responsible for obtaining this improved product. Several studies present data that refute a causal relationship between these factors, and none at present establishes causality.*

The effect of the last two factors discussed is that there is a reliance on technology in lieu of obstetrical expertise. The technology may indeed be necessary for a safe outcome; whether it is routinely necessary is both unproved and at issue.

Changing indications, the fifth factor to be discussed, are frequently cited as a reason for the increased cesarean rate. Indications may be absolute or relative, and the data suggest that the relative indications have not really changed but rather that more women are being identified as having "old" indications. For women the effect is that more births are classified as complicated (see Chapter 1), and technological intervention is presumed warranted. In connection with this, the question must be raised as to how much a climate accepting of cesarean section in and of itself promotes more cesareans. As Douglas and others[76,140,167] have noted, when the quality of a physician's obstetrical practice was judged by how low his cesarean rate was, and when each cesarean performed had to be justified, the surgical intervention was undertaken only after considerable deliberation.

One of the difficulties in evaluating this fifth factor in the rising rate is that there are no uniform criteria for the indications for a cesarean. It is perhaps significant that the most commonly reported indications are conditions that cannot be evaluated after a delivery in the same way an EFM tracing can be assessed for signs of fetal distress which may have warranted intervention. Cephalopelvic disproportion (CPD)—which in some institutions encompasses fetopelvic disproportion (FPD)—dystocia, "failure to progress," or prolonged labor, accounted for 28% of all PAS cesareans in 1974,[199] and these appear to have become "catch-all" diagnoses. In this regard, many authors cite the declining use of forceps[61] as a reason for more cesareans yet some data suggest that use of some types of forceps and vacuum extractors is increasing.

The use of cesarean section for the indication of breech presentation has increased. In the 1974 PAS study, breech presentation was the third most common indication at 7.7%,[199] but many institutions currently report that 60% to 90% of their breech presentations are delivered by this method. Mortality data suggest that cesarean breech delivery as opposed to vaginal breech delivery does seem

---

*References 81, 125, 189, 336, 337, 341.

warranted for very small or very large babies. However, experience in other countries with successful vaginal breech delivery suggests that perhaps the superior results with cesarean delivery in the United States are due to the fact that cesarean breech data are being compared with data of vaginal breech deliveries managed by persons increasingly unskilled at such deliveries. Many physicians commented, for example, that breech presentations were more safely handled by cesarean section because few physicians had sufficient experience with vaginal breech deliveries. A discussant of a recent paper on breech management noted:

Recently, I had two breeches close together, assisted at each delivery by a first- or second-year resident. . . . I discovered that these fellows knew practically nothing about breech delivery . . . their first thought was—a breech; we do a Caesarean.

It seemed to me that that was too much science and not enough art. They knew all about ultrasonic monitoring, scalp sampling, all the ultrascientific things, but nothing about the actual technique and art of delivering a breech.[347]

Considering that breech presentations comprise only about 3% to 4% of all deliveries, paucity of experience in the face of almost universal use of cesarean section for this indication is scarcely surprising. Los Angeles County – University of Southern California Women's Hospital recently completed a study demonstrating that with careful selection, vaginal term frank breech deliveries were not associated with perinatal death. The authors noted that "although perinatal morbidity occurs with vaginal breech delivery, the significant maternal complications of elective C-section make C-section for term frank breech infants an unattractive policy."[60]

The sixth contributing factor concerns shifts in age, parity, and fertility characteristics of the childbearing population. Older women and primiparous women, both of whom have a higher risk of cesarean section, have increased in the childbearing population (see Chapter 1). For example, the number of women over 30 years of age, having their first babies, has risen from 39,500 in 1966 to 76,500 in 1977, whereas primiparous births, as a percentage of all births, have steadily increased from 34% in 1966 to 42% in 1977.[225] More women potentially at risk are therefore exposed to childbirth and the possibilities of cesareans.

The seventh factor concerns economic incentives. Although the data are consistent with other findings that economic incentive contributes to surgical rates,[39] they do not definitively establish a causal relationship. Combinations of economic factors can lead toward the more profitable—in this case, surgical—approach, and it should not be inferred that cesareans are performed in a deliberate effort to make money. A decreasing number of births, an increasing number of obstetricians (the ratio of live births per obstetrician dropped from 260.7 in 1963 to 144.9 in 1975),* third-party reimbursement, the longer length of hospital stay, the predictable time involvement in the birth, and physician fear of a malpractice suit may all combine to exert an economic influence on the rate of cesareans and

---

*Data from National Center for Health Statistics: Vital statistics of the United States, vol. 1, 1977; and American Medical Association: Distribution of physicians in the United States, 1963-1975. (See also Miller, C. A. in Additional Readings.)

to decrease incentives to persist with a vaginal delivery in the face of any complications. For women the effects of this factor are higher financial outlay: a cesarean section costs approximately two-thirds more than a vaginal delivery.

The particular effects of specific obstetrical technologies and their relationship to cesarean section have already been discussed. Although inexperience with these technologies undoubtedly leads to some false positive findings, and subsequent cesareans[241] (see also literature on EFM), the data suggest that the use of technology is in and of itself conducive to using more technology and that cesareans are a logical outcome of this perspective.

Other factors contributing to the rising rate are the availability of technology for the salvage of tiny (1000 to 2500 g) babies, for the medical management of women with severe physical conditions so that they can carry an infant to term, and the increase in herpes II. In most circumstances the presence of any of these conditions is indication for cesarean section.

The concept of informed consent has been cited as providing protection for the woman from unwanted technology. Such protection is particularly pertinent in the case of cesarean birth. With cesarean birth the maternal mortality is estimated to be 1 per 1000 live births as opposed to 11.2 per 100,000 for all live births in 1977. Morbidity and general discomfort are much higher than with vaginal delivery, and the risk of respiratory distress syndrome in an immature infant is great. The cost and length of stay may be double that with a vaginal delivery.* The assertion that women are protected by the requirement of informed consent ignores the practice of many hospitals and physicians of insisting, for example, on EFM. It also does not take into account that no matter how well informed of risks and benefits she may be, a woman confronted with the statement, "What we will do will save you or your baby" is in a dilemma. When pressured to accept EFM, induced labor, amniocentesis, or a cesarean section during pregnancy, labor, or delivery, she is unlikely to refuse. The intimation that "women want the security"† of obstetrical technology should be considered from this perspective.

Birthing rooms. Many women are opting for a change from prevailing technological birth and decide to deliver at a birth center, at home (see Chapter 2), or in a hospital-based birthing room. Although it may seem inappropriate to consider birthing rooms (combination labor and delivery rooms) in hospitals in this discussion of obstetrical technology, they are, in fact, a technological answer to technology.

Birthing rooms and birth centers strive to create a homelike atmosphere, promote early discharge, and encourage bonding[176] between parents and infant. Father and other family members (rarely children) in attendance, cheerful surroundings, a comfortable bed, and a relaxed atmosphere are uniform characteristics. Many birthing rooms use a minimum of obstetrical interventions, avoiding,

---

*References 40, 70, 86, 168, 199, 256, 281, 295.
†See *Patient Care*, Feb. 15, 1978, and Feb. 28, 1978; and Testimony of the American College of Obstetrics and Gynecology on current obstetrical practice in the United States before the Subcommittee on Health and Scientific Research, U.S. Senate Committee on Human Resources, April 17, 1978.

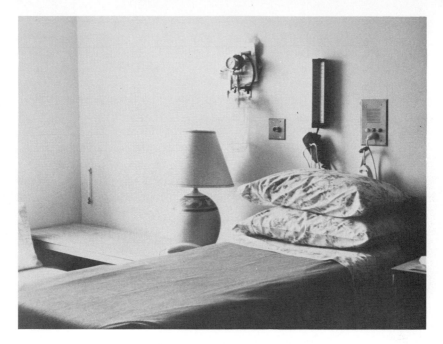

Fig. 7-5. Birthing room. (Courtesy M. A. Maurer.)

for example, shaving, enemas, EFM, episiotomy, and analgesia. Midwives are often in attendance. Delivery usually takes place with the woman flat on a large bed. Emergency equipment is on hand but is not routinely used. Many birthing rooms, however (perhaps because of fear of malpractice suits), use prevailing obstetrical technology but in a homelike manner, permitting family member attendance and encouraging bonding.[9,307,308,319]

Birthing rooms and birth centers have come about as a result of consumer demand and an economic response to a declining birthrate and underused obstetrical facilities—they make sense in terms of economic benefit and consumer satisfaction. Generally, one effect is to provide a cheaper delivery. Another effect on women, however, is perhaps to obscure the issue of the appropriateness of obstetrical technology. By emphasizing needs for intimacy and emotional warmth surrounding childbirth, the fundamental issue of whether obstetrical technology contributes to the goal of optimal maternal and infant outcome—surely the purpose of obstetrical management—remains untested and unquestioned.

MAMMOGRAPHY
Historical background

Because breast cancer is the leading cause of death among women 40 to 44 years of age, and because the average American woman has 1 chance in 14 of developing breast cancer at some time in her life, this disease in particular has been the subject of many technological developments for screening, diagnosis, and treatment.

Mammography is a procedure that usually involves two to three x-ray examinations of each breast and may be used both as a screening procedure and as a diagnostic tool. There is little controversy over the latter clinical application; substantial controversy exists over the use of mammography as a screening technique.

Following the first use of mammography in 1913, the technique was gradually improved and was in widespread use by the 1960s. After studies at the M. D. Anderson Hospital in Houston during the 1960s, mammography was found to have a false positive rate of 7% and a false negative rate of 6%; its use as a screening technique was established.[18,56] Further study supported this course of action, and the research of Shapiro et al. in the mid-1960s (the HIP study) was believed to confirm by controlled clinical trial, at least for women over 50, that "repetitive screening with clinical examination and mammography leads to at least a short term reduction in mortality from breast cancer."[294] They found that in the 7-year study of 60,000 women, there were 70 deaths from breast cancer in the study group as compared with 108 breast cancer deaths in the control group.

Current controversy

Recently the risk-benefit ratio of mammography has been questioned,[16] although some researchers remain convinced of its efficacy.[213] The controversy focuses on whether the amount of radiation to which an asymptomatic woman under 50 is exposed through routine screening mammography presents a cancer risk itself, a risk that exceeds the benefit of possibly detecting an unknown cancerous condition. To settle the controversy, three expert committees were appointed in 1976 by the National Cancer Institute (NCI) and the American Cancer Society (ACS).[35,312,322] Their functions were to review the HIP mid-1960s data and other epidemiology and statistics to decide whether radiation to the breast is carcinogenic and to study the pathology of breast cancer.

Deciding that in large enough dosage (and most observers report excessive radiation dose in community use) radiation could cause cancer, the three groups together made the following recommendations[324]:

1. Rigorous attempts should be made to keep radiation dose under 1 rad per screening examination
2. Mammography for routine screening of women under 50 years of age should be discontinued
3. The NCI should support a clinical trial of mammography to furnish more conclusive evidence of its usefulness

As a result of these reports, the NCI and the ACS restrained the use of mammography in the Breast Cancer Diagnosis Demonstration Projects (BCDDP). These projects, which they had pushed through in 1973 over many objections of NCI experts (as evidenced by files obtained under the Freedom of Information Act),[79,121] were now instructed to use mammographic screening on women with personal or family histories of breast cancer and were advised that currently the project's directors could not "recommend the routine use of mammography in screening asymptomatic women ages 35 to 50."[90] Since beginning in 1973, the BCDDP has reportedly involved some 270,000 women ranging in age

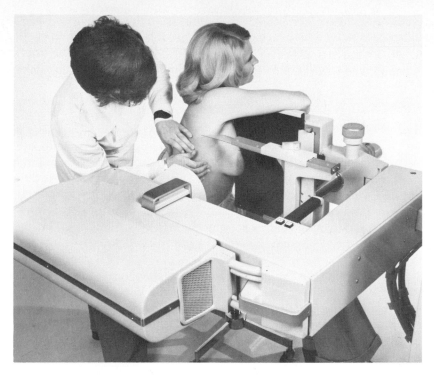

Fig. 7-6. Mammography. (Courtesy General Electric.)

from 35 to 74 years from 29 participating screening centers nationwide. The total cost in fiscal year 1977 was $9.5 million; by 1976, about 1800 cases of breast cancer had been discovered at an approximate cost of $11,000 per case.[18]

For women the effect of this technology again has been to expose them to a relatively hastily studied procedure, which, although recent improvements may make the radiation exposure safer, is nonetheless of questionable or no benefit to hundreds of asymptomatic women under 50 years of age with no family history of breast cancer. Possibly, hundreds of thousands of women have been needlessly exposed; since the publicity of breast cancer in 1974 from Ford and Rockefeller, many women, in addition to the 270,000 in the BCDDP study, have sought breast cancer detection. There may also have been unnecessary surgery as a result of the false positive rates and/or the exposure. Over physician objections, the NCI insisted that women operated on be told,[46,57] although after subsequent legal opinion was obtained, it was decided that informing women would be left to the individual physicians responsible.[182] There is the additional financial cost, especially since mammography for screening as opposed to diagnostic purposes, is not normally covered by third-party payment. Also, there is now the anxiety of women not knowing what is in the best interests of their health.

The controversy remains unsettled and is equaled by debates over which type of breast cancer surgery[4] ensures the greatest longevity and the value of breast self-examination.[95,122,221] New screening techniques for breast cancer, an immunological skin test[11] and a coagulation blood test,[231] are being developed and reported in the popular press. Although these methods may be potentially less risky, the experience with and controversy about mammography underscores the need for caution.

PAPANICOLAOU (PAP) SMEAR
Historical background

The Pap smear was developed in 1943 by George N. Papanicolaou and is designed to detect early cancer of the cervix by examining tissue scrapings from the cervix and cervical os. Widely accepted when first introduced, the Pap test received massive publicity when the ACS sponsored the first interdisciplinary conference in 1945 and pushed for the establishment of cytology screening programs and cancer detection centers nationwide.[34] In 1957 "Uterine Cancer Year" was launched by the ACS, and the annual use of the Pap test was widely publicized.

By 1973, the National Center for Health Statistics figures indicated that "75 percent of U.S. women over the age of 17 had had a Pap smear at least once and nearly half had had one in the year prior to the survey."[18] Today, federally funded health agencies mandate annual Pap tests on women requesting family planning services, and Foltz and Kelsey[93] report that in many parts of the country, hospitals are required to carry out a Pap test on any woman admitted who has not had one during the previous 3 years.

Current controversy

When the Pap test was first introduced, its accuracy was not questioned. No efforts were made to conduct randomized clinical trials, and as one researcher noted, "now because of its widespread acceptance as a diagnostic tool, it is no longer possible to do so."[293] Accuracy of the test is today one aspect of the controversy, together with debate over the natural course of the disease and the efficacy of Pap test screening in lowering cervical cancer mortality rates.

Accuracy of the Pap test has been stated at 95% by the ACS,[6] but as Banta and Behney[18] note, "in any condition with a low prevalence, such as cancer of the cervix, this statistic can hide a proportion of missed lesions (false negatives rate)." Furthermore, they note that cytologists also interpret tests differently, and this variable also affects accuracy.

Pap test results are generally reported in five classes ranging from class I (normal) to class V (invasive carcinoma). These are presumed to correspond to the stages of cervical cancer, but there is some evidence to suggest that these classes may not represent the true progression of the disease.[155,203,279,303]

Efficacy, which could be established only by a controlled clinical trial, has not been proved, it being argued that it is unethical to deny the "well-known benefits" to some women in order to have controls. Moreover, the time intervals at which Pap smears should be performed to be efficacious are also not established, and there is wide variation, particularly in countries other than the United States. On the other hand, it can be argued that it is unethical to continue presuming efficacy and a 95% accuracy rate, promoting a policy of an annual Pap smear with its subsequent treatment costs, both financial and physical, without incontrovertible evidence that the Pap test is to women's benefit. Apparently the ACS has now had second thoughts because in early 1980 they recommended "all women over 20 and sexually active women under 20 to have the test at three-year intervals once they have had two negative tests a year apart."[214a]

INFANT FORMULAS
Historical background

In most cultures breast-feeding is the normal practice. In the nineteenth and early twentieth centuries it was also the norm in the United States, done either by the mother herself, if she was from the lower or middle class, or by a wet-nurse if the mother was wealthy. As the supply of wet-nurses diminished (more money could be earned in factories) and as cow's milk was introduced with apparent success for feeding abandoned babies, wealthy families turned to bottle-feeding. This method soon acquired status and prestige, and as changing social expectations made it increasingly more difficult for women to breast-feed, bottle-feeding became the norm.

Difficulties that infants experienced with cow's milk were soon said to be counteracted by the development of infant formulas. Claimed to be "just like mother's milk," formulas are in fact different.[128,160] By 1956 La Leche League International had formed and sought to counteract the hard-sell tactics of the formula companies. It provided support and encouragement for mothers who wanted to nurse and was soon joined by tropical pediatric nutritionists who were concerned at the increase in infant marasmus and diarrhea in Third World countries where formula was being marketed.[159] Today breast-feeding is regaining popularity, particularly among well-educated urban women; at best, however, only 30% of North American women breast-feed.

Current controversy

There is presently controversy about the influence of the formula manufacturers and the reticence, until recently, of a major group in organized medicine to state their whole-hearted support for breast-feeding. In October, 1978, the American Academy of Pediatrics issued a policy stating that unless the child or mother has some specific prohibitive condition, all babies should be breast-fed.[62] Despite the pediatricians' statement, the obstetricians, who through prenatal care and delivery have significant maternal contact and could influence a mother's breast-feeding decision, have failed as an organization to take such a stand.

The benefits to the infant of human milk and breast-feeding are numerous, including the provision of protection against infection, antiallergic properties, balanced nutrition, and mother-baby interaction.[47,111,161,208] Breast-feeding is also economical, hygienic, and has contraceptive effects, and, if the mother is adequately nourished, milk is readily available.

Although decried by the World Health Organization and other international agencies, use of infant formula is still gaining ground. Employing tactics such as use of free promotional samples, massive advertising, "milk nurses" in uniforms who are really salespersons, and hospital promotional visits, major formula manufacturers have been charged with the responsibility for increasing infant mortality in the Third World. The effect of convincing women to use formula has been the abandonment of breast-feeding in an environment where contaminated water, extreme poverty that prevents purchase of adequate formula supplies, illiteracy, and poor sanitation make life-sustaining formula use an impossibility. In North America where bottle-feeding is a possibility, the health advantages of breast-feeding for both mother and infant have been obscured.

OTHER TECHNOLOGICAL INNOVATIONS
Pregnancy self-testing kit

The early pregnancy test (e.p.t.), a self-testing kit, using the immunological method for detecting human chorionic gonadotropin, was first distributed on a limited basis in the United States in 1976. Not subject to FDA approval because it was developed prior to the ruling governing the FDA's Bureau of Medical Devices, the test is marketed as a "private little revolution any woman can easily buy at her drugstore."[84] Although the test comes with clear instructions, is easy to use, and provides opportunities for women to determine their pregnancies in private, thereby affording them a degree of control over their anatomy, it may not be the "revolution" it is advertised to be. At present it is relatively expensive (dearer than tests at many clinics and Planned Parenthood facilities), is good for only one test, and, more important, even according to the manufacturers, has a high false negative rate (20%), especially with very early tests. On the other hand, the test has a 97% true positive rate and its use enables women to initiate proper self- and prenatal care very early in pregnancy.[36,214,253]

In vitro fertilization

In England in July, 1978, the first baby was born as a result of in vitro fertilization and reimplantation of an egg into the mother's uterus. Reports of such births in India, Scotland, and Australia soon followed. The infants are popularly termed "test-tube babies." Their births were said to have raised the hopes of the approximately 15% of couples who are involuntarily childless.

Many issues have been raised by this event, both in the popular press and in government hearings.[150,210,327] One question has been the extent to which the artificial process of this technological feat may be extended. For example, critics fear that a "rent-a-womb concept" may develop in which a couple's embryo would be implanted in the uterus of a second woman, not unlike the "surrogate mother" situation in which an unrelated woman is impregnated by the male partner of a couple and carries their child to term.[338] Concerns have been voiced about the possibility that in vitro fertilization would be used by single women (Women's Liberation members in particular were cited) "to achieve a child without a man"[327] or by lesbian women, already said to use artificial insemination, both self-administered and physician assisted.[68,191]

Equally of concern to critics is the potential that in the attempt to duplicate the delicate conception and implantation processes, genetic errors may occur.

Because of the impossibility of providing animal models to test the in vitro fertilization process, opponents stress that women will be experimented on by stimulation of their ovaries to release fertilizable eggs and of their uteri to receive the products of conception.[78] (Both processes reportedly have been abandoned by the main developers, Drs. Steptoe and Edwards of England.) It is said the children so produced are also the subjects of experimentation.[150] Critics also argue that the process introduces the possibility of genetic engineering.[119]

Another concern centers on the issue of when life begins and questions the disposition of unneeded or defective fertilized eggs. Proponents of in vitro fertilization argue that nature discards possibly up to 50% of embryos in the earliest stages of development. Proponents also believe that in vitro fertilization will make possible studies on congenital anomalies and disease transmission.

A National Ethics Advisory Board of seven physicians, three attorneys, and one clergyman has been formed by the National Institutes of Health (NIH) and in mid-March of 1979 decided that general support for in vitro research is acceptable from an ethical standpoint under certain specified circumstances for specified purposes. Research had been prohibited by an NIH ban in August, 1975, and was strengthened by the Buckley Amendment to the 1974 National Research Act, which denied Department of Health, Education and Welfare financial support of "research on living human fetuses, before or after abortion."[119]

Vaginal surgery

Surgery on the sexual organs of women is not a new technological innovation. The sexual surgery prevalent in the United States in the late eighteenth and early nineteenth centuries has been extensively studied, and the medical literature of that era indicates it was generally believed to be a cure for many "women's problems."[20] (See Chapter 1.) Various types of female genital operations—circumcision, excision, infibulation, and introcision—are still documented as being practiced in parts of Africa, Central and South America, Asia, and Australia, and among the Skoptsi (or Circumcisers), a Russian sect in Europe.[141,149,197,292,328]

In the United States sexual surgery, exclusive of hysterectomy (see Chapter 1), is generally no longer practiced. Clitoridectomy (removal of the clitoris) a type of sexual surgery first performed in the United States to cure a woman's "mental disorder," was probably last performed in 1925; circumcision (removal of the hood of the clitoris) continued to be performed for similar reasons at least until 1937.[20, Chapter 11] Recently the medical news literature has reported that an Ohio gynecologist, Dr. James C. Burt, claims to have perfected a new variation of sexual surgery that involves female circumcision and vaginal reconstruction "to make the clitoris more accessible to direct penile stimulation." The purpose is to enable a woman to have more frequent and intense orgasms. Dr. Burt is reportedly avoided (but not disciplined) by his colleagues, who cite his lack of publications on the matter in scientific journals and his lack of controlled studies proving efficacy. Also, sex therapists are angered by his resorting to surgery rather than "recommending the more benign remedy of counseling." Nonetheless, Dr. Burt has reportedly performed the operation "in all stages of its evolution—starting with a minor variation of standard episiotomy repair—on some 4000 women."[101]

SELECTED INTERNATIONAL PERSPECTIVES
Contraception

About 60 million women use the Pill worldwide, although the extent of total contraceptive utilization is difficult to assess. Millions of couples, for example, rely solely on coitus interruptus. Some data are available, however, on the distribution of contraceptives by international population agencies. These agencies include the International Planned Parenthood Federation, supported in part by the Victor Fund and the Victor-Bostrom Fund; the Population Council; Population Services International; the United Nations Fund for Population; the Ford and Rockefeller foundations; the United States Agency for International Development (USAID); and other individual countries' international aid programs such as the Swedish International Development Authority (SIDA). In addition, there are the multinational drug companies, the extent of whose sales to the public through pharmacies in various countries is unknown.

From 1965 to 1977, USAID obligated $1.8 million for population and health programs worldwide. This amount included the purchase of contraceptives for international distribution since 1967, when they were removed from USAID's list of "ineligible commodities." From 1968 to 1972 about $9.3 million was spent by USAID on the Pill, $4.0 million on condoms, $2.0 million on foam, $1.2 million on IUDs and inserters, $1.4 million on medical kits, and $500,000 on creams, diaphragms, and other related items.[262] From 1970 to 1972 the SIDA purchased for distribution 19.9 million cycles of contraceptive pills and 1.95 million gross of condoms.[246]

Underlying the work of international population agencies is the belief that control of population growth must go hand in hand with economic development for the latter to be successful. Critics argue that the goal of population agencies is simply to curb growth in developing countries so that inequities in distribution of the wealth both within each country and between the rich and developing nations, need not be addressed.

Potential markets for contraceptive users seem almost boundless, as evidenced by a 1971 survey which showed that of 46.5 million potential users in Iran, Korea, the Philippines, Thailand, Turkey, and Venezuela, actual users ranged from a low of 7.3% in Turkey to a high of 31.1% in Korea.[246] Despite the health risks, marketing of contraceptives is also aided around the world by less stringent prescription requirements than those in the United States. According to a 1973 survey of 45 developing countries, 26 countries legally required a physician's prescription for the Pill, but in 12 of those countries it was "readily" available over the counter and in 10 others was "sometimes" available. No prescription was required in 19 countries, and in 18 of those, over-the-counter Pills were "readily available."[27a]

Obstetrical technology in selected countries

Although still far behind the United States as users of obstetrical technology, several countries traditionally known for their low rates of obstetrical intervention[127] (and their low rates of maternal and infant mortality and morbidity) are beginning to experience an upward trend in those rates. Rates for use of

EFM, vacuum extractors, induction, and cesarean section are inching upward and for many of the same reasons as in the United States. Increasing availability of technology may be promoting its use. For example, Hewlett-Packard, a major manufacturer of the electronic fetal monitor, estimated that by 1978, 5200 of their products would be in use worldwide.[207a] In addition, the incidence of induced labors in England and Wales rose from 16.8% in 1967 to 38.9% in 1974. In Norway the data show an increase from 11% in 1967 to 14.8% in 1975.[52] Incidences of other obstetrical interventions are given in Tables 7-5 to 7-7 and, along with other

Table 7-5. Instrumental deliveries as a percentage of all deliveries, selected nations, 1968 to 1975*

	1968	1969	1970	1971	1972	1973	1974	1975
United States	37.6	40.6	38.6	38.2	37.3	36.3	35.1	33.5
Canada	10.2	11.8	13.4	14.6	15.9	15.5	16.4	16.7
England and Wales	7.0	7.5	7.9	8.2	10.3	10.5	NA	NA
Norway	2.8	2.8	3.2	3.6	3.7	4.1	4.3	4.9
Netherlands	2.3	2.4	2.7	3.3	3.4	3.8	4.1	4.9

*Based on data from Chalmers, I., and Richards, M. in Chard, T., and Richards, M., editors: Benefits and hazards of the new obstetrics, Philadelphia, 1977, J. B. Lippincott Co.

Table 7-6. Vacuum extractions as a percentage of all instrumental deliveries, selected nations, 1968 to 1975*

	1968	1969	1970	1971	1972	1973	1974	1975
United States	0.2	0.2	0.3	0.2	0.2	0.4	0.4	0.6
Canada	1.1	0.9	1.2	1.2	0.6	0.4	0.9	0.9
England and Wales	7.1	8.0	7.6	7.3	5.8	6.6	NA	NA
Norway	46.4	50.0	53.1	58.3	62.2	63.4	67.4	70.5
Netherlands	65.2	70.8	74.1	69.7	67.6	68.4	70.7	71.4

*Based on data from Chalmers, I., and Richards, M. in Chard, T., and Richards, M., editors: Benefits and hazards of the new obstetrics, Philadelphia, 1977, J. B. Lippincott Co.

Table 7-7. Cesarean sections as a percentage of all deliveries, selected nations, 1968 to 1975*†

	1968	1969	1970	1971	1972	1973	1974	1975
United States	5.0	NA	NA	5.6	6.7	7.5	8.7	9.9
Canada	4.8	5.1	5.7	6.4	7.2	8.0	9.0	NA
England and Wales	4.0	4.4	4.3	4.6	4.9	5.0	NA	NA
Norway	2.0	2.0	2.2	2.5	2.6	3.0	3.7	4.1
Netherlands	1.8	2.0	2.0	2.1	2.3	2.5	2.6	3.0

*Based on data from Chalmers I., and Richards, M. in Chard, T., and Richards, M., editors: Benefits and hazards of the new obstetrics, Philadelphia, 1977, J. B. Lippincott Co.
†In addition, in the United States in 1978 the rate was 15.2%[207a] and in the Netherlands it was 2.8% in 1977.[177]

data, indicate a marked preference by European countries for using vacuum extractors in lieu of forceps in instrumental deliveries.

Pap smear

Use of the Pap smear has not been as extensive in other countries as it has in the United States. This is not necessarily because of lack of funds, although costs of detecting a case of cervical cancer are such that a cost-benefit ranking of health services would preclude this service in many countries. A 1976 study by the ACS, Connecticut Division, for example, estimated that the cost per case of cancer detected was $3322;[7] in 1968 a British survey estimated that the cost of preventing a clinical carcinoma would be £1000.[179]

In Britain concerns have been voiced that unjustified hysterectomies have occurred because of improperly read specimens, and enthusiasm for the test has continued to be moderate.[38] Rather than advocating annual Pap tests, physicians have recommended that tests be given less frequently because they are thus more cost effective. Suggested frequencies range from once every 5 years, as in Aberdeen, Scotland, where a study demonstrated that mortality from cervical cancer seemed to be declining,[202] to a series of 10 tests given beginning at age 35 until age 80.[178]

In Canada doubts about the efficacy of the Pap test culminated in a 1976 government report known as the Walton Report.[45] On the basis of evidence as to effectiveness, availability, accuracy, and costs, the report recommended annual Pap tests only for high-risk women, defined as those having low income and multiple sex partners and who began sexual activity at an early age. For women at low risk and with negative smears, two tests 12 months apart were recommended, then tests at 3-year intervals until age 35, and then tests at 5-year intervals until age 60. Despite strong disagreement from obstetricians and gynecologists in Canada, the Walton Report's recommendations were publicized to Canadian women.

• • •

The various technologies reviewed in this chapter—contraception, estrogens, obstetrical procedures, mammography, the Pap test, formulas, pregnancy self-testing kits, in vitro fertilization, and vaginal surgery—all have characteristics in common. They were hastily developed and highly visibly marketed. Their widespread use is the result of the socially conditioned vulnerability of women and the prointervention conditioning of physicians, not the objective scientific evaluation of long-term controlled studies or persistent epidemiological research. At least for women in the United States, who have many less harmful alternatives, the data suggest that the impact of the technologies discussed here and the extent of their use, although helpful to some, has not in the main been positive.

SUGGESTED TOPICS FOR DISCUSSION, FURTHER RESEARCH, AND FIELD PROJECTS

1. How have developments in health technology changed the way in which women relate to the health system and their expectations of the outcomes of health care? What differences are there between expectations of outcome and real outcome related to

changes in health technology? Some suggested areas include EFM, cesarean section, Pap tests, breast examinations, mammography and other radiation therapy, and chemotherapy.

2. What effects, if any, have changes in medical technology had on employment of women, either in the health fields or in general?

3. Research the incidence of cesarean section in your local hospitals. Is routine repeat cesarean surgery a policy in these hospitals? If there are policies of individual evaluation, what have been the outcomes? Are mates allowed to attend a cesarean delivery?

4. Research natural birth control methods, for example, the Billings mucous method, rhythm, and herbal contraceptives. Evaluate these against the criteria discussed in the chapter. How do these rate compared with more traditional contraceptives? What factors would you need to consider in educating on natural birth control methods? Identify risks in natural birth control methods.

5. What are the factors that have led to the definition of menopause as a disease? Interview a sample of menopausal women. How did they feel about menopause? Was it as traumatic as medical journal advertisements indicate? What symptoms did they have? How were these treated? What alternatives to estrogen replacement therapy are there?

6. Select an example of new technology such as in vitro fertilization, amniocentesis to detect fetal congenital defects or sex and preconception efforts to determine fetal sex. What are the ethical issues involved? How should these ethical issues be managed and through what social structure? What effects could these technologies have on society at large?

7. Discuss the implications of adoption in the United States of a policy on Pap test frequency similar to that in England and Canada (i.e., not as a routine annual screen for all adult women).

8. Research the history of obstetrical technology, including the early development of obstetrical instruments. Are there any social factors in common between historical and contemporary periods in which major technological developments have occurred?

9. Would you agree with those who have suggested that there should be different factors used to consider the respective values of certain technologies—for example, contraceptive and obstetrical technologies—in the United States and in the Third World countries? If so, what are the differences?

10. What does the statement "A medicolegal climate can foster the growth and use of technology" mean? Select one aspect of women's health care and discuss the implications of this statement.

REFERENCES

1. Adams, D. B., et al.: Rise in female initiated sexual activity at ovulation and its suppression by oral contraceptives, N. Engl. J. Med. **299:**1145-1150, Nov. 23, 1978.

2. Adli, A. G., et al.: A study of the long-term effect of the intrauterine contraceptive device, Wis. Med. J. **73:**562, 1974.

3. Alderman, M., editor: Monitor every patient in labor? Patient Care **12:**136-163, Feb. 28, 1978.

4. Alpert, L.: Approaches to breast cancer—a pathologist's perspective, Women & Health **4:**269-286, Fall, 1979.

5. Amato, J. C.: Fetal monitoring in a community hospital: a statistical analysis, Obstet. Gynecol. **50:**269-274, Sept., 1977.

6. American Cancer Society: '76 Cancer facts and figures, New York, 1975, American Cancer Society.

7. American Cancer Society, Connecticut Division: Cytology services in Connecticut, 1970-1974, Woodbridge, Conn., 1976, American Cancer Society.

8. American College of Obstetricians & Gynecologists, District II (N.Y.), John F. Dwyer, Chairperson: Personal communication, May 31, 1978.

9. Anonymous: Hospitals bow to couples

wanting special births, Medical World News **18**:38-39, Oct. 3, 1977.

10. Anonymous: Contraceptive sponge fights V.D. too, Medical World News **18**:29, Oct. 17, 1977.

11. Anonymous: Cancer skin test, Newsweek, p. 121, April 17, 1978.

12. Anonymous: Under the skin, People **5**:36-37, 1978.

13. Antler, J.: Letters on maternity from Julia Lathrop, Women & Health **2**:48-49, Sept./Oct., 1977.

14. Aptekar, H.: Anjea, infanticide, abortion and contraception in savage society, New York, 1931, William Godwin.

15. Associated Press: Firm develops birth control drug for dogs, The Seattle Times, p. C. 11, June 29, 1978.

16. Bailar, J. C.: Mammography: a time for caution, J.A.M.A. **237**:997-998, 1977.

17. Banks, J. A., and Banks, O.: Feminism and family planning in Victorian England, New York, 1974, Schocken Books, Inc.

18. Banta, H. D., and Behney, C.: Assessing the efficacy and safety of medical technologies, Office of Technology Assessment, U.S. Congress, stock no. 052-003-00593-0, Washington, D.C., Sept. 1978, U.S. Government Printing Office.

19. Banta, H. D., and Thacker, S. B.: Costs and benefits of electronic fetal monitoring: a review of the literature, National Center for Health Services Research, (PHS) 79-3245, Washington, D.C., Dec., 1978, U.S. Government Printing Office.

20. Barker-Benfield, G. J. (Ben): Horrors of the half-known life, New York, 1976, Harper & Row, Publishers, Inc.

21. Bart, P., and Grossman, M.: Menopause, Women & Health **1**:3-10, May/June, 1976.

22. Beard, R. W., et al.: Intensive care of high risk fetus in labour, J. Obstet. Gynaecol. British Commonwealth **78**:882-893, 1971.

23. Beard, R. W., et al.: The significance of the changes in the continuous fetal heart rate in the first stage of labor, J. Obstet. Gynaecol. British Commonwealth **78**:865, Oct., 1971.

24. Berendes, H. W.: Testimony before the subcommittee on administrative practice and procedure, Committee on the Judiciary, U.S. Senate, Jan. 21, 1976.

25. Bernstein, G. S., et al.: Clinical experience with the Cu-7 intrauterine device, Contraception **6**:100-107, Aug. 1972.

26. Bibbo, M., et al.: Follow-up study of the male and female offspring of DES treated mothers: a preliminary report, J. Reprod. Med. **15**:29-37, 1975.

27. Bibbo, M., et al.: A twenty-five year follow-up study of women exposed to diethylstilbestrol during pregnancy, N. Engl. J. Med. **298**:763-767, April 6, 1978.

27a. Black, T. R. L.: Oral contraceptive prescription requirements and commercial availability in 45 developing countries, Stud. Fam. Plann. **5**:250-254, Aug., 1974.

28. Blajchman, M. A., et al.: Diagnostic amniocentesis and fetal maternal bleeding (letter), Lancet **1**:993, May 11, 1974.

29. Bonnar, J.: Selective induction of labour, Br. Med. J. **1**:651-652, 1976.

30. Boria, M. C., and Gordon, M.: Complications for intrauterine devices, J. Reprod. Med. **41**:251-255, 1975.

31. Bowe, E. T., et al.: Reliability of fetal blood sampling, maternal-fetal relationships, Am. J. Obstet. Gynecol. **107**:279-287, May 15, 1970.

32. Bracken, M. B., et al.: Role of oral contraception in congenital malformations of offspring, Int. J. Epidemiol. (In press.)

33. Bremner, W. J., and deKretser, D. M.: The prospects for new, reversible male contraceptives, N. Engl. J. Med. **295**:1111-1117, Nov. 11, 1976.

34. Breslow, L.: A history of cancer control in the U.S. with emphasis on the period 1946-1971, Los Angeles, 1977, University of California at Los Angeles School of Public Health.

35. Breslow, L.: Report of NCI ad hoc working group on the gross and net benefits of mammography in mass screening for the detection of breast cancer, J. National Cancer Institute **59**:475-478, Aug., 1977.

36. Brody, J. E.: Personal health, New York Times, Feb. 1, 1978.

37. Broome, D. L., et al.: Needle puncture of fetus: a complication of second trimester amniocentesis, Am. J. Obstet. Gynecol. **126**:247-252, Sept. 15, 1976.

38. Brudnell, M., et al.: The management of dysplasia, carcinoma in situ and micro-carcinoma of the cervix, J. Obstet. Gynaecol. British Commonwealth **8**:673-679, 1973.

39. Bunker, J. P.: Surgical manpower: a comparison of operations and surgeons in the United States and in England and Wales, N. Engl. J. Med. **282**:135-144, 1970.

40. Caesarean section and respiratory distress syndrome, Br. Med. J. **1**:978-979, April 24, 1976.

41. Caldeyro-Barcia, R.: Elective induction of labor: advantages and disadvantages, testimony to the Sub-Committee on Health of the U.S. Senate, April 17, 1978.

42. Caldeyro-Barcia, R., et al.: Effects of position changes on the intensity and frequency of uterine contractions during labor, Am. J. Obstet. Gynecol. **80**:284-290, Aug., 1960.

43. Caldeyro-Barcia, R., et al.: Control of the human fetal heart rate during labor. In Cassels, D. E., editor: The heart and circulation in the newborn infant, New York, 1966, Grune & Stratton, Inc.

44. Caldeyro-Barcia, R., et al.: A new approach to the treatment of acute intrapartum fetal distress. In Perinatal factors affecting human development, Sci. Pub. no. 185:248-253, Washington, D.C., 1969, Pan American Health Organization.

45. Canadian Task Force Cervical Cancer Screening (Walton Report), Can. Med. Assoc. J. **114**:1003-1033, 1976.

46. "Cancers" were benign—but patients' breasts are gone, Medical World News **18:**22, Oct. 17, 1977.

47. Cantrelle, P., and Leridon, H.: Breastfeeding, mortality and fertility in a rural zone of Senegal, Population Studies **25:**505-533, 1971.

48. Cates, W., Jr., et al.: The intrauterine device and deaths from spontaneous abortion, N. Engl. J. Med. **295:**1155-1159, Nov. 18, 1976.

49. Center for Disease Control: IUD safety: report of a nationwide physician survey, Morbidity and Mortality Weekly Report **26:**226, 231, July 5, 1974.

50. Center for Disease Control: Increased risk of hepatocellular adenoma in women with long-term use of oral contraception, Morbidity and Mortality Weekly Report **26:**293-294, Sept. 9, 1977.

51. Cetrulo, C. L., and Schifrin, B. S.: Fetal heart rate patterns preceding death in utero, Obstet. Gynecol. **48:**521-527, Nov., 1976.

52. Chalmers, I., and Richards, M.: Intervention and causal inference in obstetric practice. In Chard, T., and Richards, M., editors: Benefits and hazards of the new obstetrics, Philadelphia, 1977, J. B. Lippincott Co.

53. Chan, W. H., et al.: Intrapartum fetal monitoring, maternal and fetal morbidity and perinatal mortality, Obstet. Gynecol. **41:**7-13, Jan., 1973.

54. Chard, T., and Richards, M., editors: Benefits and hazards of the new obstetrics, Philadelphia, 1977, J. B. Lippincott Co.

55. Chayen, S., editor: An assessment of the hazards of amniocentesis, Br. J. Obstet. Gynaecol. **85**(suppl. II):1-41, 1978.

56. Clark, R. L., et al.: Reproducibility of the technic of mammography (Egan) for cancer of the breast, Am. J. Surg. **109:**127-133, Feb., 1965.

57. Cohn, V.: Victims will be notified of breast surgery errors, The Washington Post, Oct. 28, 1977.

58. Cole, R. A., et al.: Elective induction of labor: a randomized prospective trial, Lancet **1:**767-770, 1975.

59. Collaborative Group for the Study of Stroke in Young Women: Oral contraception and increased risk of cerebral ischemia or thrombosis, N. Engl. J. Med. **228:**871-878, April 26, 1973.

60. Collea, J. V., et al.: The randomized management of term frank breech presentation. Vaginal delivery vs. cesarean section, Am. J. Obstet. Gynecol. **131:**186-195, May 15, 1978.

61. Commission on Hospital and Professional Activities: Data from hospital record study, personal communication, March, 1978.

62. Committee on Nutrition, American Academy of Pediatrics: Breast feeding, Pediatrics **62:**591, Oct., 1978.

63. Concerned Rush Students: A critical look at the drug industry, New York, 1975, Health/PAC.

64. Corea, G.: The hidden malpractice, New York, 1977, Jove Press.

65. Cowan, B.: Birth control. Women's health care: resources, writings, bibliographies, Ann Arbor, Mich., 1977, Anshen Publishing.

66. Cragin, E. B.: Conservatism in obstetrics, N. Y. J. Med. **104:**1-3, 1916.

67. Crystle, L. D., and Rigsby, W. C.: Amniocentesis: experience in complications, Am. J. Obstet. Gynecol. **106:**310-311, Jan. 15, 1970.

68. Curie-Cohen, M., et al.: Current practice of artificial insemination by donor in the United States, N. Engl. J. Med. **300:**585-

590, March 15, 1979. (See also editorial by S. J. Behrman.)

69. Cutter, I. S., and Viets, H. R.: A short history of midwifery, Philadelphia, 1964, W. B. Saunders Co.

70. Department of Health and Social Security: Report on confidential enquiries into maternal deaths in England and Wales, 1970-1972, Report on Health and Social Subjects, No. 11, London, 1975.

71. Devereux, G.: A study of abortion in primitive societies, New York, 1976, International Universities Press, Inc.

72. Devitt, N. The statistical case for the elimination of the midwife, Women & Health **4**:81-96, 169-186, Spring/Summer, 1979.

73. Dieckmann, W. J., et al.: Does the administration of DES during pregnancy have therapeutic value? Am. J. Obstet. Gynecol. **66**: 1062-1084, Nov., 1953.

74. Digest: Ectopics are least common with combined pills; are most common with non-medicated IUDs, Fam. Plann. Perspect. **9**:87, March/April, 1977.

75. Digest: 356-hospital survey confirms pill/benign liver tumor link, Fam. Plann. Perspect. **9**:90, March/April, 1977.

76. Douglas, R. G., et al.: Pregnancy and labor following cesarean section, Am. J. Obstet. Gynecol. **86**:961-971, Aug. 1, 1963.

77. Dowie, M., and Johnston, T.: A case of corporate malpractice, Mother Jones: 37-50, Nov., 1976.

78. Dr. Steptoe's full report—at last, Medical World News **20**:10-19, Feb. 19, 1979.

79. D. S. G. Breast x-rays: files yield a disturbing tale, Science and Government Report, Vol. VI, No. 16, Oct. 1, 1976.

80. Edington, P. T., et al.: Influence on clinical practice of routine intrapartum fetal monitoring, Br. Med. J. **3**:341-343, Aug. 9, 1975.

81. Eisner, V., et al.: Improvement in infant and perinatal mortality in the United States, 1965-1973. I. Priorities for intervention, Am. J. Public Health **68**:359-366, April, 1978.

82. Encare Oval (editorial), Mod. Med. **46**:11, 15, Jan. 30, 1978.

83. Enkin, M.: Having a section is having a baby, Birth and the Family Journal **4**:99-102, Fall, 1977.

84. The e.p.t. Do-it-yourself early pregnancy test, Medical Letter **20**:39-40, April 21, 1978.

85. Ettner, F.: Hospital obstetrics 1977: do the benefits outweigh the risks? Women & Health **2**:17-23, Sept./Oct., 1977.

86. Evrard, J. R. and Gold, E. M.: Cesarean section and maternal mortality in Rhode Island. Incidence and risk factors, 1965-1975, Obstet. Gynecol. **50**:594-597, Nov., 1977.

87. Feder, H. M., et al.: Scalp abscess secondary to fetal scalp electrode, J. Pediatr. **89**: 808-809, Nov., 1976.

88. Fernandez-Rocha, L., and Oullette, R.: Fetal bleeding: an unusual complication of fetal monitoring, Am. J. Obstet. Gynecol. **125**:1153-1155, Aug. 15, 1976.

89. Findley, P.: Priests of Lucina: the story of obstetrics, Boston, 1939, Little, Brown & Co.

90. Fink, D. J., and Holleb, A. I.: Letter to project directors and coordinators of the breast cancer detection demonstration projects, Aug. 23, 1976.

91. Flynn, A. M.: Cervical mucus and identification of the fertile phase of the menstrual cycle, Br. J. Obstet. Gynecol. **83**:656-659, 1976.

92. Fogg, S.: Menopause: incapacitating disease? Los Angeles Times, Part IV, March 25, 1973.

93. Foltz, A. M., and Kelsey, J. L.: The annual Pap test: a dubious policy success, Milbank Memorial Fund Quarterly/Health and Society **56**:426-462, 1978. (Contains extensive bibliography.)

94. Food and Drug Administration: Estrogens and endometrial cancer, Drug Bulletin **6**: 18-20, Feb./March, 1976.

95. Foster, R. S.: Breast self-examination practices and breast cancer stage, N. Engl. J. Med. **299**:265-270, Aug. 10, 1978.

96. Freeman, R. K.: Use of the oxytocin challenge test for antepartum clinical evaluations of uteroplacental respiratory function, Am. J. Obstet. Gynecol. **121**:481-489, Feb. 15, 1975.

97. Freeman, R. K., et al.: An evaluation of the significance of a positive oxytocin challenge test, Obstet. Gynecol. **47**:8-13, Jan., 1976.

98. Frost & Sullivan Inc., New York: Fetal neonatal monitoring, News, Jan. 31, 1977.

99. Fuchs, F., Chairperson, Department of Obstetrics and Gynecology, Cornell Uni-

versity Medical College: Personal communication, May 23, 1978.

100. Fuchs, V.: Who shall live? New York, 1974, Basic Books, Inc., Publishers.

101. Furor over vaginal surgery for anorgasmy, Medical World News **19:**15-16, April 17, 1978.

102. Gabert, H., and Stenchever, M.: Continuous electronic monitoring of fetal heart rate during labor, Am. J. Obstet. Gynecol. **115:**919-923, April 1, 1973.

103. Gabert, H., and Stenchever, M.: The results of a five-year study of continuous fetal monitoring on an obstetric service, Obstet. Gynecol. **50:**275-279, Sept., 1977.

104. Gassner, C. B., and Ledger, W. J.: The relationship of hospital-acquired maternal infection to invasive intrapartum monitoring techniques, Am. J. Obstet. Gynecol. **126:**33-37, Sept. 13, 1976.

105. Geist, S. H., et al.: Are estrogens carcinogenic in the human female? II. Atypical endometrial proliferation in a patient treated with estrogens, Am. J. Obstet. Gynecol. **42:**242-248, Aug., 1941.

106. Gibbs, R. S., et al.: The effect of internal fetal monitoring on maternal infection following caesarean section. Obstet. Gynecol. **48:**653-658, Dec., 1976.

107. Gibbs, R. S., et al.: Internal fetal monitoring and maternal infection following caesarean section: a prospective study, Obstet. Gynecol. **52:**193-197, Aug., 1978.

108. Gill, W. B.: Structural and functional abnormalities in the sex organs of male offspring of mothers treated with diethylstilbestrol (DES), J. Reprod. Med. **16:**147, 1976.

109. Gill, W. B., et al.: Transplacental effects of diethylstilbestrol on the human male fetus: abnormal semen and anatomical lesions of the male genital tract, presented at the Conference on Women and the Workplace, Society for Occupational and Environmental Health, June 17-19, 1976, Washington, D.C.

110. Gluck, L.: Iatrogenic RDS and amniocentesis (editorial), Hosp. Pract. **12:**16-17, March, 1977.

111. Goldman, A. S., and Smith, C. W.: Host resistance factors in human milk, J. Pediatr. **82:**1082-1090, 1973.

112. Goodlin, R. C.: Fetal heart rate patterns (letter), J.A.M.A. **220:**1015, 1972.

113. Goodlin, R. C., and Clewell, W. H.: Sudden fetal death following diagnostic amniocentesis, Am. J. Obstet. Gynecol. **118:**285-288, Jan. 15, 1974.

114. Goodlin, R. C., and Haesslein, H. C.: When is it fetal distress? Am. J. Obstet. Gynecol. **128:**440-447, June 15, 1977.

115. Goodlin, R. C., and Harrod, I. R.: Letter, Lancet, **1:**559, March 10, 1973.

116. Gordon, J., et al.: Estrogen and endometrial carcinoma: an independent pathology review supporting original risk estimate, N. Engl. J. Med. **297:**570-571, Sept. 15, 1977.

117. Gordon, L.: Woman's body, woman's right, New York, 1976, The Viking Press.

118. Government challenges 12 medical practices, Medical World News **19:**7-8, Oct. 16, 1978.

119. Grabel, W.: 'Abortion' part of U.S. row over test-tube babies, Medical Tribune, Sept. 13, 1978.

120. Gray, L. A., et al.: Estrogens and endometrial carcinoma, Obstet. Gynecol. **49:**385-392, April, 1977.

121. Greenberg, D. S.: X-ray mammography: silent treatment for a troublesome report, N. Engl. J. Med. **296:**1015-1016, April 28, 1977.

122. Greenwald, P., et al.: Estimated effect on breast self-examination and routine physician examinations on breast cancer mortality, N. Engl. J. Med. **299:**271-273, Aug. 10, 1978.

123. Gusberg, S. B.: Precursors of corpus carcinoma estrogens and adenomatous hyperplasia, Am. J. Obstet. Gynecol. **54:**905-927, Dec., 1947.

124. Guttmacher, A. F.: The role of planned parenthood, The Pharos of Alpha Omega Alpha, July, 1965.

125. Haddad, H., and Lundy, L. E.: Changing indications for cesarean section: a 38-year experience at a community hospital, Obstet. Gynecol. **51:**133-137, Feb., 1978.

126. Hagen, D.: Maternal febrile morbidity associated with fetal monitoring and cesarean section, Obstet. Gynecol. **46:**260-262, Sept., 1975.

127. Haire, D.: The cultural warping of childbirth. Special report, Seattle, 1972, International Childbirth Education Association, 1414 N.W. 85th St., Seattle, Wash., 98117.

128. Hambraeus, L.: Proprietary milk versus

human milk in infant feeding, Pediatr. Clin. North Am. **24:**17-36, 1977.

129. Hanley, B. J.: Amniotomy for elective induction of labor at or near term, West. J. Surg. **59:**262, 1951.

130. Harrison, R., et al.: Risks of fetomaternal hemorrhage resulting from amniocentesis with and without ultrasound placental localization, Obstet. Gynecol. **46:**389-391, Oct., 1975.

131. Haverkamp, A. D., et al.: The evaluation of continuous fetal heart rate monitoring in high-risk pregnancy, Am. J. Obstet. Gynecol. **125:**310-320, June 1, 1976.

132. Haverkamp, A. D., et al.: A controlled trial of the differential effects of intrapartum monitoring, Am. J. Obstet. Gynecol. **134:**399-412, June 15, 1979.

133. Heinonen, O. P., et al.: Cardiovascular birth defects and antenatal exposure to female sex hormones, N. Engl. J. Med. **296:**67-70, Jan. 13, 1977.

134. Heldfond, A. J., et al.: Do we need fetal monitoring in a community hospital? Trans. Pac. Coast Obstet. Gynecol. Soc. **43:**25-30, 1976.

135. Herbert, T. J., et al.: Recurrent pneumococcal peritonitis associated with an intrauterine contraceptive device, Br. J. Surg. **61:**901-902, 1974.

136. Herbst, A. L., and Scully, R. E.: Adenocarcinoma of the vagina in adolescence, Cancer **25:**745, 1970.

137. Herbst, A. L., et al.: Adenocarcinoma of the vagina: association of maternal stilbestrol therapy with tumor appearance in young women, N. Engl. J. Med. **284:**878-881, April 22, 1971.

138. Herbst, A. L., et al.: Clear-cell adenocarcinoma of the vagina and cervix in girls: analysis of 170 registry cases, Am. J. Obstet. Gynecol. **119:**713-724, July 1, 1974.

139. Herbst, A. L., et al.: Prenatal exposure to stilbestrol. A prospective comparison of exposed female offspring with unexposed controls, N. Engl. J. Med. **292:**334-339, Feb. 13, 1975.

140. Hibbard, L. T.: Changing trends in cesarean section, Am. J. Obstet. Gynecol. **125:**798-804, July 15, 1976.

141. Hill, R.: On the frontiers of Islam, Oxford, England, 1970, Clarendon Press.

142. Himes, N.: Medical history of contraception, New York, 1963, Gamut Press.

143. Hochuli, E., et al.: The effect of moderate intensive monitoring in obstetrics on infant mortality and the incidence of hypoxia and acidosis, J. Perinat. Med. **4:**78-84, 1976.

144. Hon, E. H.: Fetal heart rate monitoring for evaluation of fetal well-being, Postgrad. Med. **61:**139-145, April, 1977.

145. Hon, E. H., and Lee, S. T.: Electronic evaluation of the fetal heart rate. VIII. Patterns preceding fetal death, further observations, Am. J. Obstet. Gynecol. **87:**814-826, Nov. 15, 1963.

146. Hon, E. H., et al.: The neonatal value of fetal monitoring, Am. J. Obstet. Gynecol. **122:**508-519, June 15, 1975.

147. Hoover, R., et al.: Menopausal estrogens and breast cancer, N. Engl. J. Med. **295:**401-405, Aug. 19, 1976.

148. Horwitz, R. I., and Feinstein, A. R.: Alternative analytic methods for case-control studies of estrogens and endometrial cancer, N. Engl. J. Med. **299:**1089-1094, Nov. 16, 1978.

149. Hosken, F.: Female circumcision and fertility, Women & Health, **1:**3-11, Nov./Dec., 1976.

150. Hubbard, R.: Testimony before the Ethics Advisory Board Hearing of DHEW, Oct. 13, 1978, Boston, Mass.

151. Hukkinen, K., et al.: Instantaneous fetal heart rate monitoring by electromagnetic methods, Am. J. Obstet. Gynecol. **125:**1115-1120, Aug. 15, 1976.

152. Hurd-Mead, K.: A history of women in medicine from the earliest times to the beginning of the nineteenth century, Connecticut, 1938, The Haddam Press.

153. Hutchinson, G. G., and Rothman, K. J.: Correcting a bias? (editorial), N. Engl. J. Med. **229:**1129-1130, Nov. 16, 1978.

154. Intrapartum fetal monitoring for all? (editorial), Br. Med. J. **2:**1466, Dec. 18, 1976.

155. Jafari, K.: False-negative Pap smear in uterine malignancy, Gynecol. Oncol. **6:**76-82, 1978.

156. Jaffe, F. S.: The pill: a perspective for assessing risks and benefits. N. Engl. J. Med. **297:**612-613, Sept. 15, 1977.

157. Jain, A. K.: Cigarette smoking, use of oral contraceptives and myocardial infarction, Am. J. Obstet. Gynecol. **126:**301-307, Oct. 1, 1976.

158. Janerich, D. T., et al.: Oral contraceptives

and congenital limb reduction defects, N. Engl. J. Med. **291:**697-700, Oct. 3, 1974.

159. Jelliffe, D. B., and Jelliffe, E. F. P.: Current concepts in nutrition, "breast is best": modern meanings, N. Engl. J. Med. (Medical Intelligence section) **297:**912-915, Oct. 27, 1977.

160. Jelliffe, D. B., and Jelliffe, E. F. P.: Human milk in the modern world, London, 1977, Oxford University Press.

161. Jelliffe, D. B., et al.: Human milk, nutrition and the world resource crisis, Science **188:** 557-561, 1975.

162. Jern, H. Z.: Hormone therapy of the menopause, J. Am. Med. Wom. Assoc. **30:**491-493, Dec. 1975.

163. Jick, H., et al.: Replacement estrogens and endometrial cancer, N. Engl. J. Med. **300:** 218-222, Feb. 1, 1979.

164. Johnson, A.: Consumers and drug safety. In Wertheimer, A. I., and Bush, P. J. editors: Perspectives on medicine in society, Hamilton, Ill., 1977, Drug Intelligence Publications.

165. Johnson, A.: The risks of sex hormones as drugs, Women & Health **2:**8-11, July/Aug., 1977.

166. Johnstone, F. D., et al.: Has continuous intrapartum monitoring made any impact on fetal outcome? Lancet **2:**1298-1300, June 17, 1978.

167. Jones, O. H.: Cesarean section in present-day obstetrics, Am. J. Obstet. Gynecol. **126:**521-530, Nov. 1, 1976.

168. Kafka, H., et al.: Perinatal mortality associated with cesarean section, Am. J. Obstet. Gynecol. **105:**589-596, Oct. 15, 1969.

169. Kahn, H. S., and Tyler, C. W., Jr.: An association between the Dalkon shield and complicated pregnancies among women hospitalized for intrauterine contraceptive device–related disorders, Am. J. Obstet. Gynecol. **125:**83-86, May 1, 1976.

170. Keettel, W. C.: Elective induction of labor. In Reid, D. E., and Barton, T. C., editors: Controversy in obstetrics and gynecology, Philadelphia, 1969, W. B. Saunders Co.

171. Keettel, W. C., et al.: The hazards of elective induction of labor, Am. J. Obstet. Gynecol. **75:**496-505, March, 1958.

172. Kelso, I. M., et al.: An assessment of continuous fetal heart rate monitoring in labor—a randomized trial, Am. J. Obstet. Gynecol. **131:**526-532, July 1, 1978.

173. Kennedy, D.: Testimony before the Subcommittee on Health and Scientific Research, The Committee on Human Resources, U.S. Senate, April 17, 1978.

174. Kennedy, D.: Testimony before the House Select Committee on Population Hearings on Depo-Provera, Aug. 8, 1978.

175. Kirschen, E. J., and Benirschke, K.: Fetal exsanguination after amniocentesis, Obstet. Gynecol. **42:**615-616, Oct., 1973.

176. Klaus, M. H., and Kennell, J. H.: Maternal-infant bonding, St. Louis, 1976, The C. V. Mosby Co.

177. Kloosterman, G. J.: Personal communication, July 14, 1978.

178. Knox, E. G.: Ages and frequencies for cervical cancer screening, Br. J. Cancer **34:**444-452, 1976.

179. Knox, E. G.: Cervical cancer. Screening for medical care. In Nuffield Provincial Hospitals Trust, Oxford, England, 1968, Oxford University Press.

180. Knox, R. A.: Nasal spray: birth control of the future? Boston Globe, June 16, 1978.

181. Koh, K. S., et al.: Experience and fetal monitoring in a university teaching hospital, Can. Med. Assoc. J. **112:**455-460, Feb. 22, 1975.

182. Kushner, R.: Unnecessary mastectomies, National Women's Health Network News **4:**5, April/May, 1979.

183. Labarthe, D., et al.: Design and preliminary observations of national cooperative diethylstilbestrol adenosis (DESAD) project, Obstet. Gynecol. **51:**453-458, April, 1978.

184. Lane, M. E., et al.: Successful use of the diaphragm and jelly by a young population: report of a clinical study, Fam. Plann. Perspect. **8:**81-86, March/April, 1976.

185. Larsen, J. W., et al.: Intrauterine infection on an obstetric service, Obstet. Gynecol. **43:**838-843, June, 1974.

186. Lauersen, N. H., et al.: Evaluation of the accuracy of a new ultrasonic fetal heart rate monitor, Am. J. Obstet. Gynecol. **125:** 1125-1135, Aug. 15, 1976.

187. Ledger, W. J.: Complications associated with invasive monitoring, Semin. Perinatol. **2:**187-194, April, 1978.

188. Lee, B. O., et al.: Ultrasonic determination of fetal maturity at repeat cesarean section, Obstet. Gynecol. **38:**294-297, Aug., 1971.

189. Lee, K.-S., et al.: Determinants of the neonatal mortality, Am. J. Dis. Child. **130:** 842-845, 1976.

190. Lee, W. K., and Baggish, M. S.: The effect of unselected intrapartum fetal monitoring, Obstet. Gynecol. **47:**516-520, May, 1976.

191. Lesbian births stir parliament debate, Medical World News **19:**7-8, Feb. 6, 1978.

192. Lieberman, S.: But you'll make such a feminine corpse, Majority Report, March 4, 1977.

193. Liley, A. W.: Technique and complications of amniocentesis, N. Z. Med. J. **59:** 581, 1960.

194. Lindsay, R., et al.: Bone response to termination of estrogen treatment, Lancet **1:** 1325-1327, June 24, 1978.

195. Lipman, A. G.: Drug interactions with oral contraceptives, Mod. Med. **46:**173, Sept. 30-Oct. 15, 1978.

196. LiVolsi, V. A.: Fibrocystic breast disease in oral contraceptive users, N. Engl. J. Med. **299:**381-385, Aug. 24, 1978.

197. Longo, L. D.: Sociocultural practices relating to obstetrics and gynecology in a community in West Africa, Am. J. Obstet. Gynecol. **89:**470-475, June 15, 1964.

198. Low, J. A., et al.: The rate of fetal heart rate patterns in the recognition of fetal asphyxia with metabolic acidosis, Am. J. Obstet. Gynecol. **109:**922-929, March 15, 1971.

199. Lowe, J. A., et al.: Caesarean sections in U.S. PAS hospitals, PAS reporter **14,** Dec., 1976.

200. Lubic, R. W.: Fetal electronic monitoring vs. home delivery, presented at the 25th Annual National Health Forum, The Third Century: Resources, Limits and Trade-offs in Developing America's Health Policy, March 23, 1977, New York.

201. MacCormack, F. A., et al.: Oral contraceptive use: epidemiology, N.Y. State J. Med. **77:**200-202, 1977.

202. MacGregor, J. E.: Evaluation of mass screening programs for cervical cancer in N.E. Scotland, Tumori **62:**287, 1976.

203. MacGregor, J. E., and Teper, S.: Uterine cervical cytology and young women, Lancet **1:**1029-1031, 1978.

204. Mack, T. M., et al.: Estrogens and endometrial cancer in a retirement community, N. Engl. J. Med. **294:**1262-1267, June 3, 1976.

205. MacKay, E. V.: Management of isoimmunized pregnant women with particular reference to amniocentesis, Aust. N.Z. J. Obstet. Gynaecol. **76:**1226, 1958.

206. Mann, J., et al.: Myocardial infarction in young women with special reference to oral contraceptive practice, Br. Med. J. **2:** 241, May 3, 1975.

207. Mann, J., et al.: Oral contraceptives— myocardial infarction in young women: a further report, Br. Med. J. **3:**631, Sept. 13, 1975.

207a. Marieskind, H. I.: An evaluation of Caesarean section in the United States, Washington, D.C., 1979, U.S. Department of Health, Education and Welfare.

208. Mathew, D. J., et al.: Prevention of eczema, Lancet **1:**321-324, 1977.

209. Mazzi, E., et al.: Prevention of scalp abscesses secondary to fetal scalp monitoring (letter), J. Pediatr. **90:**664-665, April, 1977.

210. McCormick, R. A.: Life in the test tube, The New York Times, Aug. 6, 1978.

211. McGarry, J. A.: The management of patients previously delivered by caesarean section, J. Obstet. Gynecol. British Commonwealth **76:**137-143, Feb., 1969.

212. McKinlay, S. M., and McKinlay, J. B.: Selected studies of the menopause, J. Biosoc. Sci. **5:**533-555, Oct., 1973. (Contains annotated bibliography of major reports on menopause.)

213. McLelland, R.: Mammography in the detection, diagnosis and management of carcinoma of the breast, Surg. Gynecol. Obstet. **146:**735-740, May, 1978.

214. McManus, O.: Is she or isn't she? Mixed reviews for pregnancy test, Boston Sunday Globe, April 16, 1978.

214a. Medical World News **21:**29-33, April 14, 1980.

215. Merkin, D. H.: Pregnancy as a disease: the pill in society, New York, 1976, National University Publications.

216. Merrill, B. S., and Gibbs, C. E.: Planned vaginal delivery following caesarean section, Obstet. Gynecol. **52:**50-52, July, 1978.

217. Millican, E., et al.: The clinical value of fetal electrocardiography, phonocardiography and heart rate monitoring, Am. J. Obstet. Gynecol. **96:**565-567, Oct. 15, 1966.

218. Mintz, M.: The pill: an alarming report, Boston, 1969, Beacon Press.

219. Misenheimer, H. R.: Fetal hemorrhage associated with amniocentesis, Am. J. Obstet. Gynecol. **94:**1133-1135, April 15, 1966.

220. Modanlou, H., et al.: Fetal and neonatal biochemistry and Apgar scores, Am. J. Obstet. Gynecol. **117:**942-951, Dec. 1, 1973.

221. Moore, F. D.: Breast self-examination, N. Engl. J. Med. **299:**304-305, Aug. 10, 1978.

222. Morewood, G. A., et al.: Vaginal delivery after cesarean section, Obstet. Gynecol. **42:**589-595, Oct., 1973.

223. Mothner, I.: Beyond the Pill, Rockefeller Foundation Illustrated, Sept., 1978.

224. National Association of Insurance Commissioners: Malpractice claims (closed claims study), vol. 4, May, 1977.

225. National Center for Health Statistics: Final natality statistics, 1966-1976, Washington, D.C., 1976, U.S. Government Printing Office.

226. National Center for Health Statistics: Use of intrauterine contraceptive devices in the United States, Advance Data, no. 43, Dec. 12, 1978.

227. National Disease and Therapeutic Index, Ambler, Pa., 1975, IMS America, Ltd.

228. The Nation's Health, p. 8, Dec., 1978.

229. Nelson, G. H., et al.: A complication of fetal scalp blood sampling, Am. J. Obstet. Gynecol. **110:**737-738, July 1, 1971.

230. Neutra, R. R., et al.: Effect of fetal monitoring on neonatal death rates, N. Engl. J. Med. **299:**324-326, Aug. 17, 1978.

231. New blood test for breast cancer, Mod. Med. **46:**14, May 15, 1978.

232. New York Times, p. 1, Dec. 4, 1975.

233. Niswander, K. R., and Gordon, M.: The women and their pregnancies. The collaborative perinatal study, Philadelphia, 1972, W. B. Saunders Co.

234. Odd-shaped uteri mark daughters of DES women, Medical Tribune, July 19, 1978.

235. O'Driscoll, K., et al.: Selective management of labour, Br. Med. J. **4:**727-729, 1975.

236. Okada, D. M., and Chow, A. W.: Newborn scalp abscess following intrapartum fetal monitoring: prospective comparison of two spiral electrodes, Am. J. Obstet. Gynecol. **127:**875-878, April 15, 1977.

237. Okada, D. M., et al.: Neonatal scalp abscess and fetal monitoring: factors associated with infection, Am. J. Obstet. Gynecol. **129:**185-189, Sept. 15, 1977.

238. OTC contraceptives and other vaginal drug products review panel: Memorandum to Commissioner Donald Kennedy, Feb. 9, 1978.

239. Ott, W. J., et al.: Analysis of variables affecting perinatal mortality, St. Louis City Hospital, 1969-1975, Obstet. Gynecol. **49:**481-485, April, 1977.

240. Paul, R. H.: Intrapartum fetal monitoring: current status and the future, Obstet. Gynecol. Surv. **28:**453-459, June, 1973.

241. Paul, R. H.: Personal communication, July, 1979.

242. Paul, R. H., and Hon, E. H.: A clinical fetal monitor, Obstet. Gynecol. **35:**161-168, Feb., 1970.

243. Paul, R. H., and Hon, E. H.: Clinical fetal monitoring. V. Effect on perinatal outcome, Am. J. Obstet. Gynecol. **118:**529-533, Feb. 15, 1974.

244. Paul, R. H., et al.: Clinical fetal monitoring. VII. The evaluation and significance of intrapartum baseline FHR variability, Am. J. Obstet. Gynecol. **123:**206-210, Sept. 15, 1975.

245. Paul, R. H., et al.: Clinical fetal monitoring, its effect on caesarean section rate and perinatal mortality: five-year trends, Postgrad. Med. **61:**160-166, April, 1977.

246. Piotrow, P. R., and Sullivan, T. X., editors: SIDA and contraceptives. Commercial distribution of contraceptives. Report no. 16, Washington, D.C., Winter, 1972-1973, The Victor-Bostrom Fund for International Planned Parenthood Federation.

247. Plavidal, F. J., and Werch, A.: Fetal scalp abscess secondary to intrauterine monitoring, Am. J. Obstet. Gynecol. **125:**65-70, May 1, 1976.

248. Population Reports: Barrier methods. The modern condom: a quality product for effective contraception, series H, no. 2, May, 1974.

249. Population Reports: Injectables and Implants, Series K, no. 1, March, 1975.

250. Population Reports: The diaphragm and other intravaginal barriers—a review, series 11, no. 4, Jan., 1976.

251. Population Reports: Debate on oral contraceptives and neoplasia continues; an-

swers remain elusive, series A, no. 4, May, 1977.

252. Potts, D. M.: Testimony before the House Select Committee on Population Hearings on Depo-Provera, Aug. 8, 1978 (International Fertility Research Program funded by USAID).

253. Pregnancy test kit needs no FDA approval now, Medical World News **19**:24, 29, March 6, 1978.

254. Presser, H. B.: Guessing and misinformation about pregnancy risk among urban mothers, Fam. Plann. Perspect. **19**:111-115, May/June, 1977.

255. Progestasert—a new intrauterine device, Medical Letter **18**:65-66, July 30, 1976.

256. PSRO hospital discharge data sets, Jan.-June, 1977, Office of Professional Standards Review Organization, HCFA, Washington, D.C., 1978-1979, U.S. Government Printing Office.

257. Queenan, J. T.: Editorial, Contemporary OB/GYN, **12**, Dec., 1978.

258. Quilligan, E. J.: The obstetrical intensive care unit, Hosp. Pract. **7**:67-69, 1972.

259. Quilligan, E. J., and Collea, J. V.: Fetal monitoring in pregnancy, Adv. Pediatr. **22**:83-112, 1976.

260. Quilligan, E. J., and Paul, R. H.: Fetal monitoring: is it worth it? Obstet. Gynecol. **45**:96-100, Jan., 1975.

261. Ranney, B., and Stanage, W. F.: Advantages of local anesthesia for cesarean section, Obstet. Gynecol. **45**:163-167, Feb., 1975.

262. Ravenholt, R. T.: Need, knowledge and opportunity: AID population assistance, Commercial Distribution of Contraceptives, report no. 16, Washington, D.C., Winter 1972-1973, The Victor-Bostrom Fund for The International Planned Parenthood Federation. See also Family planning programs: Population Reports, series J, nos. 14-16, pp. 253-320, March, 1977.

263. Renou, P., and Wood, C.: Interpretation of the continuous fetal heart rate record. In Beard, R. W., editor: Clinics in obstetrics and gynecology, vol. 1, no. 1, London, 1974, W. B. Saunders Co. Ltd.

264. Renou, P., et al.: Controlled trial of fetal intensive care, Am. J. Obstet. Gynecol. **126**:470-476, Oct. 15, 1976.

265. Rheingold, P. D.: The Dalkon Shield litigation, Women & Health **1**:31-32, July/Aug., 1976.

266. Rheingold, P. D.: Litigation involving DES, Women & Health **1**:26-27, Sept./Oct., 1976.

267. Rindfuss, R. R., and Ladinsky, J. L.: Patterns of births: implications for the incidence of elective induction, Med. Care **14**:685-693, Aug., 1976.

268. Riva, H. L., and Teich, J. C.: Vaginal delivery after cesarean section, Am. J. Obstet. Gynecol. **81**:501-510, March, 1961.

269. Robboy, S. J., et al.: Pathology of vaginal and cervical abnormalities associated with prenatal exposure to diethylstilbestrol (DES), J. Reprod. Med. **15**:13-18, 1975.

270. Robboy, S. J., et al.: Vaginal and cervical abnormalities related to prenatal exposure to diethylstilbestrol (DES). In Blaustein, A., editor: Pathology of the female genital tract, New York, 1977, Springer-Verlag New York, Inc.

271. Robboy, S. J., et al.: Squamous cell dysplasia and carcinoma in situ of the cervix and vagina after prenatal exposure to diethylstilbestrol, Obstet. Gynecol. **51**:528-535, May, 1978.

272. Roberts, K.: The intrauterine device as a health risk, Women & Health **2**:21-30, July/Aug., 1977.

273. Rongy, A. J.: Childbirth, yesterday and today, New York, 1937, Emerson Books, Inc.

274. Rothman, K. J.: Oral contraceptives and birth defects, N. Engl. J. Med. **299**:522-524, Sept. 7, 1978.

275. Roux, J. F., et al.: Labor Monitoring: a practical experience, Obstet. Gynecol. **36**:875-880, Dec., 1970.

276. Royal College of General Practitioners: Oral contraceptives and health, New York, 1974, Pitman Medical.

277. Ryan, G. T., et al.: Fetal bleeding as a major hazard of amniocentesis, Obstet. Gynecol. **40**:703-706, Nov., 1972.

278. Sai, F. T.: Testimony before the House Select Committee on Population Hearings on Depo-Provera, Aug. 8, 1978 (International Planned Parenthood Federation).

279. Sandmire, H. F., et al.: Experience with 40,000 Papanicolaou smears, Obstet. Gynecol. **48**:56-60, July, 1976.

280. Sauerhaft, S., Hill & Knowlton, Inc.: Memo to William L. Davis, President, Ayerst Laboratories, Majority Report, Feb. 19, 1977.

281. Schiffer, M. A., Jewish Hospital and Med-

ical Center, Brooklyn, N.Y.: Personal communication concerning ongoing mortality study in progress, April, 1978.

282. Schifrin, B. S., and Dame, L.: Fetal heart rate patterns: prediction of Apgar score, J.A.M.A. **219:**1322-1325, 1972.

283. Schifrin, B. S., and Suzuki, K.: Fetal surveillance during labor, Int. Anesthesiol. Clin. **11:**17-44, 1973.

284. Schmidt, A.: Testimony before the Senate Health Subcommittee, Jan. 21, 1976.

285. Schmitz, H. E., and Gajewski, C. J.: Vaginal delivery following cesarean section, Am. J. Obstet. Gynecol. **61:**1232-1242, June 15, 1951.

286. Schwarcz, R. L., et al.: Fetal heart rate patterns in labors with intact and with ruptured membranes, J. Perinat. Med. **1:**153, 1973.

287. Schwarcz, R. L., et al.: Fetal and maternal monitoring in spontaneous labors and in elective inductions: a comparative study, Am. J. Obstet. Gynecol. **120:**356-362, Oct. 1, 1974.

288. Seaman, B.: The doctors' case against the pill, New York, 1969, Wyden Books.

289. Seaman, B.: Free and female, Greenwich, Conn., 1972, Fawcett Fulfillment Service.

290. Seaman, B., and Seaman, G.: Women and the crisis in sex hormones, New York, 1978, Rawson Associates Publishers, Inc.

291. Serious adverse effects of oral contraceptives and estrogens, Medical Letter **18:**21-22, Feb. 27, 1976.

292. Shandall, A.: Circumcision and infibulation of females, Sudan Medical Journal **5:**179-212, 1967.

293. Shapiro, S.: Screening for early detection of cancer and heart disease, Bull. N.Y. Acad. Med. **51:**80-95, 1975.

294. Shapiro, S., et al.: Periodic breast cancer screening in reducing mortality from breast cancer, J.A.M.A. **215:**1777-1785, 1971.

295. Shearer, M.: Complications of cesarean to mother and infant, Birth and the Family Journal **4:**103-105, Fall, 1977.

296. Shelton, J. D.: Memorandum, Agency for International Development, March 9, 1978.

297. Shenker, L., et al.: Routine electronic monitoring of fetal heart rate and uterine activity during labor, Obstet. Gynecol. **46:**185-188, Aug., 1975.

298. Shoemaker, E. S., et al.: Estrogen treatment of post-menopausal women: benefits and risks, J.A.M.A. **238:**1524-1530, 1977.

299. Silverberg, S. G., and Makowski, E. L.: Endometrial carcinoma in young women taking oral contraceptive agents, Obstet. Gynecol. **46:**503-506, Nov., 1975.

300. Smith, D. C., et al.: Association of exogenous estrogen and endometrial carcinoma, N. Engl. J. Med. **293:**1164-1167, Dec. 4, 1975.

301. Smith, O. W.: Increased excretion of pregnanediol in pregnancy from diethylstilbestrol with special reference to the prevention of late pregnancy accidents, Am. J. Obstet. Gynecol. **51:**411, March, 1946.

302. Smith, O. W.: Diethylstilbestrol in the prevention and treatment of complications of pregnancy, Am. J. Obstet. Gynecol. **56:**821-834, Nov., 1948.

303. Spriggs, A. I.: Follow-up of untreated carcinoma-in-situ of cervix uteri, Lancet **2:**599, 1971.

304. Stadel, B. V., and Weiss, N.: Characteristics of menopausal women: a survey of King and Pierce Counties in Washington, 1973-1974, Am. J. Epidemiol. **102:**209-216, 1975.

305. Starkman, M.: Psychological responses to the use of the fetal monitor during labor, Psychosom. Med. **38:**269-277, July/Aug., 1976.

306. Stopes, M.: Mother England, London, 1929, John Bale, Sons and Danielsson Ltd.

307. Sumner, P. E., et al.: The labor-delivery bed—simplified obstetrics, J. Reprod. Med. **13:**158-161, Oct., 1974.

308. Sumner, P. E., et al.: Six years experience of prepared childbirth in a home-like labor-delivery room, Birth and The Family Journal **3:**79-82, Summer, 1976.

309. Supine called the worst position for labor and delivery, Family Practice News **5:**June 1, 1975.

310. Thadepalli, H., et al.: Gonococcal sepsis secondary to fetal monitoring, Am. J. Obstet. Gynecol. **126:**510-512, Oct. 15, 1976.

311. Thomas, G., and Blackwell, R. J.: A hazard associated with the use of spiral fetal scalp electrodes, Am. J. Obstet. Gynecol. **121:**1118-1119, April 15, 1975.

312. Thomas, L. B.: Report of NCI ad hoc pathology working group to review the gross and microscopic findings of breast cancer cases in the HIP study (Health Insurance Plan of Greater New York), J.

National Cancer Institute **59**:497-510, Aug., 1977.

313. Tietze, C.: Evaluation of intrauterine devices: ninth progress report of the cooperative statistical program, Stud. Fam. Plann. **55**:1-40, 1970.

314. Tietze, C., and Lewit, S.: Mortality and fertility control, Women & Health **2**:3-7, July/Aug., 1977.

315. Tietze, C., et al.: The effectiveness of the cervical cap as a contraceptive method, Am. J. Obstet. Gynecol. **66**:904-908, Oct., 1953.

316. A time to be born, Lancet, Nov. 16, 1974.

317. Tipton, R. H., and Lewis, B. V.: Induction of labor and perinatal mortality, Br. Med. J. **1**:391, 1975.

318. Turbeville, D. F., et al.: Complications of fetal scalp electrodes: a case report, Am. J. Obstet. Gynecol. **122**:530-531, June 15, 1975.

319. Turnock, B., and Pakter, J.: Family centered care activities by size of maternity service, Women & Health **4**:373-384, Winter, 1979.

320. Tutera, G., and Newman, R. L.: Fetal monitoring: its effect on the perinatal mortality and caesarean section rates and its complications, Am. J. Obstet. Gynecol. **122**:750-754, July 15, 1975.

321. Tyler, E. T., editor: Program in conception control, 1969, Philadelphia, 1969, J. B. Lippincott Co.

322. Upton, A. C.: Report of NCI ad hoc working group on the risks associated with mammography in mass screening for the detection of breast cancer, J. National Cancer Institute **59**:481-493, Aug., 1977.

323. U.S. Department of Health, Education and Welfare: Annual Report of Bureau of Radiological Health, Washington, D.C., March, 1977, U.S. Government Printing Office.

324. U.S. Department of Health, Education and Welfare, National Institutes of Health, National Cancer Institute: Final reports of National Cancer Institute ad hoc working groups on mammography screening for breast cancer and a summary report of their joint findings and recommendations, (NIH) 77-1400, Washington, D.C., 1977, U.S. Government Printing Office.

325. U.S. Senate Committee on the Judiciary: Kefauver subcommittee on antitrust and monopoly, Parts 22 and 23, May and June, 1960, Washington, D.C., 1960, U.S. Government Printing Office.

326. U.S. Senate Hearings before the Subcommittee on Monopoly, Select Committee on Small Business: The competitive problems in the drug industry, 90th Congress, 1st Session, 1967, 2nd Session, 1970, Washington, D.C., U.S. Government Printing Office.

327. Vecsey, G.: Religious leaders differ on implant, The New York Times, July 27, 1978.

328. Verzin, J. A.: Sequelae of female circumcision, Trop. Doct. **5**:163-169, Oct., 1975.

329. Vessey, M., et al.: A long-term follow-up study of women using different methods of contraception—an interim report, J. Biosoc. Sci. **8**:373-427, 1976.

330. Vital statistics of the United States, selected volumes, published annually, Washington, D.C., U.S. Government Printing Office.

331. Weideger, P.: Menstruation and menopause: the physiology and psychology, the myth and the reality, revised, New York, 1977, Dell Publishing Co., Inc.

332. Weiss, K.: Vaginal cancer: an iatrogenic disease? Int. J. Health Serv. **5**:235-251, Spring, 1975.

333. Weiss, N.: Risk and benefits of estrogen use (editorial), N. Engl. J. Med. **293**:1200-1202, Dec. 4, 1975.

334. Weiss, N., et al.: Increasing incidence of endometrial cancer in the United States, N. Engl. J. Med. **294**:1259-1262, June 3, 1976.

335. Welch, R., et al.: Transplacental carcinogenesis: prenatal diethylstilbestrol (DES) exposure, clear cell carcinoma and related anomalies of the genital tract in young females, presented at the Conference on Women and the Workplace, Society for Occupational and Environmental Health, June 17-19, 1976, Washington, D.C.

336. Wennberg, J. E.: Section 1502(9) and (6). In Papers on the national health guidelines: the priorities of Section 1502, pp. 79-91, Jan., 1977, U.S. Government Printing Office.

337. Wennberg, J. E.: Changing patterns of risk, medical care and perinatal mortality in Vermont, presented at the American Public Health Association Annual Meeting, Oct. 18, 1978, Los Angeles, Calif.

338. White, K.: Surrogate mother: relief to childless? The Seattle Times, p. K.2, July 9, 1978.

339. Wiechetek, W. J., et al.: Puerperal morbidity and internal fetal monitoring, Am. J. Obstet. Gynecol. **119:**230-233, May 15, 1974.

340. Wiles, P. J., and Zeiderman, A. M.: Pregnancy complicated by intrauterine contraceptive devices, Obstet. Gynecol. **44:**484-490, Oct., 1974.

341. Williams, R. L., and Petitti, D.: Cesarean section, fetal monitoring and perinatal mortality in California, Draft 7,28,78, personal communication, Aug. 1, 1978.

342. Willson, J. R.: Elective induction of labor: is it justifiable in normally pregnant women? Am. J. Obstet. Gynecol. **65:**848-858, April, 1953.

343. Wilson, R.: Feminine forever, revised, New York, 1972, Pocket Books.

344. Winkel, C. A., et al.: Scalp abscess: a complication of the spiral fetal electrode, Am. J. Obstet. Gynecol. **126:**720-722, Nov. 15, 1976.

345. Wolcott, I., editor: Federally sponsored contraception research and evaluation projects, Women and Health Round Table Report **3,** Feb., 1979.

346. Wolfe, S. M.: Testimony before FDA OB-GYN Advisory Committee. Evidence of breast cancer from DES and current prescribing of DES and other estrogens, Jan. 30, 1978.

347. Wolter, D. F.: Patterns of management with breech presentation, Am. J. Obstet. Gynecol. **125:**733-739, July 15, 1976. (For comments on training see page 738, discussion by E. F. Anderson.)

348. Young, J. H.: Caesarean section: the history and development of the operation from the earliest times, London, 1944, H. K. Lewis & Co.

349. Ziel, H. K., and Finkle, W. D.: Increased risk of endometrial carcinoma among users of conjugated estrogens, N. Engl. J. Med. **293:**1167-1170, Dec. 4, 1975.

ADDITIONAL READINGS

American College of Obstetricians and Gynecologists: Standards for obstetric-gynecologic services, Chicago, 1974, American College of Obstetricians and Gynecologists.

Antunes, C. M. F., et al.: Endometrial cancer and estrogen use. Report of a large case-control study, N. Engl. J. Med. **300:**9-13, Jan. 4, 1979.

Atypical Pap Smear in a Young Woman: Red Flag or Not? Medical World News **19:**16, 20, Nov. 27, 1978.

Barnes, B. A., et al., editors: Costs, risks and benefits of surgery, New York, 1977, Oxford University Press.

Beck, N. C., and Hall, D.: Natural childbirth: a review and analysis, Obstet. Gynecol. **52:**371-379, Sept., 1978.

Block, M., and Reynolds, W.: How vital is mammography in the diagnosis and management of breast carcinoma? Arch. Surg. **105:**588-591, 1974.

Brackbill, Y., and Berendes, H. W.: Dangers of diethylstilbestrol: review of a 1953 paper (letter), Lancet **2:**520, Sept. 2, 1978.

Brillman, J.: The cervical cap, Boston, 1978, Boston Women's Health Book Collective, Inc.

Campbell, S., et al.: Ultrasound in the diagnosis of spina bifida. Lancet **1:**1065-1068, 1975.

Carlson, B., and Sumner, P. E.: Hospital "at home" delivery: a celebration, J. Obstet. Gynecol. Neonatal Nursing **5:**21-27, Jan./Feb., 1976.

Chard, T., and Gordon, Y. B.: Risks of amniocentesis (letter), N. Engl. J. Med. **299:**101, July 12, 1978.

Committee on Perinatal Health: Toward improving the outcome of pregnancy, New York, 1977, The National Foundation – March of Dimes.

Community Sex Information and Education Service Inc.: Sex, a better understanding, New York 1971, Community Sex Information and Education Service Inc. Box 2858, Grand Central Station, New York, N.Y. 10017.

Connon, A. F.: The treatment of menopausal disorders, Drugs **6:**137-142, 1973.

Correspondence between Guerrant and Johnson, Third World Institute, Newman Center at the University of Minnesota, 1701 University Ave., S.E., Minneapolis, Minn. 55414.

Crile, G.: What women should know about the breast cancer controversy, New York, 1973, Pocket Books.

Crile, G.: Management of breast cancer: limited mastectomy, Int. J. Radiol. Oncol. Biological Physics **2:**969, 1977.

Culliton, B.: Cancer institute unilaterally issues new restrictions on mammography, Science **196:**853-857, May, 1977.

DES Task Force Report, June, 1978. Available from Bob Bowser, DES Project Officer, DCCR, NCI, Blair Building, 8300 Colesville Silver Spring, Md. 20910.

Donovan, B.: The cesarean birth experience, Boston, 1977, Beacon Press.

Fidler, H. K., et al.: Cervical cancer detection in British Columbia, J. Obstet. Gynecol. British Commonwealth **75:**392-404, 1968.

Finkle, W. D.: Testimony before the U.S. Senate Health Subcommittee, Jan. 21, 1976.

Gabbe, S. G., et al.: Umbilical cord compression associated with amniotomy: laboratory observations, Am. J. Obstet. Gynecol. **126:**353-355, Oct. 1, 1976.

Golbus, M. S., et al.: Prenatal genetic diagnosis in 3,000 amniocenteses, N. Engl. J. Med. **300:** 157-163, Jan. 25, 1979.

Gordis, L., et al.: Obstetricians' attitudes toward genetic screening. Am. J. Public Health **67:** 469-471, May, 1977.

Gordon, Y. B., et al.: Foetal wastage as a result of an alpha-fetoprotein screening programme, Lancet **1:**677-678, 1978.

Greenwald, P., et al.: Vaginal cancer after maternal treatment with synthetic estrogens, N. Engl. J. Med. **285:**390-392, Aug. 12, 1971.

Harris, H.: Prenatal diagnosis and selective abortion, Cambrdige, Mass., 1975, Harvard University Press.

Hatcher, R.: Contraceptive technology: 1976-77, New York, 1976, Halsted Press.

Herbst, A. L., et al.: Problems in the examination of the DES exposed female, Obstet. Gynecol. **46:**353-355, Sept., 1975.

Hobel, C. J.: Risk assessment in perinatal medicine, Clin. Obstet. Gynecol. **21:**287-295, June, 1978.

Ing, R., et al.: Unilateral breast-feeding and breast cancer, Lancet **2:**124-127, July 16, 1977.

Interprofessional Task Force on Health Care of Women and Children: The development of family-centered maternity/newborn care in hospitals, Chicago, 1978, American College of Obstetricians and Gynecologists.

Karel, R., editor: Regional perinatal services, special report, no. 2, Princeton, N. J., 1978, Robert Wood Johnson Foundation.

Keeping abreast: J. Hum. Nurturing and Inf. Nutr. **3,** Jan./March, 1978, P.O. Box 6861, Denver, Colo. 80206.

Kennedy, D.: Birth control in America: the career of Margaret Sanger, New Haven, Conn., 1970, Yale University Press.

Kushner, R.: Breast cancer: a personal history and an investigative report, New York, 1975, Harcourt Brace Jovanovich.

LaLeche League International, 9616 Minneapolis Ave., Franklin Park, Ill. 60134.

The Lactation Review: The Human Lactation Center, Ltd., 666 Sturges Highway, Westport, Conn. 06880.

Laws, P. W.: X-rays: more harm than good? Emmaus, Pa., 1977, Rodale Press. (See Chapter 6.)

Lindsay, H.: Natural birth control, Minneapolis, 1977, Elizabeth Blackwell Women's Health Center, 2000 S. Fifth St., Minneapolis, Minn. 55454.

Maidman, J. E.: Intrauterine diagnosis, Urban health **6:**42-56, March, 1977.

Maine, D.: Depo: the debate continues, Fam. Plann. Perspect. **10:**342-345, Nov./Dec., 1978.

Marano, H.: Breast feeding. New evidence it's far more than nutrition, Medical World News **20:**62-78, Feb. 5, 1979.

Massachusetts Department of Public Health. Papanicolaou testing—are we screening the wrong women (letter)? N. Engl. J. Med. **294:** 223, Jan. 22, 1976.

McDonald, T. W., et al.: Exogenous estrogen and endometrial carcinoma: case control and incidence study. Am. J. Obstet. Gynecol. **127:** 572-580, March 15, 1977.

Meyer, A. C., et al.: Carcinoma of the breast: a clinical study, Arch. Surg. **113:**364-367, 1978.

Miller, C. A.: What technology breeds—a review of recent U.S. experience with caesarean sections, Ann Arbor, Mich., March 20, 1978, The John Sundwall Memorial, School of Public Health, University of Michigan.

Milunsky, A.: Risk of amniocentesis for prenatal diagnosis, N. Engl. J. Med. **293:**932-933, Oct. 30, 1975.

Munsick, R.: One mother dies for 8 newborns saved with electronic monitoring, Obstetric and Gynecology News **13,** Dec. 15, 1978.

Napoli, M.: Mammography for women with no symptoms, Health Facts **1,** May 15, 1977, Center for Medical Consumers and Health Care Information, Inc., 410 E. 62nd St., New York, N.Y. 10021.

National Cancer Institute: Exposure in utero to diethylstilbestrol and related synthetic hormones, J.A.M.A. **236:**1107-1109, Sept. 6, 1976. (Contains list of all DES-type drugs.)

National Cancer Institute: Pamphlets: Vaginal and cervical cancers and other abnormalities associated with in utero exposure to diethylstilbestrol and related synthetic hormones; Information for the concerned public—questions and answers about DES exposure before birth; Information for the general public—were you or your daughter born after 1940? Office of Cancer Communications, Department 147-148-149-150, Building 31, Room 10A19, National Cancer Institute, Bethesda, Md. 20014.

National Institute of Child Health and Human Development National Registry for Amniocentesis Study Group: Mid-trimester amniocentesis for prenatal diagnosis: safety and accuracy, J.A.M.A. **236:**1471-1476, Sept. 27, 1976.

Oliva, E.: Fact sheet on daughters of DES mothers, Planned Parenthood, Alameda–San Francisco, 1660 Bush St., San Francisco, Calif. 94109.

Powledge, T. M., and Fletcher, J.: Guidelines for the ethical, social and legal issues in prenatal diagnosis, N. Engl. J. Med. **300:**168-172, Jan. 25, 1979.

Puretz, D.: Mammography, N.Y. State J. Med. **76:**1985-1991, Nov., 1976.

Raphael, Dana: The tender gift: breast-feeding, New York, 1976, Schocken Books, Inc.

Report on induced labor: London, 1978, National Childbirth Trust, 9 Queens Borough Terrace, London, W2, England.

Rindfuss, R. R., et al.: Elective induction stimulation of labor and the health of the infant, Am. J. Public Health **68:**872-878, Sept., 1978.

Rosenberg, C. L.: Is new technology being made a scapegoat? Medical Economics **5:**175-177, 180, 185-186, 191-194, March 20, 1978.

Sanger, M.: Woman and the new race, New York, 1920, Brentano's Publishing Co.

Schifrin, B. S.: The case against the fetal monitor, South. Med. J. **71:**1058-1061, Sept., 1978.

Shanklin, D. R.: Estrogens and endometrial carcinoma (letter), N. Engl. J. Med. **294:**846-847, April 8, 1976.

Simpson, N. E., et al.: Prenatal diagnosis of genetic disease in Canada: report of a collaborative study, Can. Med. Assoc. J. **115:**739-748, 1976.

Smith, J. K.: Breast-feeding means healthier babies, Medical World News **19:**108, Oct. 16, 1978.

Stern, E., et al.: Steroid contraceptive use and cervical dysplasia: increased risk of progression, Science, **196:**1460-1462, June 24, 1977.

Thier, S. O.: Breast cancer screening: a view from outside the controversy (editorial), **297:**1063-1065, Nov. 10, 1977.

Update on breast-feeding, Spring, 1978, International Childbirth Education Association Review, 1100 23rd Ave. E., Seattle, Wash. 98112.

Weiss, K.: Health Research Group Report on the Morning-After Pill and Fact Sheet. In U.S. Congress, Senate Committee on Labor and Public Welfare, Quality of Health Care—Human Experimentation, 93rd Congress, Part I, Feb. 21-22, 1973, 193-212, 300-315, 4.5, Washington, D.C., 1973, U.S. Government Printing Office.

Weiss, K.: Estrogen drugs: cancer by prescription? Women & Health **1:**3-4, March/April, 1976.

Weiss, K.: Epidemiology of vaginal adenocarcinoma and adenosis: current status, J. Am. Med. Wom. Assoc. **30:**59-63, Feb., 1978.

Westoff, C. F.: Trends in contraceptive practice: 1965-1973, Fam. Plann. Perspect. **8:**54-57, March/April, 1976.

Wolfe, S. M., and Warner, R.: Mammography: a case for informed consent, Nov., 1976, Washington, D.C., Health Research Group, 2000 P Street, N.W., Washington, D.C. 20036.

World Health Organization: Steroid contraception and the risk of neoplasia, report of a WHO Scientific Group, WHO Tech. Rep. Ser. G19, Geneva, Switzerland, 1978, World Health Organization. WHO Publications Center, U.S.A., 49 Sheridan Ave., Albany, N.Y. 12210.

Wright, N. H., et al.: Neoplasia and dysplasia of the cervix uteri and contraception: a possible protective effect of the diaphragm, Br. J. Cancer **38:**273-279, 1978.

Chapter 8

Women's health activism

HISTORICAL BACKGROUND

Women's health activism has a long history. Even though healing was very much women's work in early times, there were ancient attempts to prohibit women from medical practice. For example, such prohibitions had led to the arrest of Agnodice by Greek magistrates in 300 BC. Agnodice, masquerading as a man, had attended medical classes and practiced obstetrics and gynecology. Her arrest was quickly countered with demonstrations by Athenian women demanding her release, saying: "You are not our husbands but our enemies if you condemn our Agnodice, who saves our lives." After her acquittal, medical education in Greece was formally opened to women and the magistrates passed a new law "which gave gentlewomen leave to study and practice all parts of physick to their own sex, giving large stipends to those that did it well and carefully."[50] Although it was to be 16 centuries before widespread denial of medical education to women again occurred, other influences made women's participation in medicine cyclical and erratic (see Chapter 4).

Despite the obstacles and the general lack of recognition, many gifted practitioners were recorded. St. Bridget (453-525) practiced medicine and midwifery in Ireland and exerted sufficient influence to persuade the rulers to banish incompetent practitioners from the country.[68] Anna Comnena (1083-1148), historian, became physician-in-chief at the Pantocrator, a hospital of more than 10,000 beds in Constantinople.[48] Trotula di Ruggiero, of Salerno, Italy, in the mid–eleventh century was widely recognized as a leading obstetrician and is credited with the first description of the physical signs of syphilis. She is renowned for her advocacy, prior to the knowledge of sepsis, of the use of protective pads to avoid fecal contamination during childbirth.[99] However, both the efforts of Christiantity, church, and state to impose licensure and the development of universities as all male preserves eventually firmly confined women's participation in medicine to the roles of nurses, ecclesiastical and lay village healers, spiritualists, midwives, herb gatherers, and, occasionally, empirics, who were lay women apprenticed to university-educated practitioners (see Chapter 4).

Although edicts were issued against empirics practicing, Hurd-Mead[48, pp.257-272] notes that there seem to be no records of prosecutions. In the early fourteenth century, medical skills were relatively undefined. Public executioners were allowed to set bones, barbers to cup and bleed, and bath attendants to treat skin diseases. In 1389 the Guild of Surgeons was founded, and a few women were admitted to its membership. They were acknowledged by the guild as necessary to the provision of care for women.

By the sixteenth century, exclusion of women from the learning centers was complete and witch-hunts were rampant throughout Europe for the next two centuries. Nevertheless, there was a succession of outstanding midwives at this time, particularly in England and Germany, and an extremely competent group emerged in France. Many of these women studied the newly available gynecology texts, and they frequently wrote their own. Jane Sharp was the first English midwife to write a text, and her *The Compleat Midwife's Companion* was published in 1671. She exhorted midwives to study anatomy and was strongly opposed to the male domination of obstetrics. She expressly complained that, although it may be thought "women cannot attain so rarely to the knowledge of things as men may, who are bred up in universities . . . the art of midwifery chiefly concerns us (women), which even the best learned men will grant. . . . They are forced to borrow from us the very name they practice by . . . 'man-midwives.'"[50, pp.17-19]

The next three centuries were marked by organized opposition from the midwives to increasing technicalization and to the numbers of man-midwives, or andro-boethoynists. Andro-boethoynists was a name suggested by John Maubray of England in 1724 to counteract the criticism that the time-honored female tradition inherent in the word *obstetrix,* meaning "a female who stands before," was confirmation that male obstetricians simply could not exist.

Activism, however, whether in the form of writing, studying in organized groups, or agitating, focused not only on the male presence, but also on the quality of care provided, which is the substance of the argument in favor of natural childbirth as opposed to technological intervention. One organized and vocal opponent was Mrs. Elizabeth Cellier (seventeenth century), who encouraged midwives to organize, not just for study but also to change their work conditions. Reputedly an outstanding midwife, Mrs. Cellier compiled mortality statistics, recording between 1642 and 1662 that "six thousand English women died in childbirth, and about five thousand chrysome (newborn) infants were buried. . . . of this number, above two-thirds perished for want of due skill and care in those women who practice the art of midwifery."[48, p.398]

Mrs. Cellier presented a plan for a Royal Hospital to King James II in 1687, the guidelines of which indicated brilliant foresight. Included were staffing ratios, training and registration for nurses, homes for illegitimate babies, and fund-raising schemes, as well as basic concepts of maternal care. Her plans failed for want of enlightened public opinion, from lack of support from the timid midwives themselves, and from failure of the king to keep his word.[48] Mrs. Cellier attacked the king for this breach of faith. This act, coupled with her reputation as a fiery Papist in newly Protestant England and as an organizer of women, led to her being fined and sentenced to the pillory as well as being forced to witness the burning of her books. When she was tried a second time, Mrs. Cellier enterprisingly feigned pregnancy and miscarriage, concealing a pig's bladder filled with blood beneath her skirts.[8, pp.63-64]

The most vibrant protest and activism against "man-midwifery" came from Mrs. Elizabeth Nihell (b. 1723), wife of a surgeon apothecary. Although a Protestant, in 1747 she had obtained a dispensation by royal decree permitting her to study at the Hôtel Dieu, a famous midwifery school in Paris. After 2 years there she had opened an office with her husband in the Haymarket in London. She declared her "insuppressible indignation at the errors and pernicious innovations . . . sillily fostering a preference of men to women in the practice of midwifery; a preference first admitted by credulous fear . . . upon this so suspicious recommendation of those interested to make that fear subservient to their selfish ends."[50, p.20]

She attacked William Smellie (1697-1763), the leading obstetrician of the day, terming him a "great horse-god-mother of a he-midwife." The practice of Smellie and his colleagues of training obstetrical students (all male) by treatment of charity patients was characterized as the work of "two or three maggots (who) have produced thousands of . . . novices who watch the distress of poor pregnant women, even in private lodgings, where, under a notion of learning the business, they make these poor wretches, hired for their purpose, undergo the most inhuman vexation."[34, p.342]

Activism in the United States

Activists' concerns for both quality care and access to provider status continued, becoming most marked in the United States and coalescing there into the Popular Health Movement (see Chapter 4) of the 1830s and 1840s. Organized efforts by women in the United States to gain equitable access to most medical schools met with little success until the 1970s. Activism with a specific goal, for example, that centered on gaining admission of women to Harvard (a campaign waged from 1847 until admission was allowed in 1944) and to the Massachusetts Medical Society (resolved in 1884), provoked a range of arguments, including those of women's intellectual incompetence and biological unsuitability, as well as societal revulsion.[100]

Women's health activism concerning health care delivery in the early 1900s was characterized by the extraordinary efforts of Emma Goldman and Margaret Sanger. Both believed that women should have the freedom to gain control over their lives; they believed that contraception was basic to that right and should be implemented by providing universally accessible birth control services. Both women were jailed for speaking and for publishing material on birth control, but despite opposition, by 1917 there were national and local organizations devoted to the legalization and accessibility of contraception.[42] In 1914 Sanger had published the *Woman Rebel*, a socialist feminist newspaper that included promises to provide contraceptive information. With this publication she became the spokesperson for the birth control movement. After learning about contraceptive techniques in Europe, Sanger published and distributed in the United States, 100,000 copies of a birth control pamphlet, *Family Limitation*. To escape arrest, she went to Europe but later returned. The opening of her birth control clinic in Brownsville, Brooklyn, on October 16, 1916, was in direct conflict with the Comstock Laws, and Sanger was quickly arrested and jailed. The next decades of her life were devoted to the development of contraceptives and to providing widespread access to birth control services.[28]

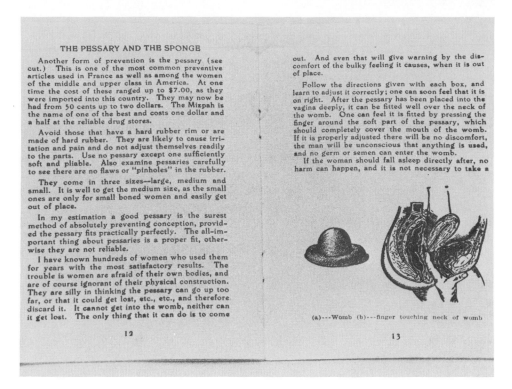

THE PESSARY AND THE SPONGE

Another form of prevention is the pessary (see cut.) This is one of the most common preventive articles used in France as well as among the women of the middle and upper class in America. At one time the cost of these ranged up to $7.00, as they were imported into this country. They may now be had from 50 cents up to two dollars. The Mizpah is the name of one of the best and costs one dollar and a half at the reliable drug stores.

Avoid those that have a hard rubber rim or are made of hard rubber. They are likely to cause irritation and pain and do not adjust themselves readily to the parts. Use no pessary except one sufficiently soft and pliable. Also examine pessaries carefully to see there are no flaws or "pinholes" in the rubber.

They come in three sizes—large, medium and small. It is well to get the medium size, as the small ones are only for small boned women and easily get out of place.

In my estimation a good pessary is the surest method of absolutely preventing conception, provided the pessary fits practically perfectly. The all-important thing about pessaries is a proper fit, otherwise they are not reliable.

I have known hundreds of women who used them for years with the most satisfactory results. The trouble is women are afraid of their own bodies, and are of course ignorant of their physical construction. They are silly in thinking the pessary can go up too far, or that it could get lost, etc., etc., and therefore discard it. It cannot get into the womb, neither can it get lost. The only thing that it can do is to come

12

out. And even that will give warning by the discomfort of the bulky feeling it causes, when it is out of place.

Follow the directions given with each box, and learn to adjust it correctly; one can soon feel that it is on right. After the pessary has been placed into the vagina deeply, it can be fitted well over the neck of the womb. One can feel it is fitted by pressing the finger around the soft part of the pessary, which should completely cover the mouth of the womb. If it is properly adjusted there will be no discomfort, the man will be unconscious that anything is used, and no germ or semen can enter the womb.

If the woman should fall asleep directly after, no harm can happen, and it is not necessary to take a

(a)---Womb (b)---finger touching neck of womb

13

Fig. 8-1. Excerpt from *Family Limitation*, 1916, by Margaret H. Sanger.

Much criticism has been leveled at Sanger because she and the birth-control movement became caught up in encouraging medical and professional control of contraception and in classist and racist eugenics arguments favoring contraceptive usage for "selective breeding." In 1919 Sanger wrote, "more children from the fit, less from the unfit — that is the chief issue of birth control."[87, pp.10-11] But the desertion of feminist and radical ideas must be weighed against the chances for success at that time had these shifts in approach not been made. Sanger's basic courage and determination in initiating the right-to-contraception fight paved the way for access to the most important tool of women's health care.

CONTEMPORARY ACTIVISM

Today women's health activism has primarily focused on issues of qualitative care and the empathetic organization and delivery of health services to women. Attempts to change health care are made by various groups with widely differing perspectives on their ability and/or their desire to effect change in the traditional structure and substance of the health care delivery system.

The Reach to Recovery program of the American Cancer Society, for example, is comprised of volunteers who provide compassionate physiological and psychological rehabilitative aid to more than 67% of all new mastectomy patients throughout the United States.[1] Initially organized by Terese Lasser in the early 1950s to meet the pressing need for providing emotional support to mastectomy patients, Reach to Recovery has continued with that objective. It does not seek changes in either the structure or process of health care delivery by, for instance, exploring the various types of breast cancer surgery or pushing for inclusion of its rehabilitative skills into routine medical services. Rather, Reach to Recovery seeks to supplement an accepted status quo with a much-needed service.

Similarly, cesarean support groups provide a valuable service to parents of babies born by cesarean section. Particularly important to the many couples who have attended prepared childbirth classes and then had a cesarean birth, the support groups enable venting of feelings of frustration, loss, or inadequacy and offer understanding and aid for the sheer physical exhaustion many women feel following the surgery. However, in meeting this important need, the groups also perpetuate the status quo. With rare exception,[17] they do not question the rising cesarean rate (see Chapter 7) nor evaluate its effect, from a cost-benefit perspective, on maternal and infant outcome.[24]

A second type of activist approach in which hundreds of women are involved is that taken by organizations such as Planned Parenthood. Essentially begun by Margaret Sanger, the organization is now widely regarded as conservative by activists seeking to restructure health care delivery. Nonetheless, while other activists have contented themselves with study groups, Planned Parenthood has in fact delivered health services to all women, including minorities, teenagers, and the poor.

Even though some of Planned Parenthood's approaches can be criticized, most notably their focus on female as opposed to male, or joint, responsibility for birth control, the stubborn reality is that in 1976 alone, Planned Parenthood provided at least one low cost and easily accessible service to 1.1 million women.[98] By using a clinic structure, by frequently locating in poorly served neighborhoods, and by using local people as volunteer or low-paid clinic personnel, Planned Parenthood has organized an alternative delivery system within traditional medicine.

Another example of alternatives organized by activists within traditional medicine is that of birth centers, either in hospitals or free standing. The usual objective of birth centers is to provide a safe and low-technology environment in which women can give birth. Usually birth centers permit mate, friend, and sibling participation at the birth, and they may utilize midwives to attend the carefully screened participants. They strive to create a homelike environment while eliminating some of the risks inherent in hospital delivery and in home birth, such as lack of emergency equipment.

Many in-hospital birth centers have also been developed, not so much as an answer to women's needs but as a selling point in a declining market for obstetrical beds.[90] Under such circumstances the concept of low technology has frequently given way to traditional obstetrics practiced in a more homelike environment (see Chapter 7).

The two forms of activism described — supplementing the status quo with a much needed service, and providing alternative processes within traditional structure—have also been criticized as performing a "safety valve" function for organized medicine.[91] Because services that meet immediate needs are readily available, pressure which might force more sweeping change is dissipated. Although these criticisms may have validity, the reality remains that vital services are provided by these alternative organizations, and frequently for groups who could not obtain them elsewhere.

WOMEN'S HEALTH MOVEMENT

Women's Health Movement activists work to change both the structure and process of health care delivery. As a long-term goal, many activists in the Women's Health Movement seek a total reorganization of health care delivery, including a redefinition of what comprises quality health care. Originating from the combination of activism for patients' rights, the 1960s' anti–Vietnamese War movement, the Community Health Movement, and the Women's Liberation Movement, the Women's Health Movement coalesced around the issue of abortion law reform. Although some women in the movement first became active in abortion law reform per se, others became interested through consciousness-raising groups, an integral component in the Women's Liberation Movement. Through these groups women question traditional social roles assigned to males and females and the institutions that determine those roles. The medical care system is seen as supporting, under the guise of science, societal sexism through its depiction of women's physical and mental capabilities and its emphasis on women's reproductive organs.

Specifically, following the Supreme Court decision on the cases of *Doe* v. *Bolton* and *Roe* v. *Wade* on January 22, 1973, it became obvious and is reinforced today (see Chapter 3) that women did not have control of accessibility to abortion; physicians, administrators, and legislators (all predominately male) were fully in charge. Although women rallied to this issue of making quality abortion services available, their interest soon expanded into other areas of women's health care, most notably gynecology and obstetrics. As more women joined and newsletters appeared, the Women's Health Movement became a nationwide identifiable force.[65]

Many of the issues raised by the movement, such as equitable access to health care, the quality of health care, and the need to end class and sex biases in the health system, are issues that also affect men. For example, the rights to abortion and to family-centered maternity care, while having their greatest effect on women, also affect men. It is therefore reasonable to ask why women are principally expressing their dissatisfaction and why it is a *women's* health movement. To date, women more than men have had the opportunity, through consciousness-raising groups and other more traditional gatherings of women, to express their dissatisfaction and recognize its collective nature. In the area of childbirth, however, men are indeed becoming organized and vocal.[9,95]

The answer to the question as to why it is a women's-health movement is more complex. Discrimination against women is derived from their "womanness": their biological differences, most notably their ability to bear children.

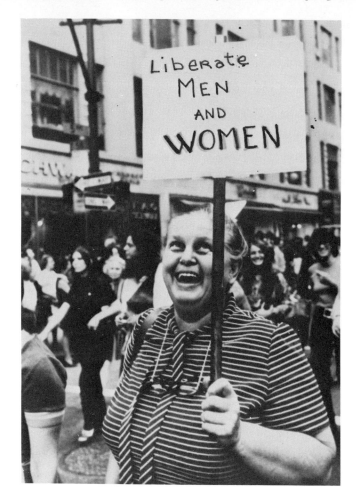

Fig. 8-2. Women's Liberation Movement rally. (Courtesy Anne Dockery, Liberation News Service.)

These differences have been used, particularly in capitalist societies, to build so-cial structures and supportive ideologies based on the concepts of female frailty, inferiority, and submissiveness, and of women's lesser rights to economic rewards and more limited abilities to earn them.[33,78]

Through its "medical" judgments about women, medicine has perpetuated this view. Women's most structured involvement with the health care system is, because of the medicalization of childbirth and contraception, uniquely female. Because of the vested interest the state has in women's reproductive capacities, this aspect of their health care, critical to equality of opportunity, is essentially externally regulated. For example, regulation may be by law, as with abortion or access to contraception. It may also be effected by prevailing medical practice.

For example, at one time the American College of Obstetricians and Gynecologists had a formula to determine if sterilization could be performed. This was indicated by whether a woman's age times the number of children she had equaled a certain number. Almost exclusive use of hospitals for births is another example. Regulation also occurs by social custom, which stresses women's innate maternal needs and (also mandated) "wifely" duties. A woman's gynecological and obstetrical experiences therefore may profoundly alter her life. If access to contraception or abortion is denied her, the result is likely to be motherhood, a status the woman may not desire, and, at the very least, for which she may be physiologically, psychologically, or economically unprepared. When breast or pelvic surgery is performed or when technological intervention is imposed during childbirth, even if medically prescribed as in the best interests of the patient, it is frequently done in opposition to the women's judgment or preference, or without her full comprehension. Her uniquely female organs, which have been both positively and negatively central to her socialization as a woman,[60,101] are not regarded as her own—their disposition is out of her hands. Therefore there are particular issues for women that are distinct from the concerns of all health consumers. The Women's Health Movement is an attempt to address these issues.

Current status and goals

It is difficult to define the Women's Health Movement because there are no universally agreed on policies or platforms, no formal means of signifying membership, and no institutional structure. Nonetheless, in a 1974 survey (updated in 1977) conducted by the Women's Health Forum–Health Right of New York City, over 1200 groups and tens of thousands of individual women were identified as considering themselves part of the Women's Health Movement.[38,39] In addition, groups are active throughout Canada, South America, Europe, Scandinavia, Australia, and New Zealand.* Activists in the Women's Health Movement are of all classes (although women's clinic clients appear not to be), all ages, and increasingly varied ethnicities. Such diversity is both a strength in terms of vitality and a liability in terms of reaching agreement for the movement, but it exemplifies the commonality of "the woman's experience."

Goals of the movement are as varied as the membership, and despite attempts to equate members with political theories, they do not readily conform to political categories.[31a] Some women seek to provide nonsexist health services to women through women's clinics, hospitals, and medical schools. Others seek to use the Women's Health Movement as a preliminary step to forcing a complete restructuring of the United States health care delivery system. Some women seek individual satisfaction from working in the movement while others may have a more global goal of humanitarian aid to all women. Specific goals may be part of the wider reorganization goal, and for many feminists the defeat of the American College of Obstetricians and Gynecologists as the authority on women's health issues is a cherished aim.

---

*References 5, 9, 12, 18, 86, 103.

Work of the Women's Health Movement falls into three main categories: struggling to change established health institutions, changing consumer and provider consciousness, and providing health-related services.

Efforts to change established health institutions take various forms and are obviously determined in part by the receptivity and flexibility of the institutions themselves. Women's health groups have sought to organize special services for women within hospitals by several means. For example, as a result of actions by its Women's Caucus, on September 22, 1973, Group Health Cooperative of Puget Sound included contraceptive coverage as a benefit, 25 years after that preventive health plan was founded. Other women's groups have conducted authorized and unauthorized "inspections" of hospitals and publicized their findings to pressure for change—for example, at Tallahassee Memorial Hospital.[80] Some women's groups have worked with local health systems agencies.*

Women's health courses have been organized, not only within the numerous women's studies programs, but also within schools of medicine and public health, for example, at the University of Michigan, which offered the course "Sex & Gender in Health" in the fall of 1978. Other women's groups have directly confronted institutions about issues such as sterilization abuse and the need for guidelines and have testified at various congressional hearings.[70]

Some institutional confrontation, however, has fallen on deaf, or at least wounded, ears. The American Medical Association asked in 1974,

What is it that caused many patients—even the more docile, soft-spoken ones—to suddenly start questioning every procedure, every prescription, to come out with shocking position statements on pre-marital sex, lesbianism, and childless marriage, and to insist on using natural childbirth, breast feeding and diaphragms, when modern medicine has provided them with much less bothersome and painless alternatives?[2]

Changing consciousness is not only done through direct consciousness-raising groups, but also through know-your-body courses or self-help clinics offered by the Women's Health Movement. Both approaches try to make available to all women easily understood information about female anatomy, bodily processes, and related health care. The self-help clinic, which is the more collectively oriented of the two approaches, should not be confused as being a physical setting. Founded in 1971 by Carol Downer of the Los Angeles Feminist Women's Health Center, a self-help clinic is a process of health education in which a group of 6 to 10 women meet together for about 10 weeks to exchange health information and experiences, to learn breast and vaginal self-examination, and to learn about common gynecological conditions. This self-help group may continue on to explore more advanced issues, for example, menstrual extraction, that require more technical knowledge.[103] Self-help groups do not provide curative care services. They are an educational process. Health care services are provided by women's clinics, which in many cases evolved from self-help clinics; where a

---

*In Boston in May, 1978, Health Service Agency IV produced the *Proposed Plan for Regionalization of Maternity and Newborn Care in Massachusetts.*

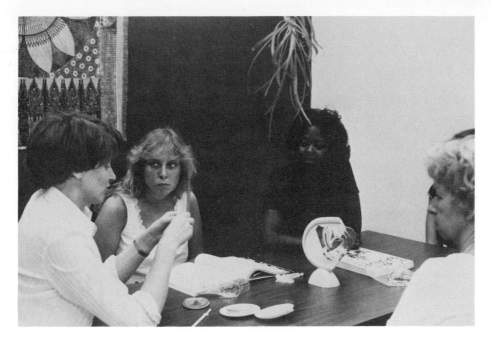

Fig. 8-3. Self-help group. (Courtesy M. A. Maurer.)

women's clinic exists, self-help groups usually continue as part of their services.[67] Two goals are common to all self-help groups: to provide health education for women and to aid women in realizing their own potential.

Women from the same or from varied socioeconomic classes may form a self-help group, but it is believed that mainly middle-class women join these groups. Socioeconomic data on the participants is usually not gathered, however, because the ethic of the groups has determined that such data collection is not in the best interests of those involved.

Because women have been shown to be misinformed and ignorant about many aspects of their health care, critics charge that self-help groups will further misinform and add more "medical mystery." But the basis of self-help is to speak from experience; in the group setting and with women questioning information that does not conform to their own experiences, the risk of acquiring misinformation is minimized. Furthermore, women are encouraged to seek clarification from other sources and to share it with the group. Self-help groups may also be special-interest groups made up, for example, of mastectomy and hysterectomy patients, pubescent adolescents, women experiencing prenatal care, or menopausal women. All groups function on the principles described.

Measuring achievement of either of the stated goals of self-help is difficult. After participating in self-help groups, most women report feelings of strength, a sense of self-worth, self-confidence, and an ability to be more assertive. Since confidence-building role playing or assertiveness training techniques are rarely consciously used by the women within the group, this feeling presumably originates from greater knowledge. Perhaps this is because the knowledge is of a part of her anatomy that is intimately intertwined with society's perceptions and expectations of her, perhaps because she now knows other women look and feel as she does, or perhaps because she now feels able to ask questions. Women soon ask why they have been ignorant, and frequently, as did the women in one survey when they could not answer the questions, express anger at their sense of helplessness.[66] The goal of realizing a woman's potential is seen in terms of alleviating this sense of helplessness or powerlessness. Questioning the health care system is seen as an appropriate beginning for women to establish control over other aspects of their lives.

There is a wide variation in the content of services provided by the more than 1200 women's health groups. Some groups are strictly educational, as outlined earlier and/or provide referrals to sympathetic and competent practitioners. Others limit their work to pregnancy screening and supportive counseling and may refer for abortions. Others are patient advocates; still others provide routine gynecological care and referral services for more complicated treatments. The Feminist Women's Health Centers, which were begun in Los Angeles and have provided the model for many others around the country, provide a full range of gynecological care, including specialist referral, and in some clinics also provide prenatal care with referrals for deliveries. A few clinics, such as Somerville Women's Health Project in Somerville, Massachusetts,[81] and the Fremont Women's Clinic in Seattle, Washington, provide routine primary care; sometimes clinics have a home-birth service as an adjunct.[37] Many other clinics that would like to provide primary care have been hampered, however, by an inability to attract physicians, male or female. The need for safe, low-cost abortions frequently has formed the basis for beginning a women's clinic and usually continues to be the economic mainstay of a clinic's operation. "Jane" — a group of about 50 women in Chicago, for example, provided 11,000 abortions in the 4 years they worked together before abortion became legal in Illinois.

Apart from education, which is discussed later, there have to date been no outcome measurements as to quality of care provided in women's clinics. Research into structure and process would suggest that competent care can be organized in a less costly and more personal manner than that traditionally provided. Research into outcomes should be encouraged. Where outcome studies have been done on physician-trained paramedics, the results have shown that quality care is being provided.[72]

Various characteristics are common to all women's health groups. All groups try to develop a minimally hierarchical structure among the clinic staff and all stress the use of paramedics, lay health workers (in conjunction with physicians), the sharing of skills and information, and the active involvement of the patient in her health care process. The Feminist Women's Health Center in Los Angeles, for example, has developed a clinic program whereby women experience care collectively. Called a "participatory clinic," a group of six to eight women collectively discuss their histories and their contraceptive and pregnancy experiences, learn to examine each other, and take routine laboratory specimens. Instead of health being a private matter, it becomes a collective effort; instead of a woman

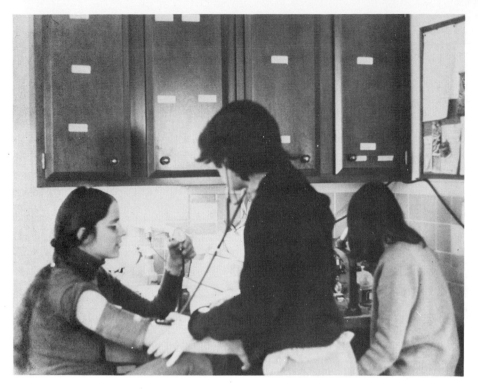

Fig. 8-4. Aradia Women's Health Center, Seattle. (Courtesy M. A. Maurer.)

believing she is an individual with a problem or a particularly unusual anatomical feature, she finds she is normal.

To varying degrees all women working in the Women's Movement continue the collective experience through which most entered and which still stands at the movement's core. Mutual support therefore is a key aspect, and regardless of their particular activities, work in the Women's Health Movement serves to bring previously isolated women a sense of unity, a sense of achievement, and, generally, through questioning of stereotypes, a sense of having autonomy in their own lives.

These collective actions demonstrate why the Women's Movement is indeed a political movement working to change power relationships. Frequently criticized by other activist groups as merely providing personal solutions for individual women's problems (although that alone would still be a valid reason for its existence), the movement is a tool that promotes collective thought and action from which radical social change can grow. Participation in the Women's Health Movement is for many women their first opportunity to be in a cooperative working and sharing relationship with other women, the first time they can see results from their group efforts, and the first time they may have "taken" knowledge for themselves. The Women's Health Movement is a practical first step to giving people power.

Selected Women's Health Movement activities

Rape support services. Evidence of the lack of support for rape victims by police, hospitals, and families led to an area of focus in the Women's Health Movement — the establishment of rape crisis centers. Frequently operated in conjunction with a women's health group or women's center, rape crisis centers seek to provide peers who will accompany a woman through the various stages of reporting a rape, offer counseling as needed, serve as an advocate during a trial, and remain in a supportive role for as long as requested.

Many groups have worked in their communities to organize educational sessions, self-defense classes, and escort services, and to pressure for legislative change to prevent mention of a victim's sex life during a trial, for better lighting — particularly on college campuses, for improved security in college dormitories, and for a "third-party reporting system" that enables victims who do not want to prosecute to give information concerning an attack to a third party who relays it to the police.[62] Also, some men in Philadelphia have formed Men Organized Against Rape (MOAR) to help partners and male family members of rape victims.

There are no data on the number of rape crisis centers, particularly since they are generally staffed by volunteers and do not receive public support. Yet a recent federally sponsored study reported these centers as being "often the first and sometimes the only contacts that victims have with community agencies."[84, p.30]

Rape support services are sorely needed. In 1976, according to the Federal Bureau of Investigation (FBI) 56,730 cases of forcible rape of females were reported to the police — one every 9 minutes. Estimating that only 20% of the actual assaults that occur are ever reported, the FBI notes that from 1967 to 1977, there was a 105.4% increase in the number of forcible rapes reported and an 88.6% increase in the rate of forcible rape of women. All these figures are exclusive of sexual assaults against males and of sex crimes such as incest and molestation against children.[31]

A 1975 study by the Law Enforcement Assistance Administration estimated that 151,000 rapes had occurred and about 56% of those had been reported.[58] Of the 69% of offenders prosecuted for rape, "42 percent were found guilty of the substantive offense, 9 percent were found guilty of a lesser offense, and 49 percent were aquitted and/or dismissed."[31,84]

Education. One goal of a self-help group, as discussed earlier, is that of providing health education, and this is also a goal inherent in the function of a women's clinic. History taking, for example, is performed as a cooperative effort between provider and recipient with explanations as to the importance of specific information. Self-care techniques are taught and encouraged, such as performing one's own pregnancy screening or pregnancy urinalysis.

Apart from verbal assurances, there are no studies that prove women's gain in knowledge after participation in a self-help group. On the other hand, women's lack of knowledge of anatomy and gynecological care has been verified. As part of her master's thesis Muriel J. Reynard tested women at a self-help clinic for their knowledge of basic anatomy and simple gynecological procedures. With a possible perfect score of 8, the sample of 100 had a mean of only 3.34[82] In a similar 1975 survey conducted among 100 women college students, respondents were asked to match names to a diagram of female reproductive organs. Only 50% could identify the uterus, 20% the vagina, 10% the fallopian tubes, 10% the urethra, and 0.5% the cervical os (the opening that leads to the uterus), but 90% could identify the clitoris.[64] In another study, with data gathered in 1974 and 1975, an attempt was made to determine gains in knowledge. With 50 in each sample, women who used a physician-staffed clinic (traditional), one staffed by physician-trained paramedics (paramedic), and a feminist facility (self-help) were tested prior to their first visit for their knowledge of basic anatomy and simple gynecological procedures and then retested after the encounter.[66] The socioeconomic characteristics are given in Table 8-1 and the scores in Table 8-2.

There are three socioeconomic factors that significantly distinguish these three groups of women and suggest possible reasons for the higher knowledge levels: age, education, and family size. Women in the traditional facility averaged 6⅓ years more in age than women from the paramedic facility and about 4½ years more than women from the self-help facility. However, most of the study samples were of comparable ages, 24, 21, and 25 years, respectively. Women in the self-help facility had a mean of 14.82 years of education as opposed to only 13.60 and 13.64 years in the other two facilities. They had 3.0 family members as opposed to 2.4 and 2.6 in the traditional and paramedic facilities, respectively.

Although a more complex data analysis must be made to establish the relationship (if any) between knowledge levels and these socioeconomic characteristics, the literature supports the impression that more education may be expected

Table 8-1. Socioeconomic characteristics and overall knowledge levels of respondents to a study using three types of facilities, 1974 to 1975

Socioeconomic variables (mean values)	Traditional facility	Paramedic facility	Self-help facility	All facilities
Age ($P < 0.05$)	31.34	24.96	26.56	27.62
Years of education ($P < 0.05$)	13.60	13.64	14.82	14.02
Ethnicity*	1.18	1.38	1.22	1.26
Income per week ($)†	2.50	2.40	2.58	2.49
Adults/children per family ($P < 0.05$)	2.44	2.60	3.00	2.68
Distance of home from facility (miles)	13.40	12.18	17.24	14.27
How heard about facility	Physician referral	Friend	Friend	Friend
Where previously obtained care	Male gynecologist	Male gynecologist	Male gynecologist	Male gynecologist
Overall knowledge levels (%)				
Before visit	50.3	53.6	65.2	55.1
After visit	52.5	61.3	72.0	61.9

*1 = White; 2 = black; 3 = Mexican-American.
†1 = 0 to 99; 2 = 100 to 199; 3 = 200 to 299.

Table 8-2. Percent of change in knowledge measurements of women after visits to three types of medical facilities, 1974 to 1975*

Test	Traditional facility	Paramedic facility	Self-help facility	All facilities
Anatomy identification (clitoris, uterus, vagina, os, fallopian tube, urethra, ovary, labia, cervix, hymen)	5.4	8.6	6.2	6.9
Definition of gynecological procedures (breast examination, Pap smear, speculum pelvic examination, D&C biopsy)	5.0	5.5	4.7	5.1
Knowledge of appropriate frequency of performing procedures	0.4	3.6	10.4	4.8
Knowledge of contraceptive contraindications (pill, IUD, diaphragm, foam, condom)	−4.8	12.8	6.0	10.4
TOTAL (ALL TESTS)	4.4	14.4	10.5	12.3

*All changes are positive unless otherwise indicated.

to produce higher knowledge levels. Common sense suggests that if the family size is greater than 2, one of the family members is often a child. The woman therefore has had more of an opportunity to familiarize herself with her anatomy. Other characteristics that were not measured in this study however, may perhaps explain the difference (e.g., whether the women attended sex education classes in school or college or whether they had read books such as *Our Bodies, Ourselves*).

The fact that an analysis of variance shows no significant difference in the overall mean of the change scores of all knowledge measurements (Table 8-1), however, suggests that the educational process within each facility may have less to do with ultimate health knowledge than do other experiences in a woman's life. It may also be possible that there is a peak level of knowledge beyond which no educational processes will have any effect.

From a preventive health perspective what is most distressing about the scores is not so much the low ability of women to accurately identify the parts of their anatomy on a diagram (in all facilities the total after the test was only 57.7%), although an ability to do so would surely increase a woman's feelings of familiarity with her body, but rather the relatively low knowledge (67%) of when to obtain techniques vitally important to maintaining good health. The extremely low scores measuring knowledge of contraceptive contraindications (33.4%) indicate that although there may be high contraceptive utilization in this country, there is low understanding of the risks of each method. These data like those of the other two studies discussed, also question the assumption that a woman gives her fully informed consent to utilize a contraceptive method—a concern expressed in recent medical literature.[35]

Advertising and textbooks. On the basis of the reasonable belief that the media, including books, are socialization agents, many women's groups are acting to curtail sexist and degrading protrayals of women. For example, Women Against Violence Against Women (WAVAW)* has been effective in curtailing the depiction of bound and whipped scantily clad women on record covers. Women's health groups have concentrated on advertising in medical journals and on unscientific textbook "facts."

Drug advertising is particularly insidious. In one study reported in the *New England Journal of Medicine,* of 24 leading medical magazines and journals, Sally Kilby, RN, noted:

Women were portrayed exclusively as sexual ornaments, as suffering housewives, or as handmaidens to the (male) doctor. Women, in all stages of seductive undress, advertise everything from antibiotics to antihypertensives, and even little girls advertise in bikinis, apparently a prescription-writing stimulus to the pediatrician. . . . Although some twenty occupations, from gastroenterologist to astronaut, appeared with male representatives, women's occupations were confined to nurse, stewardess and laboratory technician. Not one ad clearly showed a female doctor or medical student.[53]

The author concludes that these ads "could quite understandably affect doctors' attitudes toward patients."[53]

Similar feelings were expressed in 1971 about an attempt by Williams and Wilkins to publish the general medical text *The Anatomical Basis of Medical Practice.* Dr. Estelle Ramey, endocrinologist and professor of physiology and biophysics at Georgetown University School of Medicine, charged that the book violated both medical ethics and standards of professional behavior. Dr. Ramey noted that the illustrations were of provocative showgirl-type models and did not show anatomy properly, whereas the text contained many small and large errors and many jocose references to sexually attractive patients.[4] Dr. Ramey sent her comments to the publisher and many medical and scientific organizations, with the result that advertising, promotion, and printing of the book ceased.

Most critical are the depictions of women in standard widely used medical texts. In 1974 Drs. Diana Scully and Pauline Bart analyzed the contents of 27 of the 32 general gynecology texts published in the United States since 1943. They noted:

Indeed, examination of gynecology textbooks, one of the primary professional socialization agents for practitioners in the field, revealed a persistent bias toward greater concern with the patient's husband than with the patient herself. Women are consistently described as anatomically destined to reproduce, nurture and keep their husbands happy. So gynecology appears to be another of the forces committed to maintaining traditional sex-role stereotypes in the interest of men and from a male perspective.[89]

---

*c/o Feminist Women's Health Center, 6411 Hollywood Blvd., Los Angeles, Calif. 90028.

Considering just those books published since the work of Masters and Johnson appeared in the early 1960s, Scully and Bart note that:

eight of the books of that decade failed to discuss the issue of the clitoral versus vaginal orgasm. Eight continued to state, contrary to Masters and Johnson's findings, that the male sex drive was stronger; and half still maintained that procreation was the major function of sex for the female. Two said that most women were "frigid," and another stated that one-third were sexually unresponsive. Two repeated that vaginal orgasm was the only mature response.[89]

Following are samples from the texts:

The frequency of intercourse depends entirely upon the male sex drive—the bride should be advised to allow her husband's sex drive to set their pace and she should attempt to gear hers satisfactorily to his. If she finds after several months or years that this is not possible, she is advised to consult her physician as soon as she realizes there is a real problem.[71]

If like all human beings, he (the gynecologist) is made in the image of the Almighty, and if he is kind, then his kindness and concern for his patient may provide her with a glimpse of God's image.[88]

(Female orgasm) is a variegated as thumb prints and not at all contingent on mechanical and muscular stimuli but rather on how a women feels about her husband . . . The only important question to ask a women with regard to her lack of sexual satisfaction is, "Does she really love her husband?"[43]

The traits that compose the core of the female personality are feminine narcissism, masochism and passivity.[104]

There are implications for the millions of women, recently estimated to be 86%,[76] who use a gynecologist as their principal physician. These texts demonstrate that gynecologists' behavior and values are influenced by stereotypes that are disproved by scientific research even if still believed by society—and, apparently by textbook authors.

Equally of concern, considering the numbers of women undergoing mental health treatments, are the findings of the classic Broverman studies, which showed that therapists' definitions of a healthy woman's traits were comparable with those of a healthy child, whereas those of a healthy man corresponded to those of a healthy adult.[16]

With this type of socialization, it is not surprising that the physician-patient relationship is inequitable and frequently one in which the woman is not taken seriously in having her symptoms diagnosed as physical as opposed to psychological[32,59] or, as many medical sociologists have discussed, is judged incapable of understanding the nature of and necessity for the treatment of her illness.* Therefore, through both self-help groups and women's clinics, women are encouraged to maximize the physician-patient encounter, to avoid feeling intimidated, to question medications and treatment recommendations, and to undertake responsible participation in their health care process.

---

*References 11, 38, 55, 69, 74, 83, 96, 97, 106.

Classes, books, talk shows, films, and conferences. Many women's health groups have taught formalized health courses within universities. Perhaps the most radical of these was the pelvic teaching program conducted at various medical schools in Boston by the Cambridge Women's Community Health Center.[105] The other approximately 200 women's health courses being taught generally cover a wide spectrum of women's health concerns. Their approaches have ranged from a personal health informational approach at the University of Oregon[25] to viewing women's health care delivery within the context of medical care organization.*

Out of the Women's Health Movement, or in many cases to take advantage of it, have come numerous books and articles on women's health issues. As with any books, these vary widely in quality, perspective, and therefore value to women and health care providers in remedying past misconceptions of women's health needs. By far the most popular, and of great value to women, is *Our Bodies, Ourselves,* which was written by the Boston Women's Health Book Collective and first published in 1973. Now in its second revision, the book continues to be a best-seller. It is now being translated into Spanish for its large foreign audience, and other foreign language editions are forthcoming.[13]

Other topics about which much has been written, and which are not in this chapter's references or additional readings, are menopause,[20,73,79] childbirth,[7,15,19,27,51] breast cancer,[23,57,85] occupational health,[45,46,94] and general issues of women's health care.[21,30,36]

Numerous articles have been published about the Women's Health Movement. Some of the more thoughtful pieces, which have appeared both in academic journals[44,52] and in the popular press,[54,61,75,77] have tried to demonstrate positive ways in which the medical profession might respond to women's concerns. Many others have simply responded to a topical, marketable issue and have contributed little to educating women or their physicians.

Many women's health issues, for example, home versus hospital birth, hormone usage, cancer, childbirth technology, and nutrition, have been featured on talk shows. Frequently they have been discussed simply as book promotions or "miraculous" portrayals of rare medical achievements. Neither approach tends to be particularly educational, but there have been informative discussions of the issues and demonstrations of self-help techniques such as breast self-examination.†

Several women's health films have been produced. Particularly insightful of those distributed at the time of this book's publication are *Taking Our Bodies Back,‡ Rape Culture,‡ Healthcaring: From Our End of the Speculum,§ and Women Health Workers: A Slide Show.‖* Informative films on alternative child-

---

*"Women and the Health System," State University of New York College at Old Westbury, 1974-1976.

†*Not For Women Only,* WNBC, B. Walters, host, and *Turnabout,* PBS Network, G. Lange, host, are examples of television shows that have been informative.

‡Cambridge Documentary Films, Box 385, Cambridge, Mass. 02139.

§Women Make Movies, 257 W. 19th St., New York, N.Y. 10011.

‖Women's Health Collective, 5030 Newhall St., Philadelphia, Pa. 19144.

birth are *Five Women Five Births** and *The Chicago Maternity* Story.† Also commendable are several videotapes by the Feminist Women's Health Center of Los Angeles on topics ranging from self-help clinics to body building.‡

The Women's Health Movement has sponsored several nationwide conferences and now participates in more traditional conference structures as well, such as the American Public Health Association and the American Association of Planned Parenthood Physicians. In addition, the movement has several national publications, including *HealthRight*,§ a quarterly newsletter; *Women & Health*,‖ a quarterly journal; the *Monthly Extract*,¶ "an irregular periodical;" *The Federal Monitor*,# a summary of relevant legislation; and the *Women & Health Round Table Report*,** which analyzes topical legislative issues. Interest in women's issues has also produced the *Congressional Clearinghouse on Women's Rights Newsletter*.†† There are also numerous local newspapers from women's health groups around the nation.

Although not begun necessarily as an outgrowth of the Women's Health Movement, but nonetheless receiving impetus from it, are also several national health organizations organized around specific issues: DES Action‡‡ to identify all those exposed to diethylstilbestrol (see Chapter 7) and to make appropriate care available, NAPSAC (National Association of Parents and Professionals for Safe Alternatives in Childbirth),§§ ACHO (American College of Home Obstetrics),‖‖ and ICEA (International Childbirth Education Association),¶¶ all organized to improve standard obstetrical practice, NARAL (National Abortion Rights Action League, see Chapter 3),## and the NWHN (National Women's Health Network),*** organized to provide a nationwide clearinghouse of health policy and legislation.

Many other activities of the Women's Health Movement focus on medical devices, drugs, and surgery, both by offering alternatives and discussing their widespread acceptance in the face of equivocal evidence as to their benefit. These important issues are treated in greater depth in the discussion of technology in Chapter 7.

---

*Davidson Films, 132 Tunstead Ave., San Anselmo, Calif. 94960.
†Haymarket Films, 1901 W. Wellington, Chicago, Ill. 60657.
‡Feminist Women's Health Center, 6411 Hollywood Blvd., Los Angeles, Calif. 90028.
§41 Union Square, Room 206-8, New York, N.Y. 10003.
‖The Haworth Press, 149 Fifth Ave., New York, N.Y. 10010.
¶New Moon Communications, Inc., Box 3488 Ridgeway Station, Stamford, Conn. 05905.
#Gray, A., editor, Drawer Q, McLean, Va. 22101.
**2000 P St., N.W., Suite 403, Washington, D.C. 20036.
††722 House Office Bldg. Washington, D.C. 20575.
‡‡Long Island Jewish Hillside Medical Center, New Hyde Park, New York, N.Y. 11040; also DES Registry, Inc., 5426 27th St., N.W., Washington, D.C. 20015.
§§P.O. Box 1307, Chapel Hill, N.C. 27514.
‖‖664 North Michigan Ave., Suite 600, Chicago, Ill. 60611
¶¶ICEA Secretary, P.O. Box 20852, Milwaukee, Wis. 53220.
##825 15th St., N.W., Washington, D.C. 20005, 202-347-7774.
***2025 I St., N.W., Suite 105, Washington, D.C. 20006.

FACTORS AFFECTING ACTIVISM

Today's issues in the Women's Health Movement are strikingly similar to those of past centuries. The complexities may have changed, given the more advanced technology, but the fundamental conflicts around women's health care are the same. The issues of licensure, of appropriate task delegation, of hierarchy among health care providers, of whether technological intervention is superior to more natural healing methods, of the ownership of knowledge about health and healing, of mysogyny and sexism, of the rights of patients to be more autonomous in their health care decision making, of the costs of health care, and of the need for more women physicians all have their counterparts in historical health activism. This does not invalidate today's issues in any way but, rather, should show that to find solutions, even more radical measures than those taken thus far will be needed. According to historical precedent activism has not been successful in the long term. Hurd-Mead[47] delineates seven historical periods in which there was intense activity around women's health issues that subsided each time. Women should be asking why this occurred.

Obviously the answers are complex and do not apply only to women's health activism. Consumerism and natural healing have also had similar peaks as movements, only to decline without fundamentally altering the power of the health care system.* Some of the pertinent factors that are affecting the Women's Health Movement and which impede a sustained drive for change are described here.

Cooptation

For years self-help has been an essential component in, for example, diabetic and dialysis care, yet today, self-help and increased patient autonomy are suddenly fashionable.[3,41,93] Blue Cross's advertising stresses that "Good coverage is up to us, good health is up to you," and much fanfare was accorded former Secretary Califano of the Department of Health, Education and Welfare when he announced his antismoking initiative and the effort individuals could make for their own well-being.

But the practice of self-help can be controlled by allowing only limited participation. For example, without changing the substantive content of their practice, or by making only minimal changes in the physician-patient relationship and the ownership of information, gynecologists and obstetricians can and do modify the process to include self-help principles (e.g., using mirrors in self-examination, vaginal and breast self-examination, family centered care). Although obviously these features are all advantageous to the patient and should be supported, there are inherent dangers to popularizing the self-help concept. If people are viewed as being able to use self-help in all aspects of health care, a perfect excuse is provided to cut back organized services, particularly those which do not show an immediate cost benefit. In a society where exorbitant health costs must be contained, the self-help philosophy may be perceived and used as a device to cut costs. In the interests of "the good of the patient" individuals can be forced to assume respon-

---

*References 14, 22, 29, 49, 56, 92.

sibility for aspects of their health care while needed and desired services are abandoned.

When profit is the motivation for providing health care, it is tempting to have services for those who can pay and encourage self-help for those who cannot. Considering that much of self-help involves preventive and behavioral aspects of health care, a preventive self-help/curative costly high-technology dichotomy may emerge. With the history of inequitable access to health care in the United States, it is unlikely that the preventive self-help aspect of the dichotomy will be part of health care for the rich, but considering the potential risks and unproved value of much technology (see Chapter 7), such a dichotomy may not be in the best interests of the health of the upper classes.

A philosophy of self-help also can be used to deflect institutional responsibility for conditions that cause ill health, such as industrial pollution, chemical pollutants (both probably responsible for a high proportion of our cancers), social neglect, and iatrogenesis. For example, self-help knowledge of cancer's seven warning signals can only be of benefit and prolong a person's survival if it leads to early detection and treatment, but the underlying problems of the causative agents still exist and are beyond individual control. On the other hand, self-help can be a positive force in influencing and emphasizing individual responsibility, particularly regarding smoking, diet, drinking, sleep, and exercise.

Self-help has also become professionalized. For example, where groups of parents sharing common concerns such as child abuse, teenagers, alcoholism, or women's health care, have formed, new experts have appeared – in part created by the media, in part self-appointed. Self-help is also fertile ground for researchers, and various conferences have been held to dissect self-help concepts.* This is not necessarily bad, especially if the findings and skills are shared to benefit the group, but the legitimizing of the concept into the professional sphere tends to focus on the form and obscures the substance of society's responsibilities for the problem. It may also invite abuse as a problem becomes "topical," research money is made available, and a hierarchy of experts and lay persons is established. More important, such professionalization also tends to diminish the beliefs individuals have in their abilities to respond to their own needs – the fundamental ingredient in successful self-help is lost and the cycle of intimidation and sense of helplessness and lack of power begins again. For women long accustomed and conditioned to being "managed," this professionalization can be particularly insidious, all the more so because of women's lesser access to grants, conferences, and other means of promoting their "knowledge."

Fragmentation

The diversity of activities of the Women's Health Movement is both a strength and a liability – the former because of the range of possible interest areas in which women can work, and the latter because the movement becomes less of a

---

*Two examples are "Rx Self-Care" March 19-20; 1977, San Francisco, and "Self-Help and Health," June 8, 1976, New York.

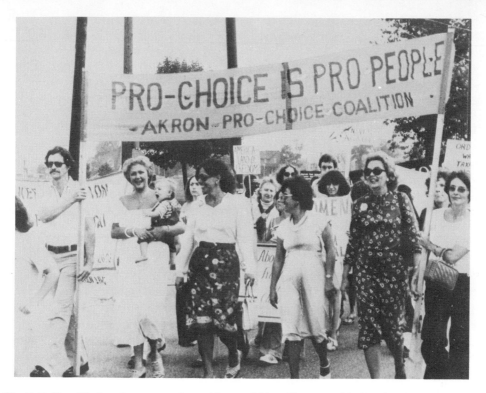

Fig. 8-5. Pro-Choice demonstration, Akron, Ohio. (Courtesy National Abortion Rights Action League, Washington, D.C.)

cohesive force. The movement becomes "spread too thin," and the diversity becomes a factor in preventing sweeping change.

This is particularly critical today when one considers the organized opposition to abortion rights—an issue of vital concern to millions of women, whether or not they are participants in the movement. Anti-abortion forces have used tactics such as setting fire to abortion clinics, following women home from clinics, telephoning women, judging all candidates for elective office by their stance on abortion, passing ordinances such as those in Akron, Ohio, which require a misleading discussion by clinic personnel of conception, pregnancy, abortion and the postoperative period, and lobbying for a Constitutional amendment.[10] These tactics demand a consolidated counteroffensive from the Women's Health Movement if it believes that women should retain the legal right to a service they have always sought and will continue to use. This service is particularly essential given the current contraceptive choices available (see Chapter 7) and the inadequate social programs available to cope with unplanned pregnancy.

One of the problems of organizing a necessary counterattack is that, unlike many minority groups, women have not responded as a cohesive unit to discrimination against them. Individual differences of class, ethnicity, professional status, age, and perceived social status have all worked to keep women apart and distrustful of each other. The traditional socialization of women, which leads to competition for physical, financial, and emotional security, still prevails, and regardless of the focus of a movement, this lack of a sense of class or community affects its success.

Reproductive focus

Although it is essential to challenge the stereotypes that have emphasized women's reproductive functions as well as the laws and institutions that have created and supported this image, this narrow focus can work against a total reorganization. For example, in believing that gynecology can be practiced more empathetically or that perhaps women's health care problems can be solved by having only women gynecologists, the movement loses perspective on the worth of reforming the entire system of laws and institutions.

The next step must be taken of asking whether the specialty of obstetrics and gynecology really is an optimal health care delivery model for women or whether this intense specialization of women's health care simply mirrors the wider social view of women.[63] If the organization of women's health care services more accurately reflected women's actual health problems — more women, for example, die of heart disease than of cancers of the reproductive tract (see Chapter 1) — some of the social control mechanisms that medical ideology and practice have reinforced would perhaps be broken.

In pursuing this line of reasoning, we are forced to confront the liability of the obstetrical/gynecological/reproductive focus of the Women's Health Movement. Although need for control over reproductive functions is a unifying and integral focal point of women's liberation, important in giving equal access to jobs and all that is implied therein, gynecological concerns cannot stand alone as the hallmark of the women's movement. To allow that buys into the very myth the movement set out to refute.

• • •

All the types of women's health activism discussed in this chapter center on providing services through alternatives to traditional medical care for women's unmet and expressed needs. The examples of women's health activism cited included the activities of Agnodice in 300 BC, the seventeenth-century English midwives, and the Popular Health Movement in the United States in the 1840s. These were followed in the United States in the twentieth century by the work of Margaret Sanger, the birth control movement, the founding of Planned Parenthood, the struggles for natural and family-centered birth, the organization of emotional support groups such as those for breast cancer patients and women who had cesarean deliveries, and the Women's Health Movement.

Whether or not the Women's Health Movement, the most politically oriented example of contemporary activism, can sustain its momentum, like activism of earlier periods, it has already left its mark. The movement has fostered the growth of services for women provided by women in areas such as rape counseling, health education, and abortion and contraceptive counseling. Most important, it has provided support and impetus for the challenge to the traditional "no need to ask questions/I'll take care of you" nature of women's encounters with the medical profession. The movement has reinforced the fact that biological differences are simply differences, despite societal and medical teaching, and are not grounds for exclusion of women from any of society's opportunities.

SUGGESTED TOPICS FOR DISCUSSION, FURTHER RESEARCH, AND FIELD PROJECTS

1. Intern at a women's health organization. Research its organizational structure and task responsibilities. Do these differ from other groups? Suggested contacts: National Women's Health Network, Parkland Building, 2025 I Street, N.W., Suite 105, Washington, D.C. 20006; HealthRight, Inc., 41 Union Square, Room 206-8, New York, N.Y. 10003; Our Bodies Ourselves Collective, Box 192, West Somerville, Mass. 02144; Feminist Women's Health Center, 6411 Hollywood Blvd. Los Angeles, Calif. 90028.
2. Research the different types of self-help groups in your area. What do they have in common? Which groups specifically are for women? How are these groups organized? To what extent do they have contact with professionals? (consider all health groups, not just gynecological ones.)
3. Research advertisements in medical journals. How are women portrayed? What percentages of ads refer to male and female patients? What are the most common categories of ads?
4. Contact a local women's health clinic. How is it organized? What is its economic base? Inquire if you can work in it. Suggested contact: Feminist Women's Health Center, 6411 Hollywood Blvd., Los Angeles, Calif. 90028.
5. Begin your own gynecological self-help group. Contact the Feminist Women's Health Center (address above) for guidelines. What are the main interests of women in your self-help group? What are the group's main achievements? In what areas do you think the group is deficient?
6. Select and research a current issue in women's health care (e.g., use of the Pill, estrogen replacement therapy, Depo-Provera, Librium, or Valium; the establishment of birth centers). When did it become an issue and for whom? What factors are preventing or encouraging resolution of this issue?
7. Design a health education program on a topic specific to women's health needs. How does your program need to be modified for maximum efficacy for different age and/ or ethnic groups? In what ways could you most effectively distribute your program?
8. Should alternative health care delivery centers such as clinics be eligible for third-party reimbursement through either private or public funds? What are the implications of allowing this reimbursement?
9. Should alternative health care centers such as women's clinics be regulated for quality control? If so, by whom and according to what and whose criteria? How should a regulating process be implemented?
10. What are the differences/similarities between contemporary and historical women's health activists? What are the differences/similarities between the social climates in which contemporary and historical activism occur?

REFERENCES

1. American Cancer Society: 1978 Cancer facts and figures, New York, 1979, American Cancer Society.
2. American Medical Association: And now the 'liberated' woman patient, American Medical News, pp. 14 ff., Oct. 7, 1974.
3. Annas, G.: The rights of hospital patients, New York, 1975, Avon Books.
4. Anonymous: Women's liberation and the practice of medicine, Medical World News **14**:33-38, June 22, 1973.
5. Anonymous: Deux americaines à Bruxelles propagent l'idée de centres de santé pour les femmes, Le Soir, Oct. 24, 1973.
6. Anonymous: High court agrees with ban on dads at cesarean births, Medical World News **19**:24, Oct. 30, 1978.
7. Arms, S.: Immaculate deception, Boston, 1975, Houghton Mifflin Co.
8. Aveling, J. H.: English midwives, their history and prospects, London, 1872, J. A. Churchill.
9. Badura, B.: Selbsthilfe und Gesundheitssicherung, Politiscke Wissenschaft, Konstanz, Germany, 1977. (Unpublished).
10. Beals, J., and NARAL: Health and public policy, Women & Health **4**:107-109, Spring, 1974.
11. Bloom, S. W., and Wilson, R. N.: Patient-practitioner relationships. In Freeman, H. E., et al., editors: Handbook of medical sociology, New Jersey, 1972, Prentice-Hall, Inc.
12. Bloomfield, C., et al.: Women's clinics, Health/PAC Bull. **34**:14, Oct., 1971.
13. Boston Women's Health Book Collective: Our bodies, ourselves, New York, 1973, Simon & Schuster, Inc.
14. Braverman, H.: Labor and monopoly capital, New York, 1974, Monthly Review Press.
15. Brewer, G. S.: Pregnancy after 30 workbook, Emmaus, Pa., 1978, Rodale Press Books.
16. Broverman, I. K., et al.: Sex-role stereotypes and clinical judgements of mental health, J. Consult. Clin. Psychol. **34**:1-7, 1970.
17. Caesarean Birth Association of Southern California: Once a cesarean always a cesarean? Santa Ana, Calif., 1978, The Association.
18. Calvert, S.: Healthy women, Broadsheet, Auckland, New Zealand, selected issues, 1977-1980.
19. Chard, T., and Richards, M., editors: Benefits and hazards of the new obstetrics, Philadelphia, 1977, J. B. Lippincott Co.
20. Clay, V. S.: Women, menopause and middle age, Pittsburgh, 1977, Know, Inc.
21. Corea, G.: Women's health care: the hidden malpractice, New York, 1977, William Morrow & Co., Inc.
22. Cray, E.: In failing health, New York, 1971, Bobbs-Merrill Co., Inc.
23. Crile, G., Jr.: What women should know about the breast cancer controversy, New York, 1974, Pocket Books.
24. C/Sec. Inc.: Manual for setting up prepared childbirth classes for cesarean parents, Boston, 1976, C/Sec, Inc.
25. Davis, L. G., and Williams, N.: The development of a women's health class from a feminist perspective, presented at the American Public Health Association Convention, Oct. 1974, New Orleans.
26. DES Action, Long Island Jewish Hillside Medical Center, New Hyde Park, New York, N.Y. 11040.
27. Donovan, B.: The caesarean birth experience, Boston, 1977, Beacon Press.
28. Douglas, E. T.: Pioneer of the future, Margaret Sanger, New York, 1970, Holt, Rinehart & Winston, Inc.
29. Ehrenreich, B., Ehrenreich, J., and Health Policy Advisory Center: The American health empire, New York, 1971, Vintage Press.
30. Ehrenreich, B., and English, D.: Complaints and disorders: the sexual politics of sickness, Old Westbury, New York, 1973, The Feminist Press.
31. Federal Bureau of Investigation: Crime in the United States, 1976, Uniform Crime Reports, stock no. 027-001-000-18-1, Washington, D.C., 1977, U.S. Government Printing Office.
31a. Fee, E.: Women and health care: a comparison of theories. In Dreifus, C., editor: Seizing our bodies, New York, 1977, Vintage Press.
32. Fidell, L.: Sex differences in health care, presented at the American Association for the Advancement of Science, 140th Annual Meeting, 1973, San Francisco.
33. Figes, E.: Patriarchal attitudes, Greenwich, Conn. 1970, Fawcett Books.
34. Findley, P.: Priests of Lucina: the story of obstetrics, Boston, 1939, Little, Brown & Co.
35. Fleckenstein, L, et al.: Oral contraceptive

patient information: a questionnaire study of attitudes, knowledge and preferred information services, J.A.M.A. **235:**1331-1336, 1976.

36. Frankfort, E.: Vaginal politics, New York, 1972, Quadrangle Books, Inc.
37. Fremont Women's Birth Collective: Lay midwifery—still an 'illegal' profession, Women & Health **2:**19-27, Nov.-Dec., 1977.
38. Friedson, E.: Patient views of medical practice, New York, 1961, Russell Sage Foundation.
39. Fruchter, R. G., et al.: The Women's Health Movement: where are we now? Health-Right **1:**1, 4, 1974.
40. Fruchter, R. G., et al.: The women's health movement: where are we now? In Claudia Dreifus, editor: Seizing our bodies, New York, 1977, Vintage Press.
41. Gartner, A., and Riessman, F.: The service society and the consumer vanguard, New York, 1974, Harper & Row, Publishers, Inc.
42. Gordon, L.: The politics of birth control, 1920-1940: the impact of professionals, Int. J. Health Serv. **5:**253-277, 1975.
43. Greenhill, J. P.: Office gynecology, Chicago, 1965, Year Book Medical Publishers, Inc.
44. Haire, D.: The cultural warping of childbirth, Special report, 1972, International Childbirth Education Association, 1414 N.W. 85th St., Seattle Wash. 98117
45. Hricko, A., with Brunt, M.: Working for your life: a woman's guide to job hazards, Berkeley, Calif., 1977, Labor Occupational Health Program.
46. Hunt, V.: Occupational health problems of pregnant women, order no. SA-5304-75, Washington, D.C., 1975, U.S. Government Printing Office.
47. Hurd-Mead, K. C.: The seven important periods in the evolution of women in medicine, address to Woman's Medical College of Pennsylvania, June 12, 1929.
48. Hurd-Mead, K. C.: A history of women in medicine from the earliest times to the beginning of the nineteenth century, Haddam, Connecticut, 1938, The Haddam Press.
49. Illich, I.: Medical nemesis, New York, 1976, Pantheon Books, Inc.
50. Jex-Blake, S: Medical women. Edinburgh, 1886, Oliphant, Anderson & Ferrier, Source Book Press.
51. Jordan, B.: Birth in 4 cultures, Quebec, 1978, Eden Press, Inc.

52. Kaiser, B. L., and Kaiser, I. H.: The challenge of the women's movement to American gynecology, Am. J. Obstet. Gynecol. **120:**652-665, Nov., 1974.
53. Kilby, S.: Androphilic, porcine ads (letter), N. Engl. J. Med. **288:**970, May 3, 1973.
54. Klemesrud, J.: Why women are losing faith in their doctors, McCall's, June 9, 1976.
55. Korsch, B., and Negrete, V.: Doctor-patient communication, Sci. Am. **277:**66-74, Aug., 1972.
56. Kotelchuck, D: Prognosis negative: crisis in the health care system, New York, 1977, Vintage Press.
57. Kushner, R.: Breast cancer: a personal and investigative report, New York, 1975, Harcourt Brace Jovanovich, Inc.
58. Law Enforcement Assistance Administration: Criminal victimization in the United States: a comparison of 1974 and 1975 findings. A national crime survey report, stock no. 027-000-00498-9, Washington, D.C., 1977, U.S. Government Printing Office.
59. Lennane, K. J., and Lennane, R. J.: Alleged psychogenic disorders in women—a possible manifestation of sexual prejudice, N. Engl. J. Med. **288:**288-292, Feb. 8, 1973.
60. Levitt, E. E., and Lubin, B.: Some personality factors associated with menstrual complaints and menstrual attitude, J. Psychosom. Res. **11:**267-270, 1967.
61. Luy, M. L.: What's behind women's wrath toward gynecologists, Modern Medicine **42:**17-21, Oct. 14, 1974.
62. Maitland, L.: Colleges acting to protect students against rape, The New York Times, Jan. 11, 1975.
63. Marieskind, H. I.: Restructuring Ob-Gyn, Social Policy **6:**48-49, Sept./Oct., 1975.
64. Marieskind, H. I.: Unpublished data, 1975.
65. Marieskind, H. I.: The women's health movement, Int. J. Health Serv. **5:**217-223, 1975.
66. Marieskind, H. I.: Gynaecological services: their historical relationships to the women's movement with recent experience of self-help clinics and other delivery modes, doctoral dissertation, University of Michigan, 1976, 762-5222-01500 Xerox University Microfilms, Ann Arbor, Mich. 48106.
67. Marieskind, H. I.: Helping oneself to health, Social Policy **7:**63-66, Sept./Oct., 1976.
68. Marks, G., and Beatty, W. K.: Women in

white, New York, 1972, Charles Scribner's Sons.

69. Martin, W.: Preferences for types of patients. In Merton, R., editor: The student physician, Cambridge, Mass., 1957, Harvard University Press.

70. National Women's Health Network: Testimony and activities by the National Women's Health Network, National Women's Health Network News 3:3, Aug./Sept., 1978.

71. Novak, E. R., et al.: Novak's textbook of gynecology, Baltimore, 1970, Williams & Wilkins Co.

72. Ostergard, D. R., et al.: A training program for allied health personnel in family planning and cancer screening, J. Reprod. Med. 7:40, July, 1971.

73. Page, J.: The other awkward age, Berkeley, Calif., 1977, Ten Speed Press.

74. Parsons, T.: The social system, New York, 1951, The Free Press.

75. Pascal, J.: A real danger, Newsday, March 15, 1974.

76. Pearson, J. W.: The obstetrician and gynecologist, primary physician for women, J.A.M.A. 231:815-816, 1975.

77. Randal, J.: Is fetal monitoring safe? The Washington Post, April 16, 1978.

78. Reed, E.: Problems of women's liberation, New York, 1971, Pathfinder Press.

79. Reitz, R.: Menopause: a positive approach, Radnor, Pa., 1977, Chilton Book Co.

80. Report on conviction: holding hospitals accountable: Feminist Women's Health Center, Tallahassee, Fla., March 7, 1977.

81. Reverby, S.: Alive and well in Somerville, Mass., HealthRight 2:1, Winter, 1975.

82. Reynard, M. J.: Gynecological self-help: an analysis of its impact on the delivery and use of medical care for women, master's thesis, SUNY/Stony Brook, 1973.

83. Richardson, W. C.: Poverty, illness and the use of health services in the United States. In Jaco, E. G., editor: Patients, physicians and illness, New York, 1972, The Free Press.

84. Rodabaugh, B.: Developing consultation and education services for sexual assault, Palo Alto, Calif., 1978, American Institutes for Research.

85. Rollin, B.: First you cry, Philadelphia, 1976, J. B. Lippincott Co.

86. Rothman, L.: Self-help clinics start in New Zealand, Her-self 3:22, April, 1974.

87. Sanger, M.: Why not birth control clinics in America? Birth Control Review 3:10-11, 1919.

88. Scott, C. R.: The world of a gynecologist, London, 1968, Oliver & Boyd.

89. Scully, D., and Bart, P.: A funny thing happened on the way to the orifice: women in gynecology textbooks, Am. J. Sociology 78: 1045-1050, Jan. 1973.

90. Sehgal, N., and Asling, J. H.: New uses for underused delivery rooms, Medical Opinion 4:78-79, 83, Feb., 1975.

91. Sidel, V., and Sidel, R.: Beyond coping, Social Policy 7:67-69, Sept./Oct., 1976.

92. Silver, G.: A spy in the house of medicine, Germantown, Md., 1976, Aspen Systems Corp.

93. Special self-help issue, Social Policy 7: 1-96, Sept./Oct., 1976.

94. Stellman, J.: Women's work, women's health, New York, 1977, Pantheon Books, Inc.

95. Stewart, D., and Stewart, L.: Safe alternatives in childbirth, Chapel Hill, N.C., 1976, NAPSAC.

96. Strauss, A.: Medical ghettos. In Jaco, E. G., editor: Patients, physicians and illness, New York, 1972, The Free Press.

97. Szasz, T. S., and Hollender, M. H.: A contribution to the philosophy of medicine: the basic models of the doctor-patient relationship, A.M.A. Arch. Intern. Med. 97:585-592, May, 1956.

98. Torres, A.: Organized family planning services in the United States, 1968-1976, Fam. Plan. Perspect. 10:83-88, March/April, 1978.

99. VonSiebold, E. C. J.: History of obstetrics, Tübingen, 1839, F. Pietzcker.

100. Walsh, M. R.: "Doctors wanted; no women need apply." Sexual barriers in the medical profession 1835-1975, New Haven, Conn. 1977, Yale University Press.

101. Weideger, P.: Menstruation and menopause: the physiology and psychology, the myth and the reality, New York, 1977, Dell Publishing Co., Inc.

102. West Coast Sisters: How to start your self-help clinic, Los Angeles, 1971, Feminist Women's Health Center.

103. West Coast Sisters: Self-help clinic, Los Angeles, 1971, Feminist Women's Health Center.

104. Willson, J. R., and Carrington, E. R.: Obstetrics and gynecology, ed. 6, St. Louis, 1979, The C. V. Mosby Co.

105. Women's Community Health Center, Inc.:

Experiences of a pelvic teaching group, Women & Health **1:**19-23, July/Aug., 1976.

106. Zola, I.: Problems of communication, diagnosis and patient care: the interplay of patient, physician and clinic organization, J. Med. Educ. **38:**829-838, Oct. 1963.

ADDITIONAL READINGS

Barker-Benfield, G. J. (Ben): Horrors of the half-known life, New York, 1976, Harper & Row, Publishers.

Boston Women's Health Book Collective: Monthly packet (a collection of relevant clippings and resources), Box 192, West Somerville, Mass. 02144.

Burgess, A. W., and Holmstrom, L. L.: Rape: victims of crisis, Bowie, Md., 1974, Robert J. Brady.

Campbell, E., and Ziegler, V.: Circle one: a woman's beginning guide to self-health and sexuality, Pittsburgh, 1973, Know, Inc., Box 86031, Pittsburgh, Pa. 15221.

Delaney, J., et al.: The curse: a cultural history of menstruation, New York, 1976, E. P. Dutton & Co., Inc.

Dreifus, C., editor: Seizing our bodies: the politics of women's health, New York, 1977, Vintage Books.

Ehrenreich, B.: Gender and objectivity in medicine, Int. J. Health Services **4:**617-623, Fall, 1974.

Emerson, J. P.: Behavior in private places: sustaining definitions of reality in gynecological examinations. In Dreitsel, H., editor: Recent sociology no. 2., London, 1970, MacMillan Co.

Field, H. S., and Barnett, N. J.: Forcible rape: an updated bibliography, J. Criminal Law and Criminology **68:**146-159, 1977.

Friedan, B.: The feminine mystique, New York, 1963, W. W. Norton & Co., Inc., Publishers.

Gordon, L.: Women's body, women's right, New York, 1976, Grossman Press.

Hornstein, F., et al.: Gynecological self-help, In Self-help and health: a report, Sept., 1976, New Human Services Institute, Queens College/CUNY.

Howell, M.: What medical schools teach about women, N. Engl. J. Med. **291:**303, Aug. 8, 1974.

Howell, M.: Healing at home, Boston, 1978, Beacon Press.

Kleiber, N., and Light, L.: Caring for ourselves: an alternative structure for health care, Vancouver, April, 1978, School of Nursing, University of British Columbia, 2075 Wesbrook Crescent, Vancouver, B.C., Canada, V6T 1W5.

Rape Crisis Center: How to start a rape crisis center, Washington, D.C., 1976, Rape Crisis Center in Washington, D.C., P.O. Box 21005, Washington, D.C.

Rennie, S., and Grimstad, K.: The new woman's survival sourcebook, New York, 1975, Alfred A. Knopf, Inc.

Rothman, L.: Self-help clinic: paramedic politics. In Alleyn, M., editor: The witch's os, Stamford, Conn., 1972, New Moon Communications.

Ruzek, S.: Women and health care: a bibliography, Program on Women 1976, Northwestern University, Evanston, Ill.

Sanger, M.: Margaret Sanger: an autobiography, New York, 1938, W. W. Norton & Co., Inc., Publishers.

Seaman, B.: Doctors case against the Pill, New York, 1969, Wyden Books.

Seaman, B.: Free and female, Greenwich, Conn., 1972, Fawcett Publications, Inc.

Stopes, M.: Mother England, London, 1929, John Bale, Sons and Danielsson.

Vancouver Women's Clinic: Vancouver women's health booklet, Vancouver, B.C., 1972, Press Gang Publishers.

Chapter 9

Toward a national health policy for women's health

A national health policy that adequately serves women must be one in which women's dual roles as reproducers and workers, both in and out of the home, are recognized. Acknowledgment of these would lead to a realization that when reproductive-related needs are excluded, men's and women's health needs are similar. Both sexes are increasingly exposed to occupational hazards (see Chapter 5) and chronic illnesses such as cancer, hypertension, and heart disease (see Chapter 1), and both experience a comparable incidence of acute illnesses needing primary care, such as upper respiratory tract infections (see Chapter 2). Despite the similarities, there are nonetheless some issues that still distinctly affect women and which deserve recognition when national health policy is formed.

Many books, reports, and articles[4,6,7,12,14] have offered suggestions for overhauling and analyzing the health care system and for restructuring national health policy. Although the data presented on women's health status and services would not disagree with this approach, it is beyond the scope of this book and this chapter to outline such a restructuring in detail. It is also beyond the scope of this book to address the inequities of class—a recognized fundamental issue to be resolved before many aspects of health status and health services for women or men can be improved. Although this overall goal is not refuted, several immediate concerns specific to women's current health status are delineated here, with the objective of creating interest for their inclusion in efforts to reshape national health policy.

POLICY CONSIDERATIONS
Goals for health status

As the data in this book demonstrate, one of the pressing health status goals concerning women in the United States is to improve the morbidity and mortality rates of minority women. Among minority women, maternal mortality, for example, is almost four times that of white women[21] (see Chapter 1). Although the rate among whites should also be reduced, lowering of the minority rate is a priority.

The reduction of obesity and the promotion of exercise and physical activity among women of all ages and ethnicities should also be a goal of a national health policy because of the effect obesity has on much other morbidity, notably heart disease and stroke. Women aged 25 to 44, for example, make almost double the rate of physician visits for obesity, and are found to be obese on examination, than men.[22, pp.202,215]

Similar scrutiny and policy actions are needed for the extremely high rate of physician visits by women for neuroses and nonpsychotic disorders—a rate in 1977 of 121.8 per 1000 women aged 25 to 44 years[22, pp.276-277] (see Chapter 2). Related mental health goals must focus on the rate of smoking, drinking, drug consumption (both prescription and illicit), and suicide (see Chapter 1) among women, with the objective of lowering these rates also.

Reduction of the rates of surgery is another health status goal, as is reduction of the incidence of recorded complicated births that require surgical intervention. This objective, as discussed later, requires the development of criteria against which perceived health status can be measured.

Another important and attainable health goal is the absolute reduction of morbidity and mortality associated with contraceptive use. Because the need to manage fertility is so fundamental to women's health, and for at least 30 years of their lives, so pervasive, it is critical that contraceptive policies and contraceptives be developed that will not in any way impinge on women's health status.

A more difficult health goal, but one critical to women's welfare, is to reduce the morbidity caused by socially promoted factors such as cosmetic use, cosmetic surgery, and diets. Achievement of this goal requires forces to counter the advertising and media portrayals of women and the uncritical willingness of providers (in these instances) to serve women's perceived needs.

Health status goals for young women do not substantially differ from those for all women, since adolescent women increasingly experience "adult" problems (see Chapter 6). Of critical importance, however, is the need for a consistent goal to reduce the incidence and effects of teenage pregnancy. This must include, as mentioned in the discussion of health services goals, preventive programs, including sex education and the provision of contraception and abortion services in conjunction with school and community programs for young people.

For elderly women, health status goals in a national policy must address such fundamental needs as enabling the elderly to chew[22, p.213] and therefore nourish themselves adequately, to walk and therefore be mobile and provide at least a degree of self-care, and to maintain their cognitive skills through meaningful social contacts and purposeful activity. This latter is particularly pertinent for older women, who, because of their greater longevity (see Chapter 1), are more apt to be widowed and left alone, frequently without resources to alleviate their isolation.

Many other health status concerns for consideration in national health policy will become apparent as improved data collection and analysis techniques are developed. Women's occupational health status, for example, is only beginning to be of national interest as the immensity of the problem for all workers becomes apparent (see Chapter 5). A rational health policy, then, must be one that has a degree of flexibility and is able to adjust and rapidly develop appropriate programs to meet dynamic health needs.

Goals for health services organization

Examination of the data suggests that a fundamental organizational goal for women in national health policy is to shift the conceptualization of women's health care as only related to reproduction, and therefore primarily under the domain of obstetrician-gynecologists, to recognizing that most of women's health needs are similar to those of men and require more generally trained providers.

As discussed in Chapter 2, women's perceptions of their health needs and their physicians' assessments of the reason for physician visits, do not appear to be most appropriately served by the specialty of obstetrics and gynecology. Women's needs also do not appear to be best served through the maternal and child health orientation of many government-funded special programs.[17]

By the same token, it does not seem that obstetrician-gynecologists' highly specialized training appropriately equips them to respond to the relatively mundane bulk of women's health needs, which include routine tests, prenatal care for predominantly normal pregnancies, and treatment of upper respiratory tract infections, hypertension, neuroses and nonpsychotic disorders, and arthritis and rheumatism.[22, pp. 276-277]

Women's health needs might be more appropriately served (and at lower cost to the nation) through a health care model that utilizes family or general practitioners, working in conjunction with midwives for the obstetrical and contraceptive needs of the woman, and referring as necessary to a network of highly trained

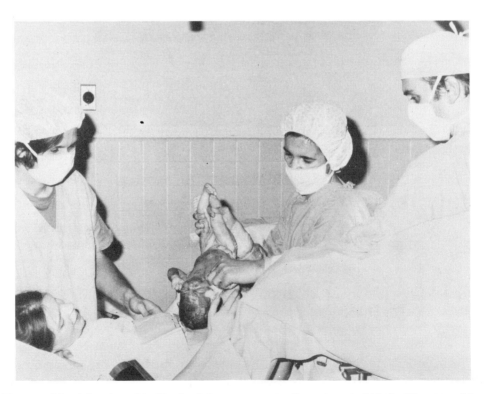

Fig. 9-1. Need for the midwife-physician team: attending a hospital birth. (Courtesy Maternity Center Association, New York.)

internists and obstetrician-gynecologists with surgical experience.[16] A health care delivery model of this type would not only assemble the expertise needed to cover the range of women's health needs, but would also demonstrate a conceptualization of women's health that acknowledges the increasingly minor role of reproductive concerns in a woman's life span.

Similarly, while special maternity-oriented governmental programs have undoubtedly met a pressing need of millions of women through their provision of obstetrical and reproductive services, women involved in these programs have experienced the frustration of receiving limited care for only a specified pregnancy or fertility-related period; when these women stop being reproducers, benefits cease.[5] The need for continuity is pressing.

Considering that many of the recipients of these special maternity programs are minority women who may suffer from other non–pregnancy-related conditions, some of which—for example, hypertension, poor nutrition, and diabetes—may be exacerbated by the pregnancy, the narrow focus of governmental aid can be doubly frustrating and may also be self-defeating. In addition, when services are for the indigent only, the concept of a two-class system of care is promoted.

The basic organizational goals of health insurance coverage must be addressed in a national health policy. As discussed in Chapter 2, many women have inadequate coverage because it is spouse- and/or employment-related and therefore dependent on the presence of either. Women must have equitable health coverage in their own right; this will also help reduce a two-class system of care.

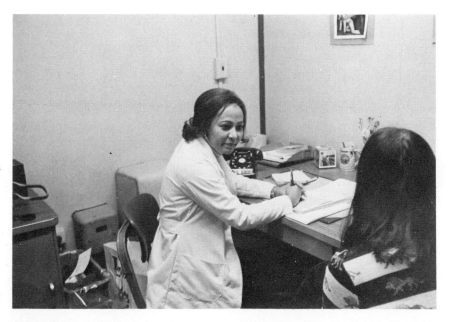

Fig 9-2. Need for Spanish-speaking personnel for Spanish-speaking clients. (Courtesy National Union of Hospital and Health Care Employees, Local 1199.)

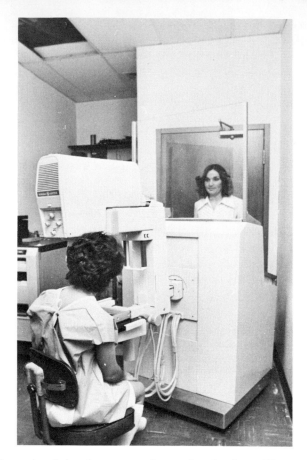

Fig. 9-3. Need for rational development and use of technology. (Courtesy General Electric.)

Other basic issues of access, such as transportation; flexible, reasonably booked office hours that respect patients' time and enable working women and women with small children to visit the physician without undue hardship; and the provision of personnel who are culturally empathetic with clients and proficient in an appropriate language, all must be addressed for satisfactory health service delivery.

Additional organizational goals concern the necessity for careful evaluation and development of criteria that determine, for example, the need for surgery, particularly hysterectomy; that delineate those births which are truly complicated and warrant surgical intervention; and that assess the menopausal conditions meriting medical management. Such goals must be an integral component in a national health policy both for cost-containment reasons and from the perspective of establishing responsible health care for women.

Related to this is the need for empowering federal agencies to review and halt, if necessary, planned medical procedures and developments before they are widely disseminated. The new National Center for Health Care Technology* will have the power to review the efficacy of currently used technology. The tragedies of diethylstilbestrol (DES) use[23]; the questionable use of mammography,[19] the Pap test,[9] cesarean section,[15] and electronic fetal monitoring[2] (see Chapter 7); and numerous other rapidly developed, quickly adopted medical practices demonstrate the need for agencies with proscriptive powers (at least for cost containment if not for health).

Similarly, evaluation of the appropriateness of specific providers for specific services and the degree of training necessary (e.g., to be a competent nurse) is an essential goal for determining a rational use of health manpower resources. For example, if midwives are assessed to provide obstetrical care as competently as obstetricians and if physicians' assistants or pediatric nurse practitioners can provide as adequate care in some areas as other specialists, then national health policy should, in the interests of cost containment, facilitate use of these practitioners. This can be achieved through modifying licensing and third-party coverage policies.

In this same vein, if alternative clinics or programs such as community health centers, home delivery services, or women's clinics can achieve outcomes comparable with those of traditional medicine (or, in the case of obstetrics, of the established[3,10,13] but disputed[8] regionalization plan), yet with higher client satisfaction and at lower cost, national health policy should facilitate their function.

The need for organizations that can impartially assume the responsibility of careful evaluation free from the constraints of lobbying, political interest, and economic pressures is reinforced.

The data in this book demonstrate that specific health service goals are also needed. Beginning in their early teen years, women must have equitable and easy access to contraception and abortion services.[1] There must be school programs for young parents that facilitate appropriate parenting while developing academic and marketable skills. Even more important, and under a broad interpretation of health, there must be programs that promote a sense of worth and self-fulfillment, negating the tremendous social influences that produce adolescent ennui and contribute to alcoholism, prostitution, drug abuse, pregnancy, and suicide in adolescent young women (see Chapter 6).

A needed goal for women employed in the work force is effective monitoring of the workplace and development of coherent and consistent labor policies that do not present a choice between safety and/or fertility maintenance and employment.[11]

Specific health services goals for the elderly include the establishment of programs and financial support systems that would enable them to stay in their homes, to socialize, and, in nursing homes, to continue as normal a routine as possible, including cohabitation if desired.

---

*Public Law 95-623, 95th Congress, second session, Nov. 9, 1978.

Related policy issues

Many other considerations are needed for a comprehensive national health policy. As this book notes, an accurate data collection system is essential for establishing a base on which relevant programs, plans, and services can be developed. Data must be race and age specific, taking into account the numerous variables discussed that affect women's health, such as education, employment status, parity, and income.[18]

In the interests of health, substantial curtailment of irresponsible, pernicious, and readily believed advertising by the medical-industrial complex must be achieved. The enormous influence this advertising has both in inducing harmful health behavior by consumers, and in shaping physician perceptions, and therefore treatment of women, is readily demonstrated through prescribing patterns and the development of standard medical practice. Undoubtedly some benefits have come from this, but the costs appear to have largely outweighed them.

The need for a national day care policy is suggested by the rapidly increasing numbers of mothers entering the work force;[24] provision of this service is critical

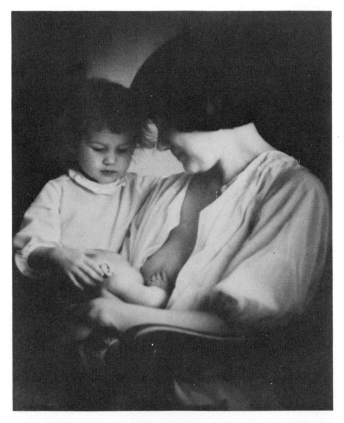

Fig. 9-4. Need to facilitate combining breast-feeding and work. (Courtesy La Leche League International, Inc., Franklin Park, Ill.)

to the well-being of both women and children. Similarly, facilitating breast-feeding by working women promotes the health of new generations of babies and also would help reduce many of the conflicts and much of the stress experienced by women who must work.

A national health policy should also address fair employment of health workers and their rights to unionize and to strike. This is particularly important for women health workers, who, as noted in Chapter 4, are predominant in the lowest ranks of the health care work force, with consequent low pay, lack of job security, lack of upward mobility, little job satisfaction, and most important, no resources other than the power to strike to effect meaningful change in their job structure.

Provision must also be made under national health policy for the poorest "paid" health worker of all—the female family member who provides care in the home.[20] The present health care system is dependent on these women to care for parents, spouses, and particularly sick children; as women expand their numbers in the job market, fewer are readily available or willing to assume this role. Satisfactory alternatives must be developed that allow women to continue needed employment without financial penalty or suffering from guilt feelings and stress.

A health policy that is rationally developed must also establish its goals for

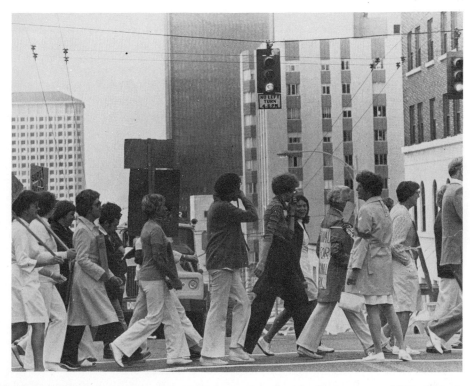

Fig. 9-5. Right to unionize and to strike: nurses in Seattle, late summer, 1976. (Courtesy The Seattle Times, Seattle.)

women from a consensus of the women involved; too often health policy has been developed by "experts" far removed from experiencing the health services they propose or design. Women can be effective advocates and spokespersons for themselves.

• • •

Adequate recognition of women's reproductive and work force roles with appropriate policy implementation would do much to reduce women's dissatisfaction with the health care system and promote equity for women both in terms of reported morbidity and actual incidence. The development of supportive services indirectly related to but affecting health, such as child care and job placement programs, and the promotion of the concept of shared child-rearing and household responsibilities would alleviate much of the underlying stress faced by women today, which undoubtedly contributes, if not partially causes, aspects of the morbidity reported.

Most important, in shaping health policy, women must recognize the validity of their health needs and the importance of planning their health services within a coordinated structure that encompasses the range of these needs, and they must strive for the opportunity to speak for themselves.

SUGGESTED TOPICS FOR DISCUSSION, FURTHER RESEARCH, AND FIELD PROJECTS

1. What is the regionalization plan for obstetrical services? How was it established? Who developed it? What are the pros and cons?
2. What are the issues involved in working women breast-feeding? Have there been any suits in your area similar to the Iowa firefighter's case (check your local newspapers about March 1, 1979). Do any local employers have breast-feeding policies? What is their reaction when you call to inquire?
3. Research several proposed plans for overhauling or analyses of the structure of the health care system. Do they address women's health concerns? If not, what effects would these proposals have on women's health?
4. What changes in women's health services might you anticipate if there were open competition (i.e., a true free enterprise system) in the health care industry? In the long run would open competition be to women's advantage or disadvantage? Would the situation differ in the short run?
5. Why should women have health coverage in their own right? Would you extend this principle to covering children in their own right? What are the costs and benefits of health insurance related to employment, spouse, or family?
6. Who should take care of the sick children and family members of working women? If you do not think the women should, how would you organize an alternative? Who should pay for this?
7. What is implied by the term "restructuring the health care system"? What aspects of health care delivery may restructuring affect? What are the pros and cons of privately financed versus publicly financed restructuring proposals?
8. Select one health status goal discussed or choose one of your own. How would you develop a policy, program, or service to improve this status? What barriers, if any, would you encounter in achieving your goal? Are there any political considerations to confront?

9. If you could reallocate federal funds for women's health, would you alter their current allocations? If so, how? What would you expect to be the changes in women's health status from your new programs?

10. How would you organize a watchdog agency or agencies that would have the power to stop medical practices of dubious benefit before they spread? In whom or what and how would you invest proscriptive power? What checks could you institute in the system to prevent abuses by agencies?

REFERENCES

1. Alan Guttmacher Institute: 11 Million teenagers, New York, 1976, Planned Parenthood Federation of America, Inc.

2. Banta, H. D., and Thacker, S. B.: Costs and benefits of electronic fetal monitoring: a review of the literature, no. (PHS) 79-3245, National Center for Health Services Research, Washington, D.C., 1979, U.S. Government Printing Office.

3. Barnes, F. E. F., editor: Ambulatory maternal health care and family planning services: policies, principles, practices, Washington, D.C., 1978, American Public Health Association.

4. Carlson, R. J.: The end of medicine, New York, 1975, John Wiley & Sons, Inc.

5. Deschin, C. S.: The need to extend medical services beyond the hospital if maternal and infant care is to become comprehensive, Am. J. Public Health **58:**1230-1236, July, 1968.

6. Enthoven, A. C.: Consumer choice health plan. I. Inflation and inequity in health care today, N. Engl. J. Med. **298:**650-658, March 23, 1978.

7. Enthoven, A. C.: Consumer choice health plan. II. Alternatives for cost control and an analysis of proposals for national health insurance, N. Engl. J. Med. **298:**709-720, March 30, 1978.

8. Fleck, A. C., et al.: Hospital size and outcomes of pregnancy, New York, 1977, Division of Child Health, New York State Department of Health.

9. Foltz, A.-M., and Kelsey, J. L.: The annual Pap test: a dubious policy success, Milbank Memorial Quarterly/Health and Society **56:** 426-462, 1978.

10. House of Representatives: Maternal and Child Health Care Act-1976, Supplemental hearing before the Subcommittee on Health and the Environment, Committee on Interstate and Foreign Commerce, 94th Congress, second session on HR 12937, HR 14309, and HR 14822—bills to establish a national system of maternal and child health care, and on HR 14497—bill to establish a national health insurance system for maternal and child health care, Sept. 13, 1976, Washington, D.C., 1976, U.S. Government Printing Office (serial no. 94-117).

11. Hricko, A., with Brunt, M.: Working for your life—a woman's guide to job health hazards, Berkeley, Calif., 1977, Labor Occupational Health Program (LOHP), University of California, 2521 Channing Way, Berkeley, Calif. 94720.

12. Illich, I.: Medical nemesis, New York, 1976, Pantheon Books.

13. Karel, F., editor: Regionalized prenatal services, Princeton, N.J., 1978, The Robert Wood Johnson Foundation.

14. Kennedy, E.: In critical condition, New York, 1973, Simon & Schuster, Inc.

15. Marieskind, H. I.: An evaluation of cesarean section in the U.S.A., Washington, D.C., 1979, Office of the Assistant Secretary of Planning and Evaluation/Health, U.S. Government Printing Office.

16. Marieskind, H. I.: New roles for women in health care delivery, Urban Health **6:**24-27, 48, April, 1977.

17. Marieskind, H. I.: Restructuring Ob-Gyn, Social Policy **6:**48-49, Sept./Oct., 1975.

18. Muller, C.: Women and health statistics: areas of deficient data collection and integration, Women & Health **4:**37-59, Spring, 1979.

19. National Cancer Institute: Final report of ad hoc working groups on mammography screening for breast cancer and a summary report of their joint findings and recommendations, no. (NIH) 77-1400, Washington, D.C., 1977, U.S. Government Printing Office.

20. Polansky, E.: The social and economic impact on the family members who care for the chronically ill at home, doctoral dissertation, Columbia University School of Social Work, New York, 1980.

21. U.S. Department of Health, Education and Welfare: Final mortality statistics, 1977,

National Center for Health Statistics, Washington, D.C., 1979.

22. U.S. Department of Health, Education and Welfare: Health, United States, 1978, no. (PHS) 78-1232, Washington, D.C., 1978, U.S. Government Printing Office.

23. Weiss, K.: Vaginal cancer: an iatrogenic disease? Int. J. Health Serv. 5:235-251, Spring, 1975.

24. Women's Bureau: 1975 Handbook on women workers, U.S. Department of Labor, stock no. 029-016-00037-2, Washington, D.C., 1975, U.S. Government Printing Office.

Bibliographies*

GENERAL

Ash, J.: Health: a multimedia source guide, New York, 1976, Bowker.

Cowan, B.: Women's health care: resources, writings, bibliographies, Ann Arbor, Mich. 1977, Anshen Publishing Co.

Culyer, A. J.: An annotated bibliography of health economics, New York, 1977, St. Martin's Press.

Harrison, C. E.: Women's movement media: a source guide, New York, 1975, R. R. Bowker Co.

Jacobs, S.-E.: Women in perspective: a guide for cross-cultural studies, Urbana, 1974, University of Illinois Press.

Rosenberg, K.: Politics of health care: a bibliography, Somerville, Mass. 1973, New England Free Press.

Rosenberg, M. B., and Bergstrom, L.: Women and society: a critical review of the literature with a selected annotated bibliography, vols. 1 and 2, Beverly Hills, Calif., 1975-1978, Sage Publications, Inc.

Ruzek, S. K.: Women and health care: a bibliography with selected annotations, Evanston, Ill. 1975, Northwestern University, Program on Women.

Sprague, J. B.: Women and health bookshelf, Am. J. Public Health **65:**741-746, July, 1975.

Wheeler, H. R.: Womanhood media supplement, Metuchen, N. J. 1975, Scarecrow Press.

Williams, K. N.: Health and development: an annotated, indexed bibliography, Baltimore, 1972, Department of International Health.

Women and the health system: selected annotated references: Health planning bibliography, series no. 4, HRA no. 78629, Hyattsville, Md., 1978, National Health Planning Information Center.

Women studies abstracts: Rush, N.Y., 1972, Rush Publishing Co.

Women's guide to books, 3 vols., New York, 1975, available from Mss Information Corp., P.O. Box 985, Edison, N.J. 08817.

Woods, R. L.: Government guides to health and nutrition, New York, 1975, Pyramid.

ABORTION

Af Geijerstam, G. K.: An annotated bibliography of induced abortion, Ann Arbor, Mich., 1969, Center for Population Planning.

Dollen, C. J.: Abortion in context: a select bibliography, Metuchen, N.J., 1970, Scarecrow Press.

Floyd, M. K.: Abortion bibliography for 1975, Troy, N.Y., 1976, Whitson Publishing Co.

Moore-Cavar, E. C.: International inventory of information on induced abortion, New York, 1974, International Institute for the Study of Human Reproduction, Columbia University.

Potts, M.: Bibliography (with reviews) on outpatient abortion. Bibliography Reproductions **19:**753, Cambridge, England.

ALCOHOL AND ADDICTIONS

Advena, J. C.: Drug abuse bibliography for 1973, Troy, N. Y., 1975, Whitson Publishing Co.

Bibliography on women and drug related issues, STASH Library, Grassroots (supp.), pp. 19-34, Aug., 1974.

Health Education: Drugs and alcohol—an annotated bibliography, Washington, D.C., 1975, National Education Association.

Lindbeck, V. L.: The woman alcoholic—a review of the literature, Int. J. Addict. **7:**567-580, 1972.

Women alcohol abusers: subject area bibliography, Rockville, Md., 1974, National Clearinghouse for Alcohol Information.

Women and drug concerns: bibliography, Washington, D.C., 1974, Department of Drug and Alcohol Concerns, United Methodist Church,

*From S. Meyer: Bibliography of bibliographies, Women & Health **4:**203-207, Summer, 1979.

100 Maryland Ave., N.E., Washington, D.C. 20002.

Women and drugs: An annotated bibliography, Rockville, Md. 1975, National Clearinghouse for Drug Abuse Information.

ALTERNATIVE LIFE STYLES

Bullough, V. L., et al.: An annotated bibliography of homosexuality, New York, 1976, Garland Publishing, Inc.

A gay bibliography, ed. 5, Philadelphia, 1975, ALA/SSRT.

A gay bibliography: eight bibliographies on lesbian and male homosexuality, New York, 1975, Arno Press.

Lesbian health issues: an annotated bibliography, Santa Cruz, Calif., c. 1978, Santa Cruz Women's Health Center.

BEREAVEMENT

Archuleta, M. J., and Archuleta, A. J.: Sudden infant death syndrome: an annotated bibliography for the layman, San Diego, 1975, Current Bibliography Series.

Kutscher, A. H., and Kutscher, M.: A bibliography of books on death, bereavement, loss and grief, 1968-1972 (supp. I), New York, 1974, Health Sciences Publishing Corp.

Strugnell, C.: Adjustment to widowhood and some related problems: a selective and annotated bibliography, New York, 1974, Health Sciences Publishing Corp.

BIRTH CONTROL AND FERTILITY

Birdsall, N.: An introduction to the social science literature on "woman's place" and fertility in the developing world. Annotated bibliography, vol. 2, no. 1. Washington, D.C., 1975, Interdisciplinary Communications Programs, Smithsonian Institution.

Freedman, R.: Sociology of human fertility: an annotated bibliography, Englewood Cliffs, N. J., 1974, Prentice-Hall, Inc.

Goode, S. H.: Population and the population explosion: a bibliography for 1972, Troy, NY., 1974, Whitson Publishing Co.

Marieskind, H. I.: Gynecological services: their historical relationship to the women's movement with recent experience of self-help clinics and other delivery modes, doctoral dissertation, University of Michigan, 1976, order no. 762-5222-01500, Ann Arbor, Mich., University Microfilms.

Marshall, J. M.: Studies relating women's non-

familial activity and fertility. Bibliography series 1. Chapel Hill, N.C., 1972, Carolina Population Center.

Sundstrom, C.: A bookshelf of family planning, Am. J. Public Health **64:**666-673, July, 1974.

MENOPAUSE

McKinlay, S. M.: Annotated bibliography: selected studies of the menopause. J. Biosoc. Sci. **5:**533-555, 1973.

PROSTITUTION

Bullough, V. L., et al.: A bibliography on prostitution. New York, 1977, Garland Publishing, Inc.

PSYCHOLOGY AND MENTAL HEALTH

Cromwell, P. E.: Women and mental health: selected annotated references, 1970-1973, Washington, D.C., 1974, National Institute of Mental Health.

Walstedt, J. J.: Psychology of women: a partially annotated bibliography, Pittsburgh, 1973, Know, Inc.

RAPE

Barnes, D. L.: Rape: a bibliography, 1965-1975, Troy, N.Y., 1977, Whitson Publishing Co.

Kemmer, E. J.: Rape and rape-related issues: an annotated bibliography, New York, 1977, Garland Publishing, Inc.

RESEARCH

American Alliance for Health, Physical Education and Recreation: Bibliography of research involving female subjects, Washington, D.C., 1975, AAHPER.

VENEREAL DISEASE

Goode, S. H.: Venereal disease bibliography for 1973, New York, 1975, Whitson Publishing Co.

WOMEN'S ROLES

Aldous, J.: International bibliography of research in marriage and family, 2 vols., Minneapolis, 1967-1974, University of Minnesota Press.

Astin, H. S., Parelman, A., and Fisher, A.: Sex roles: a research bibliography, Washington, D.C., 1975, Center for Human Services.

Chaff, S. L., et al.: Women in medicine; a bibliography of the literature on women physicians, Metuchen, N.J., 1977, Scarecrow Press.

Davis, A. B.: Bibliography on women: with special emphasis on their roles in science and society, New York, 1974, Science History Publications.

Schlacter, G., and Belli, D.: The changing role of women in America: a selected annotated bibliography of reference sources, Monticello, Ill., 1975, Council of Planning Librarians.

AGING

Bibliography on older women, 1978, available from the Publications Office, Andrus Gerontology Center, University of Southern California, Los Angeles, Calif. 90007.

The Older Women's Rights Committee (formerly the NOW Task Force on Older Women, Oakland, Calif.): Age is becoming: an annotated bibliography on women and aging, Berkeley, Interface Bibliographers, 3018 Hillegass Ave., Berkeley, Calif. 94705.

Index

326

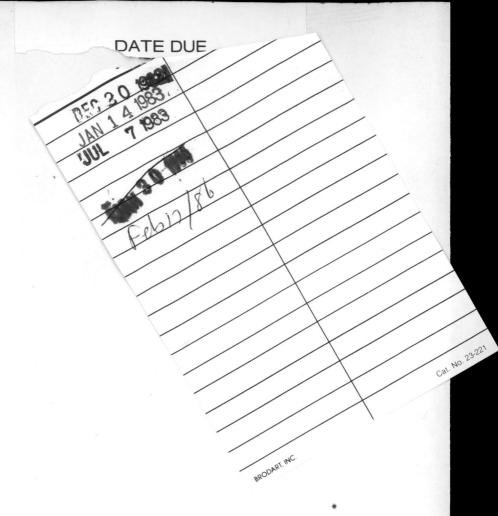